AF183904

Noninvasive Ventilation. The Essentials

Series Editor
Antonio M. Esquinas, Hospital Morales Meseguer
Murcia, Spain

Nowadays, Noninvasive Ventilation (NIV) is widely accepted in medical practice. This Series, titled "Noninvasive Ventilation: Clinical and Practice," is a culmination of extensive prior publications on the topic. It aims to define current clinical developments in NIV technologies, including equipment and ventilator modes, and provide practical recommendations primarily in Critical Care (CC), Pulmonary, Emergency, and Sleep Medicine.

Building on previous publications, a group of experienced Editors and top international contributors aim to present new books that take a multidisciplinary approach and provide a comprehensive overview of Non-invasive Ventilation. The main goals of this Series are as follows:

Establish a scientific reference for NIV clinical practice, covering pathophysiology, clinical indications, and evidence-based concepts.

Present significant advances in CC, pneumology, anesthesiology, sleep medicine, pediatrics, and healthcare organization in acute and chronic respiratory failure.

Analyze technological advancements and complementary procedures associated with NIV, such as aerosol therapy, humidification, and airway clearance, crucial for effective NIV techniques.

Serve as a valuable teaching reference for healthcare professionals, including residents, consultants, and allied healthcare professionals, as well as undergraduate and postgraduate students and fellowship participants.

The Series will produce focused thematic volumes, led by internationally recognized guest editors, providing comprehensive coverage of specific areas of NIV advancement in CC, emergency medicine, pulmonary, and sleep medicine.

Kunal Panda
Szymon Skoczyński • Mostafa Elshazly
Editors

Noninvasive Ventilatory Approaches in Interventional Procedures

Rationale and Clinical Applications

Springer

Editors
Kunal Panda
Department of Anesthesiology and Perioperative Medicine, University of Rochester School of Medicine & Dentistry, Rochester, NY, USA

Szymon Skoczyński
Department of Lung Diseases and Tuberculosis, Faculty of Medical Sciences in Zabrze, Medical University of Silesia in Katowice
Zabrze, Poland

Mostafa Elshazly
Chest Department
Cairo University Hospitals
Cairo, Egypt

ISSN 2948-2747 ISSN 2948-2755 (electronic)
Noninvasive Ventilation. The Essentials
ISBN 978-3-032-05327-5 ISBN 978-3-032-05328-2 (eBook)
https://doi.org/10.1007/978-3-032-05328-2

© The Editor(s) (if applicable) and The Author(s), under exclusive license to Springer Nature Switzerland AG 2025

This work is subject to copyright. All rights are solely and exclusively licensed by the Publisher, whether the whole or part of the material is concerned, specifically the rights of translation, reprinting, reuse of illustrations, recitation, broadcasting, reproduction on microfilms or in any other physical way, and transmission or information storage and retrieval, electronic adaptation, computer software, or by similar or dissimilar methodology now known or hereafter developed.
The use of general descriptive names, registered names, trademarks, service marks, etc. in this publication does not imply, even in the absence of a specific statement, that such names are exempt from the relevant protective laws and regulations and therefore free for general use.
The publisher, the authors and the editors are safe to assume that the advice and information in this book are believed to be true and accurate at the date of publication. Neither the publisher nor the authors or the editors give a warranty, expressed or implied, with respect to the material contained herein or for any errors or omissions that may have been made. The publisher remains neutral with regard to jurisdictional claims in published maps and institutional affiliations.

This Springer imprint is published by the registered company Springer Nature Switzerland AG
The registered company address is: Gewerbestrasse 11, 6330 Cham, Switzerland

If disposing of this product, please recycle the paper.

I would like dedicate it to young physicians and allied healthcare professionals to encourage them in new or better introductions of NIV to facilitate safety and possibility to perform Interventional Procedures even in high-risk patients.

– ***Szymon Skoczyński***

Contents

About the Editors

Kunal Panda, MD is Associate Professor of Anesthesiology and Perioperative Medicine, the Program Director of Critical Care Medicine Fellowship in the Department of Anesthesiology and Perioperative Medicine at the University of Rochester School of Medicine and Dentistry, USA. He has authored scientific papers in international medical journals as well as book chapters, serves as a reviewer for the medical journals, and has given podium presentations at international medical conferences. His research interests include mechanical circulatory support devices, ECMO, and noninvasive ventilation.

Szymon Skoczyński, MD, PhD Professor at The Medical University of Silesia, is Head of the Department of Lung Diseases and Tuberculosis, Faculty of Medical Sciences in Zabrze, Medical University of Silesia in Katowice, Zabrze, Poland. He is a specialist in internal medicine, adult respiratory medicine, and critical care medicine. His main fields of interest are high flow nasal therapy, noninvasive mechanical ventilation, and ECMO procedures in patients with respiratory failure with special interest in respiratory support in bronchofiberoscopic procedures.

Mostafa Elshazly, MD was Medical Director of Covid Designation hospital, led and managed medical operations for a dedicated COVID-19 hospital, ensuring high-quality patient care during critical public health crisis, and oversaw the implementation of clinical protocols and resource allocation to optimize patient outcomes. He also provided advanced medical education and training to undergraduate and postgraduate students, conducted cutting-edge research in pulmonary diseases and tuberculosis and delivers expert clinical care to patients with complex respiratory conditions. He was director of Pulmonary Hypertension Unit at Kasr Alaini School of Medicine, where he directed research initiatives focused on pulmonary hypertension, contributing to advancements in diagnosis and treatment, mentored junior researchers, and fostered a collaborative research environment. He also established and led the sleep research unit, conducting studies on sleep disorders and their impact on respiratory health, and developed comprehensive diagnostic and treatment programs for sleep-related breathing disorders. Currently, he is chief of respiratory critical care unit at Chest Department, Cairo University hospitals, where he leads and supervises the critical care team, ensuring optimal management of patients with severe respiratory failure, and develops and implements protocols for respiratory critical care.

Part I

Rationale For Applications

Evolution of Noninvasive Ventilation: Epidemiology and Current Practice

1

Mostafa Elshazly and Gehan Saad

The concept of noninvasive ventilation (NIV) began early in the 1800s. In fact, NIV preceded the era of advanced invasive mechanical ventilation techniques known today. The earliest noninvasive ventilators were the "body ventilators," which applied negative or positive pressure to various parts of the body. In 1864, Alfred F. Jones patented the first American tank respirator in the iron lung, known as noninvasive negative pressure ventilation [1, 2].

Due to the enormous size and immobility of early tank ventilators, more portable negative pressure devices were designed, including the chest shell "cuirass" ventilator and wrap (or raincoat) ventilator. In 1876, Ignez von Hauke introduced the first cuirass comprising an iron shell covering the anterior chest wall, with a tight seal. The year 1949 witnessed the first mass production of chest shells after R. Eisenmenger developed the first mechanical one in 1927, the "Biomotor," which was used onward for respiratory paralysis. A few years later, the wrap ventilator "Tunnicliffe breathing jacket" was described. The first widely used electrically powered body ventilator "the iron lung" was invented in 1928 by Philip Drinker; then, Emerson built a simpler and quieter version in 1931 [3].

The polio epidemics stimulated other approaches to noninvasive ventilation, including the rocking bed and the intermittent abdominal pressure ventilator, the "pneumobelt." In the 1930s, Bragg made a pneumatic belt from a rubber football bladder that was strapped around the lower chest and abdomen and was inflated by a pump, compressing the viscera during expiration. Robert Paul modified the belt, to the so-called Bragg-Paul pulsator. The device was used extensively during the 1950s because of improved convenience and portability.

M. Elshazly (✉) · G. Saad
Chest Department, Faculty of Medicine, Cairo University, Cairo, Giza, Egypt
e-mail: melshazly@kasralainy.edu.eg; Gihan_saad@cu.edu.eg

© The Author(s), under exclusive license to Springer Nature Switzerland AG 2025

K. Panda et al. (eds.), *Noninvasive Ventilatory Approaches in Interventional Procedures*, Noninvasive Ventilation. The Essentials,
https://doi.org/10.1007/978-3-032-05328-2_1

In 1952, a large outbreak of polio occurred in Denmark, during which a great revolution in the concept occurred. Due to the enormous number of patients exceeding the available negative pressure ventilators, invasive positive pressure resuscitators—initially used for anesthesia—were used. Survival rates during their use were higher than those of negative pressure ventilators, due to better secretions control and airway protection from aspiration. Owing to this, a shift to invasive positive pressure ventilation occurred, and during the 1960s, the appearance of intensive care units with more simple and cheaper positive pressure ventilators enhanced this shift.

In fact, noninvasive application of positive pressure began in the 1930s, when studies by Alvan 'Barach showed the continuous positive airway pressure (CPAP) aided during treatment of acute pulmonary edema [4]. Intermittent positive pressure ventilation (IPPV) via a mouthpiece, first described in 1947, was widely used till the early 1980s to deliver nebulized bronchodilators in patients with airway diseases but was also assessed in many studies as noninvasive ventilatory support [5].

The introduction of nasal CPAP mask for the treatment of obstructive sleep apnea in the early 1980s represented as a starting point to a new era in noninvasive ventilation. In 1984, Rideau and colleagues suggested the use of those masks with positive pressure ventilators for nocturnal ventilation of patients with Duchenne muscular dystrophy. Advantages of nasal masks such as comfort, tolerance, and efficiency led to gradual replacement of negative pressure ventilation by noninvasive positive pressure ventilation (NIPPV). Rapidly, the NIPPV became the best treatment option for patients with respiratory failure due to neuromuscular and chest wall diseases or other causes of hypoventilation, such as obesity [4].

In 1992, BiPAP®, a bilevel ventilator first designed for patients with obstructive sleep apnea syndrome who could not tolerate CPAP, was introduced by Respironics. In 1999, the Consensus Conference on the clinical indications for NIPPV in chronic respiratory failure due to restrictive lung disease, chronic obstructive pulmonary disease, and nocturnal hypoventilation was published establishing the criteria for home NIPPV. Following a few years, NIPPV emerged as the widely accepted and most effective treatment for acute exacerbations of chronic obstructive pulmonary disease. The Global Initiative for Chronic Obstructive Lung Disease (GOLD) then set specific criteria for the use of NIPPV in this context. In 2001, the American Thoracic Society published the International Consensus Conference on NIPPV in acute respiratory failure [4].

The main factors attracting people to NPPV are its benefits over invasive mechanical ventilation. Research has demonstrated that this approach can effectively reduce resource consumption and avoid several consequences linked to invasive mechanical ventilation, including but not limited to upper airway injuries, ventilator-associated infections, and speech and swallowing impairments [6, 7]. Nonetheless, NPPV needs to be viewed as a substitute for invasive mechanical ventilation in certain circumstances rather than as a replacement for it [8].

Careful patient selection and a well-designed clinical procedure are essential for the efficacy of NPPV and for the improvement of the clinical outcomes of patients with acute respiratory failure, as the failure of NPPV simply postpones potentially more definitive therapy with invasive ventilation.

The increasing evidence supporting NIV's efficacy has boosted its use in clinical practice over time, as indicated by observational studies based on on-site data collection at selected hospitals rather than physicians' estimations of use in response to questionnaires.

Numerous surveys have investigated the use and awareness of NIV among clinicians at different institutions across different regions. Overall, this research demonstrated that NIV practices vary widely across nations and have been evolving over time [9].

Only half of the 268 acute care hospitals in the United Kingdom had NIV available at the time of one of the earliest surveys, which was conducted in 1998 and evaluated the device's use and availability (particularly in the intensive care unit) and, when they were accessible, were underutilized (used by more than 60 patients annually in only 7% of medical facilities). Also, in North America, the utilization of NIV was low. An analysis conducted in 2006 revealed that respiratory therapists in Massachusetts and Rhode Island, North America, had an estimated 20% utilization rate of NIV in acute care settings, with significant regional differences [9]. Another survey conducted in 2004 revealed similar findings of a limited penetration of NIV for the treatment of acute exacerbation of chronic obstructive pulmonary disease (AECOPD) throughout Canadian urban hospitals. The primary identified obstacles to the use of NIV in all these trials were equipment shortages, a lack of medical expertise, and financial constraints. In their worldwide web-based survey of intensivists published in 2007, Devlin and colleagues noted a significant regional variance in the stated usage of NIV in acute respiratory failure (ARF). In general, European doctors were more likely than North American doctors to employ NIV, especially in cases of obesity hypoventilation syndrome, congestive heart failure (CHF), and AECOPD. Conversely, they noted that, in comparison to European doctors, North American doctors were more likely to employ sedatives (41% vs 24%), analgesics (48% vs 35%), and hand restraints (27% vs 16%) during NIV treatment [10].

The original obstacles to the technique have been overcome by the remarkable spread of scientific material on the benefits of NIV, and the procedure is starting to become more generally available in hospitals. However, significant regional variations have been observed once more.

A Spanish study published in 2008 revealed a relatively high rate of NIV utilization among Spanish intensive care units (ICUs), respiratory medicine departments, and emergency departments (EDs) (100%, 88%, and 69% of respondents, respectively) and a relatively low percentage of use in internal medicine departments (37%) and other wards (11%), with a wide range of patient types, equipment types, and lack of protocols [11].

The findings of a 2009 survey of physicians and respiratory therapists (RTs) working in EDs in North America revealed that 90% of RTs and 64% of doctors said they were extremely familiar with NIV and that it is more frequently used in the ED for AECOPD and CHF. Additionally, the study validates the known obstacles to a wider use of this technique, including physician familiarity, the availability of equipment in EDs, the cost of personnel, and the significant issue of RT availability [12].

In 2010, Crimi et al. conducted a web-based survey in Europe to identify the perceived pattern of NIV utilization and the reason for choosing a specific ventilator and interface type in four common clinical scenarios: acute hypercapnic respiratory failure (AHRF), cardiogenic pulmonary edema (CPE), de novo hypoxic respiratory failure and weaning/post-extubation failure (W/PE). A response was obtained from 272 (51.3%) out of 530 selected European physicians involved in NIV practice. The NIV utilization rate was higher for pulmonologists than intensivists/anesthesiologists (p 0.05). AHRF was the most often given indication (48%) among all the physicians. Because of the ability to employ the double circuit and inspiratory oxygen fraction control, doctors were more likely to use an ICU ventilator with NIV module in de novo hypoxic respiratory failure and W/PE, as well as an NIV dedicated ventilator in AHRF and CPE. Regardless of the clinical setting, the most commonly used interface overall was the oronasal mask. They came to the conclusion that NIV use is rather common in Europe, particularly among pulmonologists and AHRF. In addition to oronasal masks, dedicated NIV ventilators and ICU ventilators with NIV modules are preferred in AHRF and de novo hypoxic respiratory failure, respectively [13].

Similar outcomes were observed in an epidemiological investigation conducted in the United States by Stefan and colleagues, who discovered a consistent rise in hospital admissions between 2001 and 2009 with a discharge diagnosis of ARF determined by the *International Classification of Diseases, Ninth Revision* (ICD-9) coding system. The study found that rates of invasive mechanical ventilation were declining, along with a notable shift toward the use of NIV, which climbed from 3.8% to 10.1% [14].

In conclusion, there has been a gradual but noticeable increase in the clinical use of NIV in ICUs, pulmonary medicine departments, and emergency departments over the past 10 years. Its application is consistent with scientific findings. Nonetheless, there are still clear distinctions between North American and European approaches; the latter are less likely to employ NIV, even in clinical settings where there is compelling evidence to support it.

The ICU is unquestionably the best environment for the efficient and secure application of NIV in acute and deadly bouts of respiratory failure, as evidenced by the bulk of studies on the subject. However, new research has shown that NIV is beneficial in a number of common clinical scenarios, including AECOPD, acute cardiogenic pulmonary edema, and acute respiratory failure in immunocompromised patients. As a result, NIV is becoming a more desirable and attractive tool in clinical practice outside of the ICU, particularly in general wards [15].

Paus-Jenssen and colleagues, in a single center in Canada, observed all consecutive patients hospitalized for ARF (AECOPD, hypoxic respiratory failure, hypercapnic respiratory failure, CHF, and patients with shortness of breath) over a 5-month period and described the feasible use of NIV outside the critical care setting. The author found no difference in outcome and mortality compared with data from controlled studies performed in more aggressively monitored patients [16].

In 2015, Cabrini and colleagues conducted a worldwide web-based survey focused on NIV use in general wards for ARF. Data on hospital and ICU characteristics, NIV application and monitoring settings and methods, estimated outcomes, technical and organizational issues, and observed complications were gathered through the development of a questionnaire. The respondents were from 51 countries from all 5 continents. NIV application in general wards was reported by 66% of the respondents. Treatments were reported as increasing in 57% of cases.

The most frequent excuses for not implementing NIV in general wards were inadequate training and staffing. The majority of responders believed that NIV typically avoided the need for tracheal intubation; the most common reasons for NIV failure were intolerance, worsening of ARF, and incapacity to control secretions. They concluded that the use of NIV in general wards was reported as effective, common, and gradually increasing. When used in general ward settings, protocols and improved staff training could make this approach safer and more widely used [17].

1.1 Emerging Applications

The use of NIPPV spread beyond ICU or intermediate care units, to its successful application in out-of-hospital situations and emergency departments.

Bruge et al. conducted 2-year prospective observational research of NIV in prehospital treatment in emergency response vehicles equipped with bi-level ventilators. The study's results were encouraging and suggested that NIV may be used even in the prehospital context [18].

In an NAEMSP (the National Association of EMS Physicians) position statement and resource document about prehospital noninvasive ventilation published recently, they recommended that noninvasive ventilation in the form of CPAP and BiPAP is safe and effective in the prehospital environment. Its use at the basic life support (BLS) level has been successfully and safely implemented in many EMS (Emergency Medical services) systems. Novel methods of noninvasive ventilation such as HFNC (High Flow Nasal Cannula) and helmet NIV are promising but require further research to determine optimal patient populations and deployment strategies [19].

Although it has been reported that using NIV during diagnostic and therapeutic bronchoscopy is a practical and safe method, more research is necessary to determine how it affects critically sick patients' mortality and intubation rate [20]. However, it should be performed only in centers with a wide experience.

Sircar and colleagues evaluated the feasibility of FOB (FiberOptic Bronchoscopy) through NIV mask in 28 patients with respiratory failure managed by NIV. They came to the conclusion that hypoxemic ICU patients can safely have basic therapeutic and diagnostic bronchoscopies performed at the bedside with NIV support, largely avoiding intubation and with low rates of complications [21].

Five patients with amyotrophic lateral sclerosis with forced vital capacity ranging from 21% to 44% of predicted during percutaneous endoscopic gastrostomy tube installation were supported with bi-level NIV by Boitano et al. without any complications [22]. The benefits of NIV have also been documented in case series. Using a modified face mask, NIV allows for the successful performance of continuous transesophageal echocardiography examination in patients with mildly sedated severe aortic valve stenosis and orthopnea without the need for intubation or general anesthesia [23].

Nava and colleagues in a prospective, multicenter, randomized study, compared the effect of NIV to that of standard medical therapy in reducing the rate of meeting the intubation criteria in patients older than 75 with AHRF. They found that NIV decreased the rate of intubation and mortality, concluding that NIV should be offered as an alternative to patients considered poor candidates for intubation and those with a DNI (Do Not Intubate) order [24].

There have been reports of the use of NIV following complex surgical operations in patients who are at high risk of developing acute respiratory failure following surgery (due to factors like obesity). In comparison to oxygen treatment, some studies suggested that it might be useful in avoiding and treating ARF following major surgery (lung and abdomen), lowering the rate of patient intubation.

Imperatore and colleagues evaluated the efficacy of NIV in a postanesthesia care unit (PACU) in reducing post-extubation acute ARF after biliointestinal bypass (BIBP) in obese patients. They found that after bariatric surgery, short-term NIV during PACU observation promotes a more rapid recovery of postoperative lung function and oxygenation in obese patients, reducing the necessity for critical care in the days following surgery. Therefore, as day-case surgery becomes more advocated even for morbid obesity, it might be considered a necessary procedure [25].

Pettenuzzo and colleagues, in their systematic review and network meta-analysis about the effects of noninvasive respiratory support in postoperative patients, found that in postoperative patients receiving noninvasive respiratory support after extubation, NIV reduced the rate of re-intubation, compared to COT (Conventional Oxygen Therapy), when used for treatment of post-extubation respiratory failure and in patients at high risk of post-extubation respiratory failure [26].

1.2 Summary

The use of NIV has increased dramatically over the last three decades. NIV can significantly alter the prognosis for certain patients suffering from respiratory failure. It is now considered the gold standard for managing ARF in a variety of diseases, including COPD (Chronic Obstructive Pulmonary Diseases) and cardiogenic pulmonary edema, and, frequently, in immunocompromised individuals. Surveys and observational studies have shown that, despite strong evidence supporting its usefulness in clinical practice, its real-world application is still varied. However, research indicates that the usage of NIV rises with physician familiarity and the availability of financial and human resources. Overall, data from the literature indicates that during the past 10 years, there has been an increase in the use of NIV in selected subgroups of respiratory failure, both inside and outside the ICU. New trends in the application of NIV appear promising, but larger studies are required to confirm its safety.

References

1. Nava S, Hill N. Non-invasive ventilation in acute respiratory failure. Lancet. 2009;374(9685):250–9.
2. Slutsky AS. History of mechanical ventilation. From vesalius to ventilator-induced lung injury. Am J Respir Crit Care Med. 2015;191(10):1106–15.
3. Braun NMT. Negative Pressure Noninvasive Ventilation (NPNIV): history, rationale, and application. In: Nocturnal Non-Invasive Ventilation. New York: Springer; 2015. p. 27–71. https://doi.org/10.1007/978-1-4899-7624-6_2. PMCID: PMC7122449.
4. Mehta S, Hill NS. Noninvasive ventilation. Am J Respir Crit Care Med. 2001;163(2):540–77.
5. Bach JR, Alba AS, Saporito LR. Intermittent positive pressure ventilation via the mouth as an alternative to tracheostomy for 257 ventilator users. Chest. 1993;103(1):174–82. https://doi.org/10.1378/chest.103.1.174. PMID: 8417874.
6. Brochard L. Mechanical ventilation: invasive versus noninvasive. Eur Respir J Suppl. 2003;47:31s–7s.
7. Ambrosino N. Ventilation techniques: invasive versus noninvasive. Monaldi Arch Chest Dis. 1994;49(6):513–5.
8. Servera E, Sancho J, Zafra MJ, Catala A, Vergara P, Marin J. Alternatives to endotracheal intubation for patients with neuromuscular diseases. Am J Phys Med Rehabil. 2005;84(11):851–7.
9. Pierson DJ. History and epidemiology of noninvasive ventilation in the acute-care setting. Respir Care. 2009;54(1):40–52.
10. Devlin JW, Nava S, Fong JJ, Bahhady I, Hill NS. Survey of sedation practices during noninvasive positive-pressure ventilation to treat acute respiratory failure. Crit Care Med. 2007;35(10):2298–302.
11. Chiner E, Llombart M, Martinez-Garcia MA, et al. Noninvasive mechanical ventilation in Valencia, Spain: from theory to practice. Arch Bronconeumol. 2009;45(3):118–22.
12. Hess DR, Pang JM, Camargo CA Jr. A survey of the use of noninvasive ventilation in academic emergency departments in the United States. Respir Care. 2009;54(10):1306–12.
13. Crimi C, Noto A, Princi P, et al. A European survey of noninvasive ventilation practices. Eur Respir J. 2010;36(2):362–9.
14. Stefan MS, Shieh MS, Pekow PS, et al. Epidemiology and outcomes of acute respiratory failure in the United States, 2001 to 2009: a national survey. J Hosp Med. 2013;8(2):76–82.
15. Boldrini R, Fasano L, Nava S. Noninvasive mechanical ventilation. Curr Opin Crit Care. 2012;18(1):48–53.
16. Paus-Jenssen ES, Reid JK, Cockcroft DW, Laframboise K, Ward HA. The use of noninvasive ventilation in acute respiratory failure at a tertiary care center. Chest. 2004;126(1):165–72.
17. Cabrini L, Esquinas A, Pasin L, et al. An international survey on noninvasive ventilation uses for acute respiratory failure in general non-monitored wards. Respir Care. 2015;60(4):586–92.
18. Bruge P, Jabre P, Dru M, Jbeili C, Lecarpentier E, Khalid M, Margenet A, Marty J, Combes X. An observational study of noninvasive positive pressure ventilation in an out-of-hospital setting. Am J Emerg Med. 2008;26(2):165–9.
19. McCoy AM, Morris D, Tanaka K, Wright A, Guyette FX, Martin-Gill C. Prehospital noninvasive ventilation: an NAEMSP position statement and resource document. Prehosp Emerg Care. 2022;26(sup1):80–7. https://doi.org/10.1080/10903127.2021.1993392.
20. Ambrosino N, Guarracino F. Unusual applications of noninvasive ventilation. Eur Respir J. 2011;38(2):440–9.
21. Sircar M, Jha OK, Chabbra GS, Bhattacharya S. Noninvasive ventilation-assisted bronchoscopy in high-risk hypoxemic patients. Indian J Crit Care Med. 2019;23(8):363–7. https://doi.org/10.5005/jp-journals-10071-23219. PMID: 31485105; PMCID: PMC6709836.
22. Boitano LJ, Jordan T, Benditt JO. Noninvasive ventilation allows gastrostomy tube placement in patients with advanced ALS. Neurology. 2001;56(3):413–4.

23. Guarracino F, Cabrini L, Baldassarri R, Petronio S, De Carlo M, Covello RD, et al. Noninvasive ventilation for awake percutaneous aortic valve implantation in high-risk respiratory patients: a case series. J Cardiothorac Vasc Anesth. 2011;25(6):1109–12.
24. Nava S, Grassi M, Fanfulla F, et al. Noninvasive ventilation in elderly patients with acute hypercapnic respiratory failure: a randomized controlled trial. Age Ageing. 2011;40:444–50.
25. Imperatore F, Gritti F, Esposito R, Giudice CD, Cafora C, Pennacchio F, Maglione F, Catauro A, Pace MC, Docimo L, Gambardella C. Non-invasive ventilation reduces postoperative respiratory failure in patients undergoing bariatric surgery: a retrospective analysis. Medicina (Kaunas). 2023;59(8):1457. https://doi.org/10.3390/medicina59081457. PMID: 37629747; PMCID: PMC10456476.
26. Pettenuzzo T, Boscolo A, Pistollato E, et al. Effects of non-invasive respiratory support in post-operative patients: a systematic review and network meta-analysis. Crit Care. 2024;28:152. https://doi.org/10.1186/s13054-024-04924-0.

Noninvasive Ventilation: Rational Physiologic Effects in Endoscopy Procedures

2

Domenica Di Costanzo, Mariano Mazza,
and Antonio M. Esquinas

2.1 Alteration of Respiratory Mechanics During Endoscopy Procedures of the Airway

Airway endoscopy procedures, i.e., fiber-optic bronchoscopy (FOB), are widely performed for the assessment, diagnosis, and treatment of patients with respiratory disease.

The execution of FOB, both flexible bronchoscopy (FB) and rigid technique, is responsible for physiological changes in respiratory mechanics.

In this chapter, we will focus on the physiological alterations induced by FOB with a flexible bronchoscope, i.e., videobronchoscopy and endobronchial ultrasound (EBUS), and on the rationale for using noninvasive respiratory supports during these procedures.

2.1.1 Reduction in the Caliber of the Airways

A flexible bronchoscope inserted in the upper airways decreases their cross-sectional area in a measure proportional to the outer diameter of the bronchoscope, thus increasing the resistance to air flow [1]. It has been estimated that the instrument occupies only about 10% of the tracheal cross-sectional area and about 15% of the

D. Di Costanzo (✉)
Ambulatorio Pneumologia, Azienda Sanitaria Locale Napoli 3 Sud, Napoli, Italy

M. Mazza
Ambulatorio Pneumologia Chronic Care Center, Azienda Sanitaria Locale Caserta, Caserta, Italy

A. M. Esquinas
Intensive Care Unit, Hospital Morales Meseguer, Murcia, Spain

© The Author(s), under exclusive license to Springer Nature Switzerland AG 2025

K. Panda et al. (eds.), *Noninvasive Ventilatory Approaches in Interventional Procedures*, Noninvasive Ventilation. The Essentials,
https://doi.org/10.1007/978-3-032-05328-2_2

cross-sectional area at the cricoid ring level, but this is sufficient to determine an increase in flow resistances in the patient's airways, resulting in an increase of the work of breathing (WOB) [2].

A more moderate and usually tolerable obstruction can be obtained by transnasal insertion of the bronchoscope in spontaneously breathing patients, which only causes small variations in the intratracheal pressure [2].

In intubated patients, the presence of the endotracheal tube itself claims space in the airway especially if the tube is cuffed, and the bronchoscope can provide further obstruction: in some studies, it has been measured that a 5.7 mm bronchoscope occupies about 40% of a 9.0-mm internal-diameter (ID) endotracheal tube and 66% of a 7.0-mm-ID endotracheal tube [3]. This condition is sufficient to significantly increase flow resistance and the WOB even more than in non-intubated patients [4].

2.1.2 Negative Tracheal Pressure

The suctioning maneuvers during FB may create a negative tracheal pressure, resulting in dramatically decreased tidal volume; these effects are due to continued use of suction when secretions are not being removed, i.e., the suction channel is filled with air.

When suctioning is applied, generally, about 200–300 mL of tidal volume is lost at each maneuver, and end-expiratory lung volume is reduced, with alveolar de-recruitment, increased vascular shunt, and venous admixture.

Further effects of FB are a possible loss of functional gas exchange surface, if bronchoalveolar lavage (BAL) is performed, and reflex bronchospasm due to stimulation of vagal receptors in the upper airways [5].

Moreover, during suctioning, there is removal of oxygen-enriched air from the lungs, which is replaced by room air enriched with more diluted oxygen because of the higher inspiratory flow rate. The higher the rate of removal of pulmonary air by suctioning, the lower the fractional concentration of oxygen in the oxygen-enriched air which replaces it [6].

These factors may cause a loss of arterial oxygen partial pressure (PaO2) in the order of about 10 to 20 mmHg during bronchoscopy, especially when BAL is added, because of the contribution of concurrent altered ventilation-perfusion ratio [7, 8]. Hypoxemia during or immediately after taking BAL is the most common complication of this procedure [9]. Moreover, after taking BAL, an elevation of arterial carbon dioxide partial pressure (PaCO2) occurs and principally reflects decreased alveolar ventilation.

Ultimately, PaCO2 can increase up to about 30%, while PaO2 can decrease up to 40% [2].

2.1.3 Upper Airway Collapse

Desaturation during bronchoscopy has also been attributed to upper airway obstruction (UAO), due to sedatives or analgesics used or the suctioning itself. Acute hypoxemia secondary to UAO despite supplemental oxygenation in patients undergoing FB under local anesthesia and sedation could be successfully treated with insertion of a nasopharyngeal tube [10].

2.1.4 Hemodynamic Changes

The execution of FB can indirectly cause significant hemodynamic changes: the increase of airway resistance and WOB theoretically leads to changes in intrathoracic pressure, which may also affect venous return and afterload, while reducing cardiac output.

However, it has been reported that cardiac output increases up to 50% secondary to sympathetic stimulation during FB, and it returns to baseline in 15 min after its completion [2, 11]. In fragile or cardiopathic patients, performing FB may cause a dangerous cardiopulmonary distress, associated with electrocardiographic alteration in up to 21% of awake patients over 60 years old [12]. This aspect should also drive the clinician to choose the more appropriate oxygenation strategy from a physiological point of view.

2.1.5 Normal Versus Damaged Lungs

The normalization of respiratory changes induced by bronchoscopy after the procedure generally may take 15 min, in a healthy lung, up to several hours, in severe parenchymal lung diseases.

FB is generally considered a safe procedure, usually without consequences in patients without a baseline hypoxemia [13], but it is well known that critically ill patients with bronchoscopy have an intrinsically higher risk of complications of all kinds, particularly the deterioration of preexisting hypoxemia, that can be transitory or not [14, 15].

When lung parenchyma is already compromised by an underlying pathologic condition, the physiological alterations induced by uncomplicated FB can be detrimental since they may worsen gas exchange, leading to the development of respiratory failure or the acute worsening of a such preexisting condition [16, 17].

2.1.6 Role of Sedation

Although some procedures may be performed with just an extensive topical anesthesia, others (e.g., EBUS) may require deep sedation obtained with different pharmacological strategies including both sedatives (e.g., midazolam, propofol, or dexmedetomidine) and analgesics (e.g., remifentanil) alone or in combination, according to the needs. However, it must be taken in account that these drugs can modify the critical closing pressure of the upper airways, inducing their collapse [18, 19], and they can affect the breathing pattern and/or the respiratory drive, due to their direct action on central nervous system. In particular, the deeper the sedation, the higher the effect [20, 21].

2.2 Effects of Different Forms of Oxygen Therapies and Ventilatory Support During Flexible Bronchoscopy

2.2.1 Conventional Oxygen Therapy During Flexible Bronchoscopy

The use of conventional oxygen therapy (COT) during FB has been investigated in several studies. Oxygen can be delivered by a cannula placed either in the nostrils or in the mouth, as the average peripheral arterial oxyhemoglobin saturation (SpO2) maintained within the procedure is similar between the two modalities, and no sinus symptoms or nasal congestion have been reported [22].

FB itself can lead to desaturation, and COT through nasal prongs is appropriate to reduce transitory procedural hypoxemia [6].

Although not always required [23], COT has shown its benefits in patients with higher risk of desaturation, including those with baseline (before procedure) SpO2 < 93% [24], an obstructive ventilatory defect [25], or a forced expiratory volume in the first second lower than 1 L [23, 26].

In hypoxemic patients, supplemental oxygen is recommended during bronchoscopy to achieve an SpO2 of at least 90% [27].

However, the inspired oxygen fraction (FiO2) cannot be predicted and might not be enough in severe cases. Severe hypoxemia (PaO2 < 60 mm Hg despite FIO2 of 0.5) in non-intubated patients is generally regarded as a contraindication to bronchoscopy, as these patients are at high risk for developing hypoxia-related cardiorespiratory complications [1].

2.2.2 High-Flow Nasal Cannula During Flexible Bronchoscopy

High-flow nasal cannula oxygen therapy (HFNCOT) utilizes higher gas flow rates than conventional low-flow oxygen systems. The devices used deliver heated and humidified mixture of air and oxygen at a flow of up to 60 L/min via dedicated nasal cannulas [15].

HFNC has been introduced in clinical practice as a valuable alternative for oxygen support during FB [28–30]. At our best knowledge, four main points support the use of HFNCOT during and after the procedure.

1. HFNCOT can provide a constant high flow up to 60 L/min, which ensures a more stable FiO2 than COT, as it is able to match the increased patient's inspiratory flow [31]. When inspiratory flow rates of the patient exceed the constant high-flow supplies, the additional flow from the surrounding air will be recruited, resulting in lower FiO2 than the delivered gas [32].
2. Although HFNCOT does not intend to provide end-expiratory positive airway pressure (EPAP), its high flow can generate positive airway pressures in the nasopharynx, depending on the flow rate, the upper airway anatomy, the breathing through the nose or mouth, and the size of the cannula in relation to the nostrils [31]. The positive airway pressures in the nasopharynx translate then to the alveoli [33]. It has been estimated that every increase in flow of 10 L/min can produce a 0.8 cm H2O increase in expiratory pressure during mouth-closed breathing [34].
3. The high flow reduces the dead space in the upper airways up to 70 mL and increases the alveolar ventilation [31].
4. The HFNC decreases the resistive breathing effort, reducing the upper airway resistance [31, 35, 36].

However, during HFNCOT, the presence of large nasal prongs prevents the possibility to use the nasal route, leading the physician to insert the FB through the mouth.

Noteworthy, the EPAP generated by HFNCOT would be significantly reduced during open-mouth breathing, losing theoretically its benefit on alveolar distending pressure and lung de-recruitment prevention [31].

However, it has been recently demonstrated that in outpatients undergoing FB with BAL, when compared to COT, HFNCOT prevents oxygenation from worsening by avoiding end-expiratory loss of lung volume and preserves the same tidal volume with a lower diaphragm activation [37].

2.2.3 Continuous Positive Airway Pressure During Flexible Bronchoscopy

The application of continuous positive airway pressure (CPAP) has also been adopted during FB. CPAP results in a positive pressure throughout the entire breathing cycle, thereby recruiting lung atelectatic regions [38], reducing venous admixture [39], and decreasing the patient's inspiratory effort [40].

2.2.4 Noninvasive Mechanical Ventilation During Flexible Bronchoscopy

Noninvasive mechanical ventilation (NIV) is used in the treatment of respiratory failure to improve gas exchange alterations [8].

In patients with respiratory failure, it has several beneficial effects: NIV provides EPAP, which prevents alveolar collapse or recruits closed alveoli [41], thus augmenting ventilation; it also provides inspiratory positive airway pressure through which it decreases the work of breathing and improves lung mechanics [42–44], thereby ameliorating gas exchange and hypoxemia in patients with respiratory failure [45].

Clinically, NIV reduces respiratory effort, dyspnea, and the activity of the accessory respiratory muscles, preventing the complications related to invasive mechanical ventilation with preservation of the airway defense mechanism [46].

As previously said, FB is associated with temporary alterations in gas exchange, hemodynamics, and lung mechanics, due to reduction in the airway size which increases airway resistance and work of breathing [47].

Several reports suggest that application of NIV, for its effects, can facilitate the performance of bronchoscopy in patients with severe respiratory failure thereby improving its tolerability and safety [48].

In studies comparing the use of NIV and HFNC, a fundamental difference between HFNC and NIV is the fact that HFNC systems maintain a fixed flow and generate variable pressures, whereas many NIV systems generate a fixed pressure by utilizing variable flow [35]. While using HFNC, as the respiratory rate and inspiratory effort increase during the procedure, the flow may not be sufficient, resulting in lower FiO2. In contrast, with the NIV mode, the flow can be adequately adjusted to reach and maintain the target inspiratory pressure and a constant FiO2 [15]. Moreover, when using HFNC during FB, EPAP has been shown to be lost when the mouth is opened [34]; due to the closed circuit of the NIV face mask, even when patients open their mouth, EPAP would be maintained instead.

Furthermore, in patients with obstructive sleep apnea, NIV is likely to counter upper airway collapse during bronchoscopy [49, 50].

However, NIV may be negatively affected by poor patient-ventilator interaction, which impairs its effectiveness [51–55] and air leaks from interfaces used, and FB can favor the onset of these complications, altering the tightness of the ventilator-patient circuit due to its very nature.

Different interfaces have been used for FB on NIV support including oronasal mask [1, 16, 56, 57], full-face mask [48, 58], and nasal mask with bite block covered by glove finger through which FB is introduced [24, 59], in order to minimize air leaks in the patient-ventilator circuit.

Helmets and face masks for CPAP or NIV have then been specifically designed to be used during FB, to allow both oral and nasal routes for bronchoscope insertion. For example, Korkmaz Ekren et al. have used a dedicated full-face mask with an interchangeable connector between the ventilator tubing and the mask that allows the insertion of the bronchoscope through a sealed hole [57]. Heunks et al. [26] have used in another study a total face mask with a dedicated sealed hole below the connector between ventilator tubing and interface, allowing the performance of the FB through the mouth during NIV. However, air leaks may occur around the interface or through the dedicated hole for FB insertion, leading to patient-ventilator asynchronies which may be difficult to manage [52, 60]. To our best knowledge, no study till date has compared different types of masks.

The use of NIV during FB has been extended to more complicated procedures, such as transbronchial lung biopsy, balloon dilation, electrocautery, and argon plasma coagulation. In keeping with the abovementioned studies, NIV guarantees a stable oxygenation and good patient tolerance, whereas minor complications, as well as the number of patients requiring intubation after the procedure, are quite low [50, 59].

Similar findings have been also reported for patients with chronic [61] and acute-on-chronic [62, 63] respiratory failure already on noninvasive ventilatory support. Since these patients have an intrinsic high risk of endotracheal intubation secondary to NIV failure, bronchoscopy should only be performed by clinicians experienced with bronchoscopy, NIV, and endotracheal intubation in an environment with a high level of monitoring of vital signs, which is required both before initiation of FB and for extended periods afterward as late complications can occur [48].

2.3 Conclusions

Flexible bronchoscopy can induce several physiological alterations of lung mechanics such as a decrease of the cross-sectional area of upper airways, the generation of a negative tracheal pressure during the suctioning maneuvers, and upper airway collapse.

These alterations can lead to hypoxemia and, when lung parenchyma is already compromised by an underlying pathologic condition, to the development of respiratory failure or worsening of such preexisting condition.

Moreover, the anesthetic or sedative drugs used can affect the respiratory physiology, together with the hemodynamic changes induced by FB itself.

The application of NIV can facilitate the performance of FB in patients with severe respiratory failure through its beneficial effects. NIV prevents alveolar collapse or recruits closed alveoli, thus augmenting ventilation; it also decreases the work of breathing and improves lung mechanics, thereby ameliorating gas exchange and hypoxemia.

NIV can facilitate both diagnostic and therapeutic bronchoscopic procedures in very severe hypoxemic patients, thus avoiding intubation, provided that it is performed by clinicians experienced with interventional procedures and mechanical ventilation in an environment with a high level of monitoring.

References

1. Agarwal R, Khan A, Aggarwal AN, Gupta D. Bronchoscopic lung biopsy using noninvasive ventilatory support: case series and review of literature of NIV-assisted bronchoscopy. Respir Care. 2012;57(11):1927–36.

2. Lindholm CE, Ollman B, Snyder JV, Millen EG, Grenvik A. Cardiorespiratory effects of flexible fiberoptic bronchoscopy in critically ill patients. Chest. 1978;74(4):362–8.
3. Campos JH. Fiberoptic bronchoscopy guidelines for the anesthesiologist. Rev Mex Anestesiol. 2011;31:S264–9.
4. Matsushima Y, Jones RL, King EG, Moysa G, Alton JD. Alterations in pulmonary mechanics and gas exchange during routine fiberoptic bronchoscopy. Chest. 1984;86(2):184–8.
5. Sircar M, Jha OK, Chabbra GS, Bhattacharya S. Noninvasive ventilation-assisted bronchoscopy in high-risk hypoxemic patients. Indian J Crit Care Med. 2019;23(8):363–7. https://doi.org/10.5005/jp-journals-10071-23219.
6. Miller EJ. Hypoxemia during fiberoptic bronchoscopy. Chest. 1979;75(1):103.
7. Herrejón A, Simó M, Pérez ME, Chiner E, Marín J. Comparison between arterial and transcutaneous oxygen pressure in fibrobronchoscopy. Arch Bronconeumol. 1989;25:80–3.
8. Mohamed AS, El-Sharawy DE. Noninvasive ventilation with add-on fiberoptic bronchoscopy in patients with chronic obstructive pulmonary disease. Egypt J Chest Dis Tuberc. 2018;67(1):26.
9. Barrett CR Jr, Vecchione JJ, Bell AL Jr. Flexible fiberoptic bronchoscopy for airway management during acute respiratory failure. Am Rev Respir Dis. 1974;109:429–34.
10. Chhajed PN, Aboyoun C, Malouf MA, Hopkins PM, Plit M, Grunstein RR, et al. Management of acute hypoxemia during flexible bronchoscopy with insertion of a nasopharyngeal tube in lung transplant recipients. Chest. 2002;121:1350–4.
11. Lundgren R, Häggmark S, Reiz S. Hemodynamic effects of flexible fiberoptic bronchoscopy performed under topical anesthesia. Chest. 1982;82(3):295–9.
12. Davies L, Mister R, Spence DP, Calverley PM, Earis JE, Pearson MG. Cardiovascular consequences of fibreoptic bronchoscopy. Eur Respir J. 1997;10(3):695–8.
13. Facciolongo N, Patelli M, Gasparini S, Lazzari Agli L, Salio M, Simonassi C, Del Prato B, Zanoni P. Incidence of complications in bronchoscopy: multicentre prospective study of 20,986 bronchoscopies. Monaldi Arch Chest Dis. 2009;71:8–14.
14. Albertini RE, Harrell JH, Kurihara N, Moser KM. Arterial hypoxemia induced by fiberoptic bronchoscopy. JAMA. 1974;230:1666–7.
15. Simon M, Braune S, Frings D, Wiontzek A-K, Klose H, Kluge S. High-flow nasal cannula oxygen versus non-invasive ventilation in patients with acute hypoxaemic respiratory failure undergoing flexible bronchoscopy, a prospective randomised trial. Crit Care. 2014;18(6):712.
16. Antonelli M, Conti G, Riccioni L, Meduri GU. Noninvasive positive-pressure ventilation via face mask during bronchoscopy with BAL in high-risk hypoxemic patients. Chest. 1996;110(3):724–8.
17. Goldstein RA, Rohatgi PK, Bergofsky EH, Block ER, Daniele RP, Dantzker DR, et al. Clinical role of bronchoalveolar lavage in adults with pulmonary disease. Am Rev Respir Dis. 1990;142(2):481–6.
18. Eastwood PR, Platt PR, Shepherd K, Maddison K, Hillman DR. Collapsibility of the upper airway at different concentrations of propofol anesthesia. Anesthesiology. 2005;103(3):470–7.
19. Shteamer JW, Dedhia RC. Sedative choice in drug-induced sleep endoscopy: a neuropharmacology-based review. Laryngoscope. 2017;127(1):273–9.
20. Costa R, Navalesi P, Cammarota G, Longhini F, Spinazzola G, Cipriani F, et al. Remifentanil effects on respiratory drive and timing during pressure support ventilation and neurally adjusted ventilatory assist. Respir Physiol Neurobiol. 2017;244:10–6.
21. Vaschetto R, Cammarota G, Colombo D, Longhini F, Grossi F, Giovanniello A, et al. Effects of propofol on patient-ventilator synchrony and interaction during pressure support ventilation and neurally adjusted ventilatory assist. Crit Care Med. 2014;42(1):74–82.
22. McCain TW, Dunagan DP, Adair NE, Chin R. Prospective randomized trial comparing oxygen administration during nasal flexible bronchoscopy: oral vs nasal delivery. Chest. 2001;120(5):1671–4.
23. Antonelli M, Pennisi MA, Conti G, Bello G, Maggiore SM, Michetti V, et al. Fiberoptic bronchoscopy during noninvasive positive pressure ventilation delivered by helmet. Intensive Care Med. 2003;29:126–9.

24. Chiner E, Llombart M, Signes-Costa J, Andreu AL, Gomez-Merino E, Pastor E, et al. Description of a new procedure for fiberoptic bronchoscopy during noninvasive ventilation through a nasal mask in patients with acute respiratory failure. Arch Bronconeumol. 2005;41:698–701.
25. Trachsel D, Erb TO, Frei FJ, Hammer J, Swiss Paediatric Respiratory Research Group. Use of continuous positive airway pressure during flexible bronchoscopy in young children. Eur Respir J. 2005;26:773–7.
26. Heunks LM, de Bruin CJ, van der Hoeven JG, van der Heijden HF. Non-invasive mechanical ventilation for diagnostic bronchoscopy using a new face mask: an observational feasibility study. Intensive Care Med. 2010;36:143–7.
27. British Thoracic Society. Guidelines on diagnostic flexible bronchoscopy. Thorax. 2001;56(Suppl 1):i1–21.
28. Pisani L, Astuto M, Prediletto I, Longhini F. High flow through nasal cannula in exacerbated COPD patients: a systematic review. Pulmonology. 2019;25(6):348–54.
29. Cortegiani A, Longhini F, Carlucci A, Scala R, Grof P, Bruni A, et al. Highflow nasal therapy versus noninvasive ventilation in COPD patients with mild-to-moderate hypercapnic acute respiratory failure: study protocol for a noninferiority randomized clinical trial. Trials. 2019;20(1):450.
30. Garofalo E, Bruni A, Pelaia C, Cammarota G, Murabito P, Biamonte E, et al. Evaluation of a new interface combining high-flow nasal cannula and CPAP. Respir Care. 2019;64(10):1231–9.
31. Renda T, Corrado A, Iskandar G, Pelaia G, Abdalla K, Navalesi P. High-flow nasal oxygen therapy in intensive care and anaesthesia. Br J Anaesth. 2018;120(1):18–27.
32. Saksitthichok B, Petnak T, So-Ngern A, Boonsarngsuk V. A prospective randomized comparative study of high-fow nasal cannula oxygen and non-invasive ventilation in hypoxemic patients undergoing diagnostic flexible bronchoscopy. J Thorac Dis. 2019;11(5):1929–39.
33. Helviz Y, Einav S. A systematic review of the high-flow nasal cannula for adult patients. Crit Care. 2018;22:71.
34. Groves N, Tobin A. High flow nasal oxygen generates positive airway pressure in adult volunteers. Aust Crit Care. 2007;20:126–31.
35. Lee JH, Rehder KJ, Williford L, Cheifetz IM, Turner DA. Use of high flow nasal cannula in critically ill infants, children, and adults: a critical review of the literature. Intensive Care Med. 2013;39:247–57.
36. Ricard J-D. High flow nasal oxygen in acute respiratory failure. Minerva Anestesiol. 2012;78:836–41. Gotera C, Díaz Lobato S, Pinto T, Winck JC. Clinical evidence on high flow oxygen therapy and active humidification in adults. Rev Port Pneumol. 2013;19:217–27.
37. Longhini F, Pelaia C, Garofalo E, Bruni A, Placida R, Iaquinta C, et al. Highflow nasal cannula oxygen therapy for outpatients undergoing flexible bronchoscopy: a randomised controlled trial. Thorax. 2022;77:58–64. https://doi.org/10.1136/thoraxjnl-2021-217116.
38. Cammarota G, Vaschetto R, Turucz E, Dellapiazza F, Colombo D, Blando C, et al. Influence of lung collapse distribution on the physiologic response to recruitment maneuvers during noninvasive continuous positive airway pressure. Intensive Care Med. 2011;37(7):1095–102.
39. Lindner KH, Lotz P, Ahnefeld FW. Continuous positive airway pressure effect on functional residual capacity, vital capacity and its subdivisions. Chest. 1987;92(1):66–70.
40. Lenique F, Habis M, Lofaso F, Dubois-Randé JL, Harf A, Brochard L. Ventilatory and hemodynamic effects of continuous positive airway pressure in left heart failure. Am J Respir Crit Care Med. 1997;155(2):500–5.
41. Jaber S, Monnin M, Girard M, et al. Apnoeic oxygenation via highflow nasal cannula oxygen combined with noninvasive ventilation preoxygenation for intubation in hypoxaemic patients in the intensive care unit: the singlecentre, blinded, randomized controlled OPTINIV trial. Intensive Care Med. 2016;42:1877–87.
42. Frat JP, Thille AW, Mercat A, et al. High-flow oxygen through nasal cannula in acute hypoxemic respiratory failure. N Engl J Med. 2015;372:2185–96.
43. Stéphan F, Barrucand B, Petit P, et al. High-flow nasal oxygen vs noninvasive positive airway pressure in hypoxemic patients after cardiothoracic surgery: a randomized clinical trial. JAMA. 2015;313:2331–9.

44. Bräunlich J, Seyfarth HJ, Wirtz H. Nasal high-flow versus non-invasive ventilation in stable hypercapnic COPD: a preliminary report. Multidiscip Respir Med. 2015;10:27.
45. Brochard L. Noninvasive ventilation for acute respiratory failure. JAMA. 2002;288(8):932–5.
46. Esquinas A, Zuil M, Scala R, Chinerd E. Bronchoscopy during non-invasive mechanical ventilation: a review of techniques and procedures. Arch Bronconeumol. 2013;49:105–12.
47. Katz AS, Michelson EL, Stawicki J, Holford FD. Cardiac arrhythmias. Frequency during fiberoptic bronchoscopy and correlation with hypoxemia. Arch Intern Med. 1981;141(5):603–6.
48. Baumann HJ, Klose H, Simon M, Ghadban T, Braune SA, Hennigs JK, et al. Fiber optic bronchoscopy in patients with acute hypoxemic respiratory failure requiring noninvasive ventilation – a feasibility study. Crit Care. 2011;15:R179.
49. Borowiecki B, Pollak CP, Weitzman ED, Rakoff S, Imperato J. Fiberoptic study of pharyngeal airway during sleep in patients with hypersomnia obstructive sleep-apnea syndrome. Laryngoscope. 1978;88:1310–3. 33.
50. Popper RA, Leidinger MJ, Williams AJ. Endoscopic observations of the pharyngeal airway during treatment of obstructive sleep apnea with nasal continuous positive airway pressure – a pneumatic splint. West J Med. 1986;144:83–5.
51. Nava S, Navalesi P, Carlucci A. Non-invasive ventilation. Minerva Anestesiol. 2009;75(1–2):31–6. 8.
52. Garofalo E, Bruni A, Pelaia C, Liparota L, Lombardo N, Longhini F, et al. Recognizing, quantifying and managing patient-ventilator asynchrony in invasive and noninvasive ventilation. Expert Rev Respir Med. 2018;12(7):557–67 + 52.
53. Longhini F, Colombo D, Pisani L, Idone F, Chun P, Doorduin J, et al. Efficacy of ventilator waveform observation for detection of patient-ventilator asynchrony during NIV: a multicentre study. ERJ Open Res. 2017;3(4):00075–2017. 53.
54. Cammarota G, Olivieri C, Costa R, Vaschetto R, Colombo D, Turucz E, et al. Noninvasive ventilation through a helmet in postextubation hypoxemic patients: physiologic comparison between neurally adjusted ventilatory assist and pressure support ventilation. Intensive Care Med. 2011;37(12):1943–50. 54.
55. Longhini F, Pan C, Xie J, Cammarota G, Bruni A, Garofalo E, et al. New setting of neurally adjusted ventilatory assist for noninvasive ventilation by facial mask: a physiologic study. Crit Care. 2017;21(1):170.
56. Antonelli M, Conti G, Rocco M, Arcangeli A, Cavaliere F, Proietti R, et al. Noninvasive positive-pressure ventilation vs. conventional oxygen supplementation in hypoxemic patients undergoing diagnostic bronchoscopy. Chest. 2002;121:1149–54.
57. Korkmaz Ekren P, Basarik Aydogan B, Gurgun A, Tasbakan MS, Bacakoglu F, Nava S. Can fiberoptic bronchoscopy be applied to critically ill patients treated with noninvasive ventilation for acute respiratory distress syndrome? Prospective observational study. BMC Pulm Med. 2016;16:89. https://doi.org/10.1186/s12890-016-0236-y.
58. Rady W, Abouelela A, Abdallah A, Youssef W. Role of bronchoscopy during nonivasive ventilation in hypercapnic respiratory failure. Egypt J Chest Dis Tuberc. 2014;63:1003–11.
59. Chiner E, Sancho-Chust JN, Llombart M, Senent C, Camarasa A, Signes-Costa J. Fiberoptic bronchoscopy during nasal non-invasive ventilation in acute respiratory failure. Respiration. 2010;80:321–6.
60. Bruni A, Garofalo E, Pelaia C, Messina A, Cammarota G, Murabito P, et al. Patient-ventilator asynchrony in adult critically ill patients. Minerva Anestesiol. 2019;85(6):676–88.
61. Bove T, Votta CD, Ciriaco P, Papalardo F, Oriani A, Frau G, et al. Bronchoscopy during non-invasive ventilation in a patient with acute respiratory distress syndrome. Signa Vitae. 2017;13:103–4.
62. Cabrini L, Nobile L, Cama E, Borghi G, Pieri M, Bocchino S, et al. Noninvasive ventilation during upper endoscopies in adult patients. A systematic review. Minerva Anestesiol. 2013;79(683–694):37.
63. Folgado MA, De la Serna C, Llorente A, Rodriguez S, Ochoa C, DiazLobato S. Utility of noninvasive ventilation in high-risk patients during endoscopic retrograde cholangiopancreatography. Lung India. 2014;31:331–5.

Upper Airways and Lung Mechanics During Endoscopy

3

Marta Duarte-Silva and Dionísio Maia

Upper gastrointestinal (GI) endoscopy is a widely performed diagnostic and therapeutic procedure that involves several factors that can influence upper airways and lung mechanics. Effective management of these factors is essential to ensure patient safety and procedural success. This chapter delves into the key considerations and strategies for managing the airway during upper GI endoscopy, including sedation, anesthesia, patient positioning, and preexisting respiratory conditions.

3.1 Sedation and Anesthesia

Sedation plays a critical role in upper GI endoscopy by providing patient comfort and facilitating the procedure. However, sedation-related complications are predominantly airway related, making it essential to maintain upper airway patency, preserve spontaneous ventilation, and suppress the cough reflex [1].

The use of propofol for sedation requires careful dose titration to maintain spontaneous ventilation and preserve laryngeal reflexes. Deep sedation, while beneficial for performing complex procedures, poses significant challenges for airway management. Understanding the upper airway anatomy is crucial to avoid adverse outcomes. During sedation, the tone of the upper airway musculature is reduced, potentially leading to airway collapse, most commonly at the velopharynx. This airway obstruction can lead to hypoxemia and thoracoabdominal asynchrony. Managing this involves several strategies such as increasing supplemental oxygen (via conventional nasal cannula or high-flow oxygen therapy); inserting a

M. Duarte-Silva (✉) · D. Maia
Unidade Local de Saúde São José – Hospital de Santa Marta, Pulmonology Department, Lisbon, Portugal
e-mail: maria.silva42@ulssjose.min-saude.pt; dionisio.maia@ulssjose.min-saude.pt

© The Author(s), under exclusive license to Springer Nature Switzerland AG 2025

K. Panda et al. (eds.), *Noninvasive Ventilatory Approaches in Interventional Procedures*, Noninvasive Ventilation. The Essentials,
https://doi.org/10.1007/978-3-032-05328-2_3

nasopharyngeal airway; performing airway maneuvers (chin lift, jaw thrust, and neck extension); withdrawing the endoscope and applying positive pressure ventilation; and inserting a laryngeal mask airway and endotracheal intubation, if necessary [2].

3.2 Patient Positioning

Positioning the patient prone or semi-prone is common during endoscopic procedures like Endoscopic Retrograde Cholangiopancreatography (ERCP), which adds further challenges, especially in an unintubated patient. Although gravitational forces prevent airway collapse, airway complication rates remain high [3]. Maneuvers such as the chin lift, jaw thrust, and neck extension widen the pharyngeal space, facilitating airway patency. Adults with obstructive sleep apnea benefit from a sniffing position (flexion of cervical spine and extension of atlanto-occipital joint) [4]. These maneuvers can only be applied after withdrawal of the endoscope; hence, timely endoscope withdrawal and efficient institution of these measures are critical to their success.

3.3 Monitoring

Monitoring is crucial to detect and manage adverse events, with hypoxemia being the most significant risk. Monitoring end-tidal carbon dioxide is recommended by the American Society of Anesthesiologists during sedation procedures, but it is often unreliable during upper GI endoscopy due to the location of the CO_2 sensor and air dilution by fresh gas. Therefore, careful observation of chest movement and the use of alternative monitoring methods, such as acoustic respiratory monitors, impedance pneumograms and oxygen reserve index, are options to improve patient safety [2].

3.4 Face Masks and Airway Devices

Different face masks and airway devices can be used to supplement oxygen and/or drive positive pressure ventilation [2, 5]. These include:

- *Panoramic face mask*: Uses a reservoir bag to deliver high inspiratory oxygen.
- *Endoscopy mask*: Includes a leak-proof cushioned seal along the facial contour that allows positive pressure ventilation.
- *DEAS endoscopic mask*: Incorporates additional monitoring features for end-tidal CO_2 and inspiratory pressure.
- *Nasopharyngeal airway*: Helps bypass upper airway obstruction.
- *Gastrolaryngeal tube*: Designed for complex procedures, it allows simultaneous use of a gastroscope and provides ventilation. The tube has two cuffs: the distal one inflates in the esophagus-preventing the regurgitation of gastric contents.

The second cuff lies proximally and inflates to block air leak via the naso/oropharynx.
- *Bite blocks*: Assist the endoscopist to introduce the gastroscope into the oral cavity and simultaneously prevent the patient from biting the scope. Various designs like Goudra's bite block and Hague airway incorporate features to prevent airway obstruction and facilitate oxygen delivery.

Any patient with risk of aspiration (bleeding, emergency, drainage of pseudocyst, gastric outlet obstruction, removal of foreign body, pharyngeal pouch) would necessitate endotracheal intubation. However, in the majority of cases, non-advanced endoscopic procedures may be safely performed with an oxygen cannula, keeping in mind that the endoscope itself can act as an upper airway stent [2].

References

1. Goudra B, Singh P. Anesthesia for gastrointestinal endoscopy: a subspecialty in evolution? Saudi J Anaesth. 2015;9:237.
2. Goudra B, Singh PM. Airway management during upper GI endoscopic procedures: state of the art review. Dig Dis Sci. 2016;62:45–53.
3. Goudra B, Nuzat A, Singh PM, Gouda GB, Carlin A, Manjunath AK. Cardiac arrests in patients undergoing gastrointestinal endoscopy: a retrospective analysis of 73,029 procedures. Saudi J Gastroenterol. 2015;21:400–11.
4. Isono S, Tanaka A, Ishikawa T, Tagaito Y, Nishino T. Sniffing position improves pharyngeal airway patency in anesthetized patients with obstructive sleep Apnea. Anesthesiology. 2005;103:489–94.
5. Bazerbachi F, White RM, Forbes N, Goudra B, Dayyeh BKA, Chandrasekhara V, Sweitzer B. Endo-anesthesia: a primer. Gastroenterol Rep. 2022;10:goac069.

Part II

Equipment for Noninvasive Ventilation Support

Nasal High-Flow Devices

4

Mostafa Elshazly and Hebatallah Hesham Ahmed

4.1 Introduction

Oxygen therapy is the first-line treatment for acute hypoxemic respiratory failure. It is traditionally delivered through a face mask (standard oxygen) or noninvasive ventilation (NIV) and, more recently, through a nasal cannula with high-flow heated and humidified oxygen, also known as high-flow nasal cannula (HFNC) therapy.

The oldest oxygen delivery method/therapy is the use of a non-rebreathing face mask, which was first documented in 1946. The maximum oxygen flow rate that can be achieved with traditional devices is 15 L/min. Meanwhile, patients experiencing respiratory failure require inspiratory flows that range significantly from 30 to 120 L/min [1]. With conventional oxygen devices, the patient's inspiratory flow and supplied flow vary significantly, and FiO_2 is inconsistent and typically lower than anticipated [2]. Also, when supplemental oxygen is given at low flow, it is typically not humidified. Even with the use of bubble humidifiers, the emergent gas's absolute humidity stays low.

During the 1990s, noninvasive ventilation was found to be superior to invasive ventilation for exacerbations of COPD, acute cardiogenic pulmonary edema, and acute respiratory failure in patients who were immunocompromised [3].

High-flow oxygen therapy (HFOT) was first patented by Transpirator Technologies, Inc. in 1988 and was developed for use in both humans and racehorses to optimize their respiratory and cardiovascular function [4]. Soon after, commercial production began, and in the last few years, the number of clinical scenarios in which HFOT is used has increased.

M. Elshazly (✉) · H. H. Ahmed
Faculty of Medicine, Cairo University, Giza, Egypt
e-mail: melshazly@kasralainy.edu.eg

© The Author(s), under exclusive license to Springer Nature Switzerland AG 2025

K. Panda et al. (eds.), *Noninvasive Ventilatory Approaches in Interventional Procedures*, Noninvasive Ventilation. The Essentials,
https://doi.org/10.1007/978-3-032-05328-2_4

HFNC is a method that provides comfort by delivering warmed and humidified gas flow via nasal prongs. It maintains high FiO2 levels and generates a low level of positive pressure in the upper airways due to a high flow of gas, which also offers washout of dead space.

HFNC therapy became popular in the 2000s as a substitute for more traditional methods of respiratory support for critically ill patients [5]. Preliminary data also indicated that HFOT could avoid tracheal intubation in individuals with severe COVID-19 [6].

The interfaces and the capacity to provide distinct inspiratory and expiratory pressures versus a constant pressure are the main distinctions between HFNC and NIV.

The process of warming and humidifying inspired gas before administering it to patients at flow rates higher than those of traditional oxygen delivery devices is known as "high-flow therapy." Numerous terms are used to allude to this idea, such as "high-flow nasal oxygen (HFNO)," "nasal high flow (NHF)," "humidified high-flow therapy (HHFT)," and "high-flow nasal cannula oxygen (HFNC) therapy."

Only a flow generator, an active heated humidifier, a single heated circuit, and a nasal cannula are needed for the straightforward HFNC system. NIV interfaces increase anatomic dead space, whereas HFNC delivery lowers dead space [7].

4.1.1 Mechanism of Action

HFNC operates by delivering oxygen at high flow rates, typically between 30 L/min and 60 L/min, through a specialized nasal cannula. This approach offers several physiological advantages [8]:

Enhanced Oxygenation By delivering oxygen at high flow rates, HFOT ensures a consistent and adequate supply of oxygen, improving oxygenation in patients with hypoxemia.

1. *Reduced work of breathing*: The high flow of oxygen helps in reducing the patient's work of breathing by providing a small amount of positive end-expiratory pressure (PEEP), keeping the airways open and reducing the effort required for inhalation. Exponential reductions in minute ventilation and work of breathing are also linked to increasing HFNC flows [9]. Increasing HFNC flow rates cause linear improvements (increases or decreases as appropriate) in end-expiratory lung volume, oxygenation, respiratory rate, and positive airway pressure [9–11].
2. *Washout of anatomical dead space*: HFOT effectively washes out carbon dioxide from the anatomical dead space in the upper airways, improving ventilation efficiency.
3. *Humidification and heating*: The humidified and heated oxygen prevents drying of the mucosa, maintaining mucociliary function and patient comfort.

4.2 The High-Flow Nasal Cannula Delivery System's Components

As previously mentioned, the flow generator, humidifier, inspiratory limb, and nasal interface make up the basic HFNC system.

Both Vapotherm and Optiflow offer significant benefits in the management of respiratory failure, with each system having unique features that cater to specific clinical needs.

4.2.1 Flow Generator

Unlike conventional oxygen delivery systems, FiO_2 and gas flow rate are separately tunable. HFNC systems that are sold commercially can provide flow rates ranging from 2 L/min to 100 L/min [12–15]. Adult patients experiencing acute respiratory failure may have respiratory flow needs ranging from 30 L/min to over 120 L/min [1].

Depending on the HFNC delivery system applied, medical gases are attached to the device, or, alternatively, air is entrained using a turbine, and supplemental oxygen is added.

The HFNC system has an advantage over normal oxygen therapy in that it can more effectively satisfy the patient's inspiratory demands—indeed, exceed them—by delivering FiO_2 more precisely and lowering inspiratory resistance.

Air-oxygen blenders, built-in flow generators, and *entrainment systems* are the three categories of standalone flow generators. The most widely used of these is the air-oxygen blender with flow meter. Stable distribution of FiO_2 and gas flow is made possible by using a mechanical air-oxygen blender, a flow meter, and air and oxygen straight from the wall supply. Air-oxygen blenders typically titrate the concentration of oxygen based on the quantity of medical gas inhaled; however, some gas is lost during the blending process. A flow generator is built in with the BioVent A Series (Fig. 4.1). Air-oxygen blender is used in Bio-Med Devices, CT (Fig. 4.2).

A MaxVenturi (Maxtec, UT) provides high flow via an air entrainment system when higher concentrations are required. Using the Venturi principle, the MaxVenturi allows users to mix ambient air and oxygen without the need for piped medical-grade air [16].

A variety of critical care ventilators are built with an HFNC capacity as standard features. In these situations, the heated humidifier that is frequently attached to the ventilator is used to adjust the flow and FiO_2. Even though they are becoming more prevalent, standalone systems are still utilized most of the time.

To choose a flow rate that corresponds with the patient's maximal inspiratory flow, careful observation is needed. By doing this, the alveoli are able to get a consistent and dependable fraction of inspired oxygen (FiO_2) without breathing in excess ambient room air. Dilution of supplementary entrained oxygen may be unavoidable in patients in acute respiratory distress, who may breathe at flow rates exceeding 100 L/min^{-1} and in whom the maximal flow rate should be selected [17].

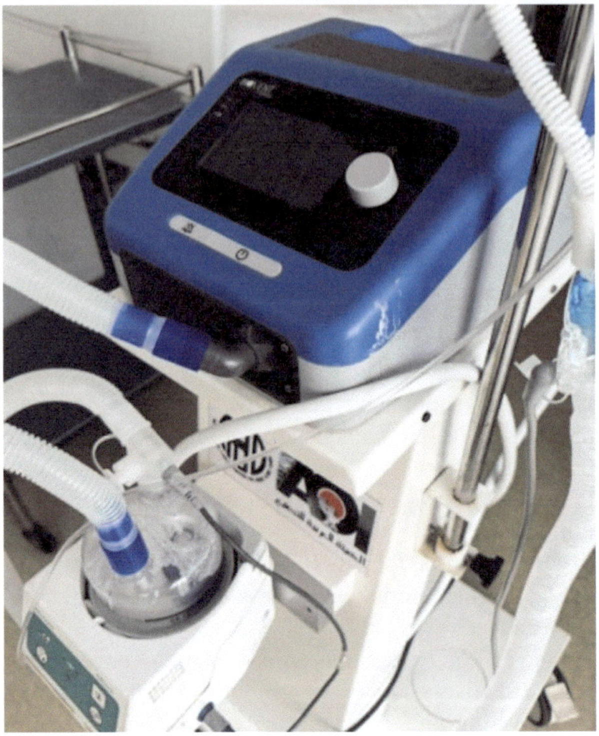

Fig. 4.1 BioVent A Series

4.2.2 Humidifying Devices

For oxygen therapy to be delivered via HFNC successfully, there must be adequate humidification. Dry gas is known to have diverse adverse effects on the respiratory system, such as mucociliary malfunction, epithelial damage, mucus plugging, ulceration of mucosa, and lung injury. To properly condition the inspired gas to 37 °C for adults and 34–37 °C for children, with 44 mg H_2O/L, HFNC delivery systems need an active heated humidifier. At flows of up to 60 L/min, HFNC delivers medical gas, usually through a heated humidifier incorporated into the delivery system. The humidifier is a traditional "pass-over heated humidifying system" [18].

To guarantee that the patient receives the ideal humidity from the start of therapy, it is imperative that enough time be given for the humidifier to reach the necessary maximum temperature before administering HFNC. High flows that are started before the gas has had enough time to heat up and become humid can cause discomfort and irritate the mucosa, which, in turn, leads to poor patient compliance with the therapy.

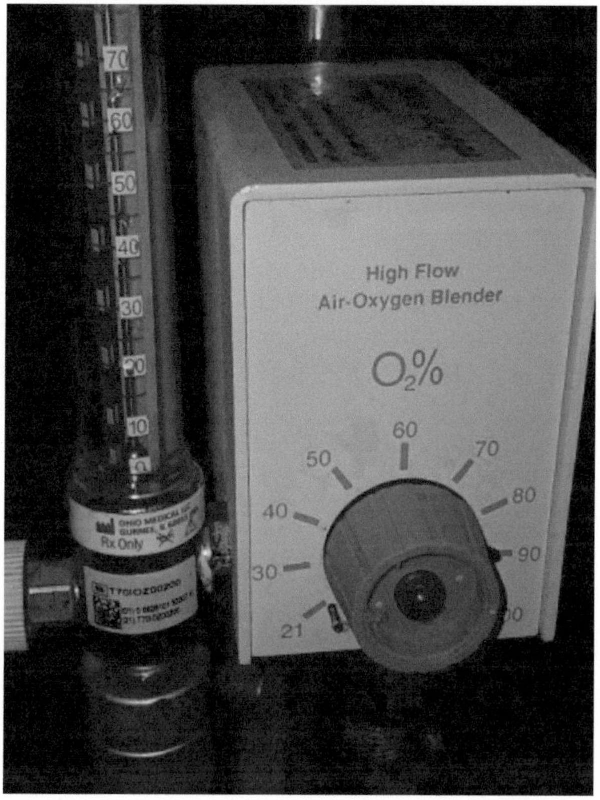

Fig. 4.2 Bio-Med Devices, CT

4.2.3 Inspiratory Limb

A single-limb heated inspiratory circuit is used to administer the warmed humidified gas to the patient. With a heater wire built in the tube wall and insulated to reduce condensation and the effects of surrounding air temperature, the circuit (or tubing) is flexible and lightweight. Like other humidified circuits, there is a potential for condensation or "rainout," which lowers humidification effectiveness and raises the risk of infection [19]. In addition to disrupting sleep, this rainout can cause desaturation and coughing. The likelihood of condensation increases with decreasing outside temperature. Condensation raises the risk of patient arousal, aspiration, irritation, and desaturation in addition to pain and a potentially clinically significant deterioration of the patient's condition. It is crucial to prevent circuit vapor loss to guarantee that patients receive medical gas that has been sufficiently humidified [18].

Manufacturers have created a variety of inspiratory circuit types with the goal of minimizing condensation; the most popular kind of these circuits is one that just has a heating wire in it. Another popular option for both invasive and noninvasive respiratory support is the heated wire circuit.

To regulate the thermal output of the heating wire placed inside the limb, the supplied electric current is servo-controlled. Heating wire placement differs, depending on the maker: A (RT202 [Fisher & Paykel]) and B (SLH [Intersurgical, Berkshire, United Kingdom]).

The SLH has a shorter heating wire than the RT202, and the temperature probe is located at a different location on the distal end of the wire.

Although only 10 cm long, the wire influences temperature control and decreases condensation; however, because of the temperature gradient from each of the heating wires to the circuit wall, some degree of condensation is inevitable and is likely to be greater with a shorter wire.

The outside limb can be protected from the colder surrounding air, and moisture can be reduced by wrapping a plastic sleeve around the circuit [5].

4.2.4 Interface

In the realm of respiratory support, expanding the use of NIV over the last 20 years has been significant [20]. However, no study revealed a success rate of 100% [21].

A primary cause of this is the discomfort or intolerance of patients toward interfaces. Initially, patients typically try wearing oronasal masks, but many find them to be excessively unpleasant. Patients tolerate HFNC better than NIV [22].

Two cannulae that fit snugly but do not entirely obstruct the nostrils are used to transfer the heated, humidified gas directly into the nose. A lot of the HFNC that are on the market look like slightly larger low-flow nasal cannula; however, two other kinds of cannulae have somewhat different designs (*Comfort Flo Plus*, Teleflex, and *Optiflow*, Fisher & Paykel) (Fig. 4.3). These devices attach to the heated inspiratory circuit using bigger diameter corrugated tubing, have wider bore silicone cannulae made of softer silicone and have a clip to secure the corrugated tubing, minimizing cannula displacement from the nose.

Depending on which commercially available device is used, the nasal cannulae are held in place with a head strap; secured behind the head; or hooked over the ears and secured under the chin. Choosing the right cannula size is crucial and should be guided by both cannula comfort and tolerability and the manufacturer's recommendations.

4.3 Vapotherm

The Precision Flow® is a system for high-flow humidified respiratory therapy by a Vapotherm-approved interface. Incorporating an electronic blender and flow controller, it integrates the basic humidification technology of Vapotherm. A detachable, disposable patient circuit incorporates both the gas and water channels.

- *The Precision Flow® consists of two parts*:

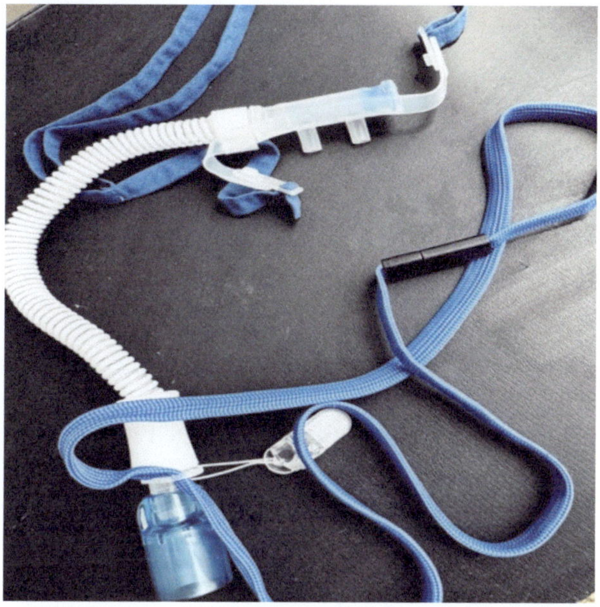

Fig. 4.3 Interface in Optiflow system

4.3.1 Main Unit

- The capital unit contains all the electrical and electronic components including the electronic blender and flow controllers and remote sensors to monitor the disposable water path. Since there are no water paths in the main unit and the gas pathway only contains dry gas at room temperature, it does not require internal cleaning or disinfection.
- Mass flow sensors monitor the flow of air and oxygen. The required flow of each is determined by the operating software to meet the operator-set target flow and oxygen %. Through the manipulation of proportional solenoid valves on the gas lines, the system regulates gas flows correspondingly. An oxygen sensor keeps track of the gas mixture and alerts the user to any deviations from the target and observed percentages. Every 24 h and at power-up, the oxygen sensor is automatically calibrated with oxygen.
- Sensors are used by firmware in the main unit to track water temperature, gas pressure, and air leakage into the disposable patient circuit (bubble detector). If any of the parameters deviate from the standard range, an alarm is raised. Additional indications display the type of installed cartridge and the low charge level of the backup battery.
- After a 2-h charging period, an internal battery backup will maintain the set flow and oxygen blend for at least 15 min without AC power.

4.3.2 Disposable Patient Circuit

- The delivery tube, vapor transfer cartridge (VTC), and disposable water path (DWP) make up the disposable patient circuit (DPC). Through the interface connecting the main unit and the disposable water channel, conditions in the circulating water and gas streams are remotely detected.
- A flow generator, an active heated humidifier, a single-limb heated circuit, and a nasal cannula make up a Vapotherm, same as in HFNC [7].

4.3.3 Flow Generator

Precise flow generators are incorporated into devices manufactured by Fisher & Paykel Healthcare (Auckland, New Zealand) and Vapotherm (NH) (Fig. 4.4). Typically, these entrain room air and employ turbines to produce high flow.

4.3.4 Humidifying Devices

Vapotherm provides a filter-type humidifying system. Humidification is generated by passing blended gas through a bundle of narrow tubes (like a fluid warmer for IV fluids) with 0.005 μ pore size. Filter systems need a larger evaporation surface than pass-over heated humidifying systems do.

Vapotherm supplies two cartridge sizes: one for flows of 5–40 L/min and the other for flows of 1–8 L/min. Both pass-over and filter-cartridge humidifying devices usually work well. Unlike most humidifiers, there is no direct contact between the water and gas streams. The gas stream leaves the cartridge saturated with vapor at the set temperature [18].

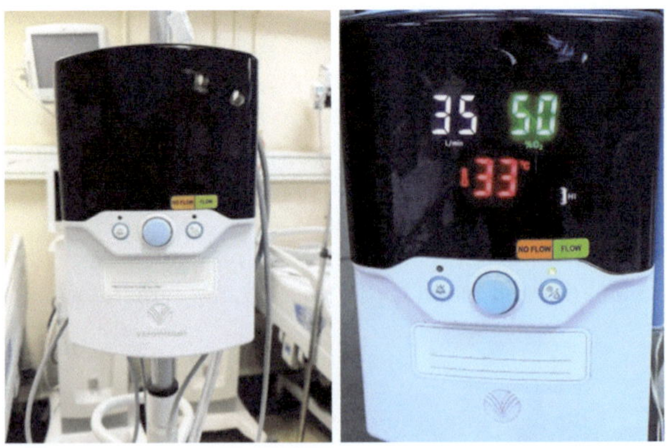

Fig. 4.4 Precision Flow Plus (Vapotherm, NH)

4.3.5 Inspiratory Limb

Patient delivery tube The triple-lumen heated delivery tube's middle is where the warmed humidified gas travels. To keep the central lumen warm and reduce rainout, two outside lumens that circulate warmed water surround the center lumen, as shown in Fig. 4.5.

The humidified breathing gas is delivered to the patient's nares via a specialized small nasal cannula that is attached to the end of the delivery tube. It is normal for non-DEHP PVC tubing to appear slightly cloudy, or yellow, especially during longer use or when operated at higher temperatures [23].

Disposable water path The disposable water path houses a water reservoir, pump, connections for the vapor transfer cartridge and delivery tube, and sensor interfaces to the main unit. Water is pumped past a heater plate through the outer lumens of the delivery tube.

Returning water passes through the outer jacket of the specially designed vapor transfer cartridge where some water is lost as vapor to the gas stream. There is no direct contact between water and gas flows. The water then returns to the pump reservoir. Heater power automatically maintains the set temperature. Water flows into the circuit from the sterile water supply to replace evaporative losses in the vapor transfer cartridge. Air is purged into the atmosphere from the circulation via a hydrophobic filter membrane.

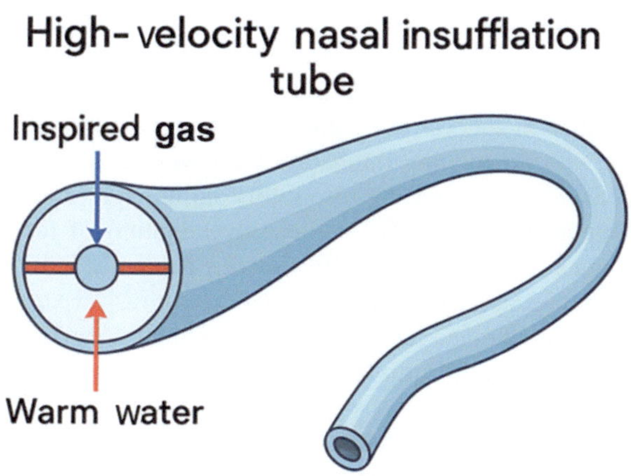

Fig. 4.5 Triple-lumen heated delivery tube

4.3.6 Interface

The high-velocity nasal insufflation system (Hi-VNI, Vapotherm) uses a slender nasal cannula similar in appearance to a regular nasal oxygen cannula. Both the internal diameter and nasal prong bore are narrow, and this results in high flow out of the nasal prongs. Moreover, via two connecting tubes, Hi-VNI delivers flow to each prong from either side [24].

4.3.7 Consumables

For single patient use, humidification chambers, heated circuits, air inlet filters, and patient interfaces should be changed on a regular basis in compliance with manufacturer's instructions.

4.4 Contraindications and Adverse Events

There is currently no consensus on the usage of HFNC; hence, there is little information available regarding contraindications. The two main reasons why using HFNC is contraindicated are upper airway problems and airway protection.

HFNC therapy is well-tolerated, and stable patients report that it is more comfortable than NIV and continuous positive airway pressure (CPAP) [25]. Patients in acute hypoxemic respiratory failure report that HFT is additionally associated with less mouth dryness and improved breathlessness than facemask oxygen [8]. Adverse event reports are uncommon in the literature. Most adverse events are associated with patient discomfort brought on by heat or a high gas delivery flow that causes rhinorrhea or discomfort in the nasal passages. No serious adverse events have been reported in the literature because of HFT [26]. In a retrospective research, Kang and colleagues [27] found that patients who needed further intubation after receiving HFNC for longer than 48 h had higher intensive care unit (ICU) mortality, worse extubation success rates, and more difficulty weaning from mechanical ventilation. As with postponing intubation with NIV [28], caution must be exercised in early detection of increasing respiratory failure symptoms and appropriate escalation of supportive treatments. In their investigation of the domiciliary usage of HFNC, Nagata and colleagues [29] noted a few mild side effects, such as sleeplessness, night sweats, nasal discharge, and a skin rash. Extended usage may result in localized skin damage (erythema and skin breakdown) in the area beneath the straps and in the nasal philtrum, but this risk is significantly lower than that of NIV or CPAP [30, 31].

It is recommended that patients and clinicians periodically check for changes in the skin and modify the interface size, strap tightness, and/or HFT settings, as necessary. The clinical indication for HFNC administered in the acute setting should be clearly documented, and patients should be closely watched for indications of treatment failure. These symptoms could include worsening oxygen saturation, as well as an increase in breathing effort and respiratory rate. Regular clinical reviews and continuous physiological monitoring lower the likelihood of postponing invasive mechanical ventilation, which is linked to a poor prognosis.

4.5 Summary

HFNC is a method that provides comfort by delivering warmed and humidified gas flow via nasal prongs. It maintains high FiO_2 levels and generates a low level of positive pressure in the upper airways due to a high flow of gas, which also offers washout of dead space. The basic HFNC system's therapeutic effects are primarily determined by temperature, flow, and oxygen content. Only a flow generator, an active heated humidifier, a single heated circuit, and a nasal cannula are needed for the straightforward HFNC system. They are easy to set up and use and well tolerated by patients and have few reported adverse events.

References

1. L'Her E, Deye N, Lellouche F, Taille S, Demoule A, Fraticelli A, et al. Physiologic effects of noninvasive ventilation during acute lung injury. Am J Respir Crit Care Med. 2005;172(9):1112–8.
2. Markovitz GH, Colthurst J, Storer TW, Cooper CB. Effective inspired oxygen concentration measured via transtracheal and oral gas analysis. Respir Care. 2010;55(4):453–9.
3. Brochard L, Mancebo J, Wysocki M, Lofaso F, Conti G, Rauss A, et al. Noninvasive ventilation for acute exacerbations of chronic obstructive pulmonary disease. N Engl J Med. 1995;333(13):817–22.
4. Transpirator Technologies, Inc. Annual report form 10-KSB 2002. https://sec.report/Document/0000950144-02-007036/.
5. Chikata Y, Unai K, Izawa M, Okuda N, Oto J, Nishimura M. Inspiratory tube condensation during high-flow nasal cannula therapy: a bench study. Respir Care. 2016;61(3):300–5.
6. Mellado-Artigas R, Ferreyro BL, Angriman F, et al. High-flow nasal oxygen in patients with COVID-19-associated acute respiratory failure. Crit Care. 2021;25(1):58.
7. Nishimura M. High-flow nasal cannula oxygen therapy in adults: physiological benefits, indication, clinical benefits, and adverse effects. Respir Care. 2016;61(4):529–41.
8. Roca O, Riera J, Torres F, Masclans JR. High-flow oxygen therapy in acute respiratory failure. Respir Care. 2010;55(4):408–13.
9. Mauri T, Alban L, Turrini C, Cambiaghi B, Carlesso E, Taccone P, et al. Optimum support by high-flow nasal cannula in acute hypoxemic respiratory failure: effects of increasing flow rates. Intensive Care Med. 2017;43:1453–63.
10. Corley A, Caruana LR, Barnett AG, Tronstad O, Fraser JF. Oxygen delivery through high-flow nasal cannulae increases end-expiratory lung volume and reduces respiratory rate in post-cardiac surgical patients. Br J Anaesth. 2011;107:998–1004.
11. Parke RL, Bloch A, McGuinness SP. Effect of very-high-flow nasal therapy on airway pressure and end-expiratory lung impedance in healthy volunteers. Respir Care. 2015;60:1397–403.
12. Franklin D, Babl FE, Schlapbach LJ, Oakley E, Craig S, Neutze J, et al. A randomized trial of high-flow oxygen therapy in infants with bronchiolitis. N Engl J Med. 2018;378:1121–31.
13. Ward JJ. High-flow oxygen administration by nasal cannula for adult and perinatal patients. Respir Care. 2013;58:98–122.
14. Wilkinson DJ, Andersen CC, Smith K, Holberton J. Pharyngeal pressure with high-flow nasal cannulae in premature infants. J Perinatol. 2008;28:42–7.

15. Mikalsen IB, Davis P, Oymar K. High flow nasal cannula in children: a literature review. Scand J Trauma Resusc Emerg Med. 2016;24:93.
16. https://www.maxtec.com/product/delivery/mixers-blenders/maxventuri/.
17. Ritchie JE, Williams AB, Gerard C, et al. Evaluation of a humidified nasal high-flow oxygen system, using oxygraphy, capnography and measurement of upper airway pressures. Anaesth Intensive Care. 2011;39:1103–10.
18. Chikata Y, Izawa M, Okuda N, Itagaki T, Nakataki E, Onodera M, et al. Humidification performance of two high-flow nasal cannula devices: a bench study. Respir Care. 2014;59(8):1186–90.
19. Klompas M, Branson R, Eichenwald EC, Greene LR, Howell MD, Lee G, et al. Strategies to prevent ventilator-associated pneumonia in acute care hospitals: 2014 update. Infect Control Hosp Epidemiol. 2014;35(Suppl 2):S133–54.
20. Patel BK, Wolfe KS, Pohlman AS, Hall JB, Kress JP. Effect of noninvasive ventilation delivered by helmet vs face mask on the rate of endotracheal intubation in patients with acute respiratory distress syndrome: a randomized clinical trial. JAMA. 2016;315(22):2435–41.
21. Ozyilmaz E, Ugurlu AO, Nava S. Timing of noninvasive ventilation failure: causes, risk factors, and potential remedies. BMC Pulm Med. 2014;14:19.
22. Calvano TP, Sill JM, Kemp KR, Chung KK. Use of a high-flow oxygen delivery system in a critically ill patient with dementia. Respir Care. 2008;53(12):1739–43.
23. Tero R, Cecich J, Sanabria O, Sun S, Batista J, Stout S, et al. Risks associated with conventional humidifiers adapted for high-flow nasal cannula therapy in human infants: results of a time and motion study. Int J Clin Pediatr. 2014;3(4):99–104.
24. Miller TL, Saberi B, Saberi S. Computational fluid dynamics modelin g of extrathoracic airway flush: evaluation of high flow cannula design elements. J Pulm Respir Med. 2016;6(5):1–7.
25. Braunlich J, Kohler M, Wirtz H. Nasal high flow improves ventilation in patients with COPD. Int J Chron Obstruct Pulmon Dis. 2016;11:1077–85.
26. Corley A, Rickard CM, Aitken LM, et al. High-flow nasal cannulae for respiratory support in adult intensive care patients. Cochrane Database Syst Rev. 2017;5(5):CD010172.
27. Kang BJ, Koh Y, Lim CM, Huh JW, Baek S, Han M, et al. Failure of high-flow nasal cannula therapy may delay intubation and increase mortality. Intensive Care Med. 2015;41:623–32.
28. Moretti M, Cilione C, Tampieri A, Fracchia C, Marchioni A, Nava S. Incidence and causes of non-invasive mechanical ventilation failure after initial success. Thorax. 2000;55:819–25.
29. Nagata K, Kikuchi T, Horie T, Shiraki A, Kitajima T, Kadowaki T, et al. Domiciliary high-flow nasal cannula oxygen therapy for patients with stable hypercapnic chronic obstructive pulmonary disease. A multicenter randomized crossover trial. Ann Am Thorac Soc. 2018;15:432–9.
30. Stéphan F, Barrucand B, Petit P, et al. High-flow nasal oxygen vs noninvasive positive airway pressure in hypoxemic patients after cardiothoracic surgery: a randomized clinical trial. JAMA. 2015;313:2331–9.
31. Hernandez G, Vaquero C, Colinas L, et al. Effect of postextubation high-flow nasal cannula vs noninvasive ventilation on reintubation and postextubation respiratory failure in high-risk patients: a randomized clinical trial. JAMA. 2016;316:1565–74.

Noninvasive Ventilator Devices

5

Konrad Mendrala and Tomasz Cyzowski

5.1 Introduction

A solid understanding of medical equipment is essential for ensuring patient safety. Incorrect installation, improper ventilation parameters, and alarm misinterpretation can be disastrous. We strongly advise reading the manufacturer's manual, even if you believe you know a similar model. Even small details can have a substantial impact. If the ventilation is ineffective or uncomfortable, the patient may reject it, or it may cause harm. In this chapter, we will discuss the general principle of ventilators in noninvasive modes and some differences between manufacturers.

We can distinguish three main types of devices that generate positive airway pressure, which is not always synonymous with noninvasive ventilation [1–3].

1. Continuous positive airway pressure (CPAP) masks: maintaining constant positive airway pressure. The simplest devices consist of a face mask designed to fit securely over the nose and/or mouth equipped with an excess pressure valve and an oxygen/air flow port. The excess of fresh gases creates positive pressure in the mask, the level of which is regulated by the valve. Respiratory support results from the constant positive pressure during the respiratory cycle. "Pure" CPAP does not support ventilation during apnea. CPAP increases functional residual capacity, reduces inspiratory work of breathing in patients with left heart failure, and reduces V/Q mismatch [1, 4].
2. HFNOT: similar to CPAP masks, this device for high-flow nasal oxygen therapy generates a constant positive airway pressure estimated at 3–5 cmH_2O, slightly

K. Mendrala (✉) · T. Cyzowski
Department of Anaesthesiology and Intensive Care, Faculty of Medical Sciences in Katowice, Medical University of Silesia, Katowice, Poland
e-mail: kmendrala@sum.edu.pl

© The Author(s), under exclusive license to Springer Nature Switzerland AG 2025

K. Panda et al. (eds.), *Noninvasive Ventilatory Approaches in Interventional Procedures*, Noninvasive Ventilation. The Essentials,
https://doi.org/10.1007/978-3-032-05328-2_5

stabilizing the upper airways and thus protecting against collapse. In addition, the high flow of fresh gases slightly reduces patients' anatomical dead space [1].

3. Ventilators: Devices for active ventilation. Unlike CPAP and HFNOT, the ventilator allows both invasive and noninvasive ventilation providing inspiration or actively supporting the patient's spontaneous breath. Modern ventilators are equipped with processors monitoring the patient's respiratory activity giving the ability to synchronize and adjust respiratory support during therapy [1–3].

5.2 Ventilators

Newly designed and manufactured ventilators allow mechanical ventilation in both invasive and noninvasive forms for children and adults [1–3]. Full-feature intensive care unit (ICU) ventilators are large, making them unfeasible to use during patient transport. Instead, they offer advanced modes of mechanical ventilation and spirometric measurements. Portable ventilators are suitable for use in healthcare facilities and homes and during patient physical activity [3]. Today, the line between good-quality new portable ventilators and older-generation stationary devices is becoming increasingly blurred. Nevertheless, the difference remains crucial when using sophisticated ventilation modes (Fig. 5.1).

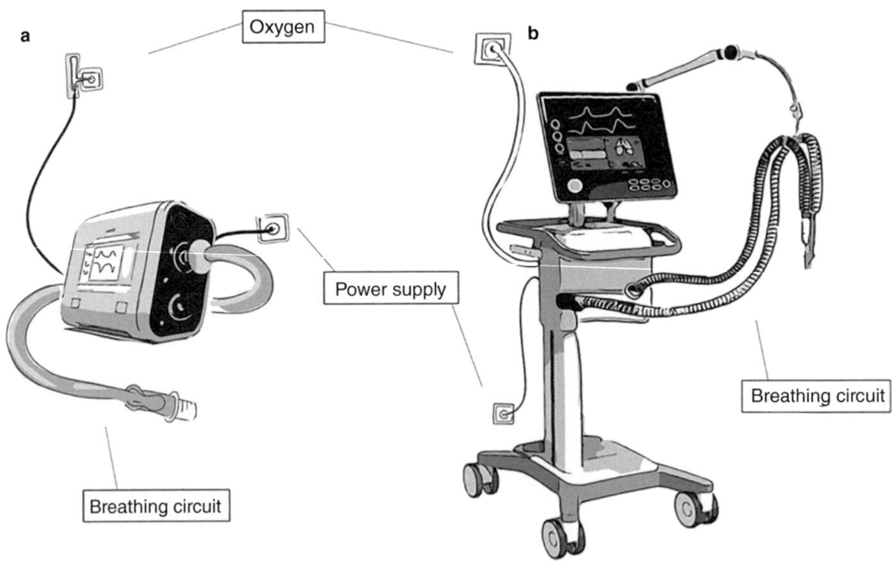

Fig. 5.1 Portable and ICU ventilators. The differences between (**a**) portable ventilators and (**b**) ICU ventilators mainly relate to dimensions, advanced ventilation modes, and spirometric measurement capabilities. (Figure source: own material)

5.2.1 Ventilation Modes

There are two ways to provide inspiration during positive-pressure ventilation: applying a predefined positive airway pressure that generates volume (so-called PCV, pressure control ventilation) or administering a predefined volume that produces a pressure increment (so-called VCV, volume control ventilation). Positive airway pressure is generated in both cases, hence the general name positive-pressure ventilation (PPV). An alternative to PPV ventilation is rarely used, i.e., negative-pressure ventilation (NPV). Surprisingly, noninvasive negative-pressure ventilation devices are back on the market.

During PCV, a predefined pressure is generated in the respiratory tract for a predefined time; this results in an unknown tidal volume, thus carrying the risk of both hypo- and hyperventilation (especially in patients whose respiratory compliance changes dynamically as, e.g., during asthma management). Contrarily, during VCV, a predefined volume is given to the patient over a predefined time, resulting in an unknown pressure increment.

Regardless of how inspiration is administered, there are various modes of PPV ventilation, differing mainly in patient synchronization and the extent of respiratory support. Unfortunately, due to the lack of unification in terminology, different manufacturers call similar ventilation modes in different ways (e.g., BiLEVEL, BiPAP, DuoPAP). The main ventilation modes are as follows [1]:

1. CMV: Controlled mechanical ventilation, a mode in which the ventilator does not synchronize with the patient but only administers a set volume/pressure at a fixed rate.
2. A/C: Assist/control, like CMV ventilator, delivers a preset volume or pressure-controlled breath at a set rate but can actively detect the patient's inspiration and give an additional (same as predefined) inspiration "on demand."
3. SIMV: Synchronized intermittent mandatory ventilation synchronizes mandatory and spontaneous breathing. This means that if the patient makes an inspiratory effort within a specific time before the planned mandatory breath, the synchronized mandatory breath replaces the initially scheduled one. Unlike A/C, patient synchronization is improved, and the physician can adapt the ventilator's response to patient-triggered inspiration via the pressure support (PS) parameter. When PS value is set to "0," the ventilator will allow the patient to perform his own inspiration without assistance between the mandatory breaths. Any other PS value will cause the ventilator to generate positive pressure when the patient inhales, providing additional respiratory support.
4. PSV: PEEP with pressure support (sometimes called CPAP+PS or just PS), exclusively pressure mode in which ventilator generates constant average positive pressure during the whole breathing cycle, but also actively detects and support the patient's own inspiration. Unlike the other modes, there is no mandatory ventilation.
5. BiLEVEL: this mode is pure pressure mode, although modifications with guaranteed inspiratory volume are becoming more common. The physician sets the

baseline pressure (expiratory positive airway pressure, EPAP) and the peak pressure created by the ventilator (inspiratory positive airway pressure, IPAP). The pressure difference causes the volume increment. Additionally, the patient can inhale and exhale during the whole respiratory cycle (both inspiration and expiration), which gives tremendous synchronization with the ventilator. BiLEVEL exhibits features of two time-varying CPAP. There is confusion with the naming of this mode both within types of ventilation and between manufacturers (BiPAP is the name of the NIV registered by Respironics, BIPAP stands for invasive ventilation used in Drager ventilators). Modes, such as Bi-Vent, Bi-phasic, and DuoPAP, are also available on the market.

The fact that a patient is ventilated noninvasively does not indicate the type of ventilation mode, but only the type of connection between the ventilator and the patient. Unlike invasive ventilation through an endotracheal tube or supraglottic device, NIV implements face masks, nasal cannulas, helmets, and other noninvasive interfaces. A physician can use all the ventilation modes available on a specific ventilator for both invasive and noninvasive ventilation. Still, the choice of ventilation mode should be based on the patient's clinical condition and neurological status. Most often, NIV ventilation is performed in conscious, cooperative patients, so CMV lacking the element of synchronization may be highly inappropriate (Fig. 5.2). The choice of ventilation mode, whether it be pressure-controlled ventilation (PCV) or volume-controlled ventilation (VCV), may also be important (Table 5.1). PCV is thought to be more physiological than VCV by generating constant pressure over time, allowing even volume distribution across various alveoli. Furthermore, PCV produces lower peak pressure than VCV for the same volume, resulting in less unintentional mask leakage. In a French epidemiologic study, PSV with or without PEEP was used to treat respiratory failure in 67% of patients, while ventilators with support volume control were used in only 15% [2]. Several clinical trials have failed to show that pressure ventilation has an advantage over volume ventilation regarding oxygenation, pCO2 retention, and serious complications [1–4].

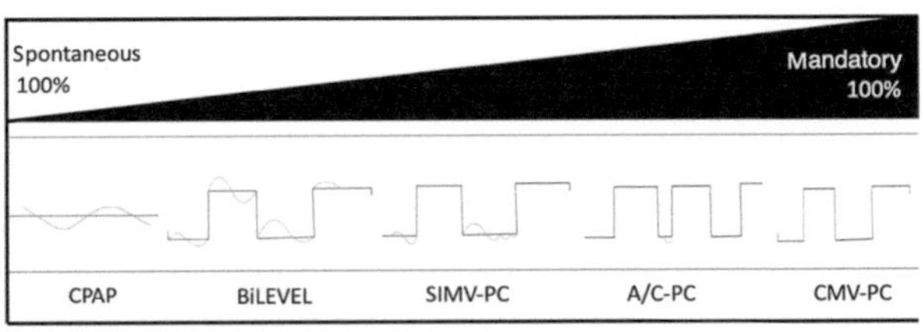

Fig. 5.2 Ventilation modes. The patient's spontaneous breathing during different ventilation modes

Table 5.1 Most commonly used noninvasive ventilation modes

Mode	Name	P/V	Definition	Inspiration	Expiration
A/C A(C)V	Assist/control	Pressure or volume	Assisted ventilation with forced respiration—breaths triggered and controlled both by patient and ventilator	Pressure or volume	PEEP
CPAP	Continuous positive airway pressure	Pressure	Only spontaneous breaths–during both inspiration and expiration the pressure is constant	CPAP	CPAP
PSV;PS	Pressure support ventilation	Pressure	A type of CPAP in which a ventilator delivers spontaneous pressure-assisted breaths. Patients trigger breaths and determine their timing and volume	PS (pressure support)	PEEP
S/T; S(T)	Spontaneous/ timed	Pressure	A type of BiLEVEL in which breaths may be spontaneous or forced. The patient(s) initiates breaths, and if there is no activity for a predefined time, the ventilator will initiate a mandatory breath (t)	IPAP	PEEP
SIMV	Synchronized intermittent mandatory ventilation	Pressure or volume	Synchronization of mandatory inspiration with the patient. The breaths triggered by the patient after the mandatory breath are spontaneous, which can be further supported by the ventilator	Pressure or volume	PEEP

(continued)

Table 5.1 (continued)

Mode	Name	P/V	Definition	Inspiration	Expiration
AVAPS-AE	Average volume-assured pressure support——automated expiratory positive airway pressure	Pressure with guaranteed volume	A type of BiLEVEL, instead of a fixed inspiratory pressure (IPAP) uses a maximum pressure (Max P) and minimum pressure (Min P) to meet target tidal volume (Vt). Also, the end-expiratory pressure is automatically adjusted by the ventilator within the specified range depending on the airway resistance	AVAPS (variable, target Vt)	EPAP (variable)
iVAPS	Intelligent volume-assured pressure support	Pressure with guaranteed volume	A type of BiLEVEL. Ventilator automatically adapts the pressure to the patient's target alveolar ventilation (Va) and respiratory rate (RR)	iVAPS (variable, target Va and RR)	PEEP
MPV	Mouthpiece ventilation	Pressure or volume	Ventilation on demand without the exhalation device. The ventilator detects the application of the mouthpiece to the patient's mouth—no patient effort is required to generate a breath	Pressure or volume	Passive by mouth

5.2.2 Trigger

The key to success is the correct synchronization of the patient with the ventilator, which depends on the ventilator's ability to detect the patient's spontaneous inspiration. This ability is called a "trigger" and can detect either a change in respiratory pressure or flow, depending on the method chosen. The inspiratory trigger's sensitivity must be balanced between two extremes: (1) an insensitive trigger increases the work of breathing and (2) oversensitive trigger results in an auto-trigger (in extreme cases, the ventilator can be triggered by an apical heart beat or a leak in the system). Both pressure and flow triggers should be selected individually for the patient and modified as necessary during therapy. In addition, patients with COPD and dynamic airway collapse may experience so-called intrinsic PEEP or autoPEEP—air trapped distally in the bronchial tree cannot be expired and results in positive pressure at the end expiration. With pressure trigger, this can make the ventilator less sensitive to the patient's respiratory effort. The external (ventilator-generated) PEEP is set to counteract the effect of intrinsic PEEP on ventilator triggering [1].

5.2.3 Flow

Another technical challenge is the ventilator's ability to fully cover the patient's demand for fresh gas mixture flow. For patients with high respiratory drive and high respiratory effort, setting the flow too low may result in a deficiency and increase the patient's work of breathing. On the other hand, too high flow rate may be perceived by the patient as uncomfortable. In both cases, poor synchronization between the patient and the ventilator may occur. Different manufacturers allow to adjust the inspiratory flow rate differently, although there is rarely a specific parameter. The flow depends on the time of inspiration, the slope of the inspiratory curve, airway resistance, lung compliance, and the given volume/pressure [1].

5.2.4 Expiration

While the manner in which inspiration is delivered is regulated precisely by the user (and patient), expiration is passive. During mechanical ventilation, the onset of expiration should be based on the clinical condition and adjusted to the patient's needs. The typical and most commonly set criterion for the transition of a respiratory cycle into expiration is a drop in inspiratory flow from peak to 25% and/or completion of the cycle after a predetermined time [1]. It is important to adjust the end-inspiratory flow threshold to achieve good expiratory synchronization. For example, in patients with COPD, prolonged expiration may force this value to be set at 30–40% of peak flow [1]. Setting a maximum inspiratory time (e.g., 3 sec) protects the patient from hyperinflation in the presence of leaks, where peak flow may not fall below the specified value.

5.2.5 PEEP and CPAP

CPAP (the "ventilation" mode, or more precisely respiratory support strategy) maintains positive pressure throughout the respiratory cycle, while PEEP (the setting of the ventilation mode) indicates positive pressure only during end expiration. CPAP and PEEP are intended to open and stabilize both alveoli and collapsed airways, thereby reducing atelectasis. The additional benefit of "pressing" the alveolus close to the vessel may reduce V/Q mismatch [4]. Both CPAP and PEEP can be beneficial in conscious patients with cardiogenic pulmonary edema. However, it should be noted that positive thoracic pressure can reduce heart preload and increase right ventricle afterload by compressing intrathoracic vessels and increasing pulmonary vascular resistance. At the same time, in systole, the left ventricular transmural pressure gradient is reduced, leading to a decrease in left ventricular stroke work. Thus, the effect of ventilation depends largely on the patient's clinical condition [1, 4].

5.2.6 Breathing Systems

The most common breathing systems in the ICU are circle systems (dual-limb) with separate inspiratory and expiratory limbs and a small (negligible) volume of the common part (Fig. 5.3). This configuration allows for precise Vt delivery and accurate measurement of system volumes, flows, and pressures during both the inspiratory and expiratory phases. However, such a configuration creates the need for dedicated ventilators and patient interfaces, as the entire system should be of minimal leak (except for technological leaks that are difficult to avoid). Single-limb systems are an alternative to these systems. Their advantage is simplicity and portability, which seems particularly important for a conscious patient [1, 3]. To allow expiration in such a system, it must have an external expiratory valve or expiratory port, allowing for intentional leakage. External valves can be electronically controlled or have an elastic diaphragm that occludes the expiratory orifice during inhalation and descends during exhalation, allowing gases to flow into the environment (plateau exhalation valve). The exhalation port is a simpler solution and can have different forms, ranging from holes in a specific diameter to more complex geometric shapes. Also, the location of exhalation ports depends on the manufacturer—some uses separate respiratory components mounted near the patient's interface (e.g., Whisper-Swivel, a fixed-resistance, variable-flow leak port), while others integrate exhalation ports into the patient interface (intentional leak through tiny holes around the mask connection or on the respiratory circuit). The basic idea is that there is a constant leak during inspiration and expiration, the amount of which depends on the flow and pressure in the system. The ventilator software takes this leakage into account. The design and control of valves also vary widely between manufacturers (Fig. 5.4). You should always read the instructions provided by the manufacturer and pay particular attention to the type of respiratory system used—manufacturers often allow different types of systems but replacing them requires the recalibration of the ventilator. Furthermore, the common circuit part for inspiration and expiration in single-limb systems is greater volume than in circle systems, increasing the potential for rebreathing and pCO2 retention. The presence of a fixed leak in the system is the solution to this problem. User modification of these components can endanger patient safety.

a b

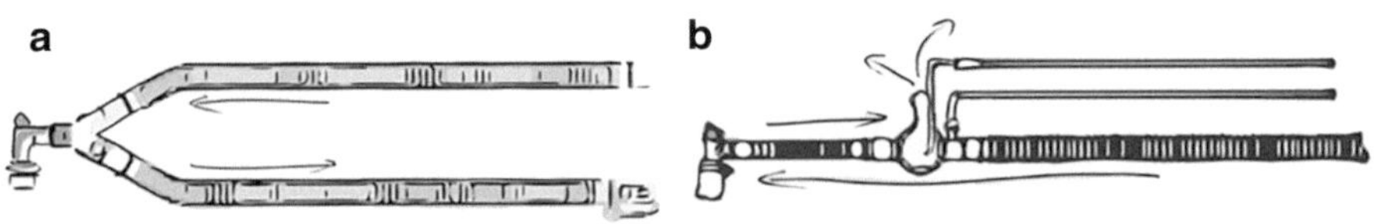

Fig. 5.3 The most common types of breathing circuits. (**a**) Dual-limb system with separate inhalation and exhalation arm (**b**) Single-limb system with expiratory valve and pressure line. (Figure source: own material)

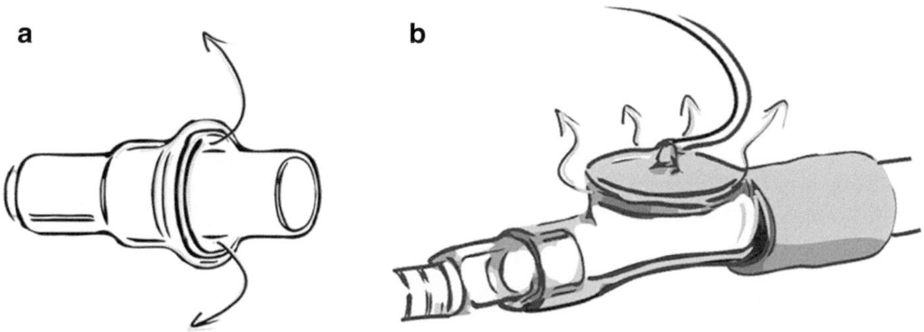

Fig. 5.4 Examples of expiratory ports. The most common exhalation ports used in single-limb systems (**a**) Whisper-Swivel, a fixed-resistance, variable-flow leak port (**b**) External expiratory valve with pressure line. (Figure source: own material)

5.2.7 Unintentional Leakage

The use of older-generation ventilators without dedicated modes for noninvasive ventilation is NOT contraindicated. However, it can be challenging, especially with mandatory modes. An additional element that affects ventilator work is the presence of leakage, which is often difficult to avoid (technological leaks are common even on well-fitted and fitted masks). This can activate ventilator alarms, hinder synchronization, and, in extreme cases, lead to patient hypoventilation. Noninvasive ventilation modes offered by modern devices are the solution to this problem. They have a leak compensation function that adjusts the basal flow to the current leak and allows proper ventilation and proper functioning of the inspiratory trigger.

5.3 Additional System Components

5.3.1 Oxygen Port

Most portable ventilators and some traditional ventilators have compressors or turbine pumps as the source of air administered to patients [1, 3]. Some models require connection to an external source of compressed air. In some scenarios, it is necessary to enrich the respiratory mixture with oxygen. For this purpose, the oxygen source is connected to the oxygen port of the ventilator. Oxygen ports can differ among manufacturers. The simplest option is connectors mounted directly to the respiratory circuit usually near the patient's mask. The amount of oxygen is regulated by a flowmeter. More advanced ventilators have oxygen delivery systems and pipeline Schrader connectors for direct connection to a hospital high-pressure oxygen source. The ventilator is equipped with a fresh gas blender, and the user sets the inspiratory fraction through device software. Also, some ventilators have sensors for the inspiratory and expiratory fractions of fresh gases. This makes it possible to control inspiratory and expiratory O_2 (less commonly CO_2).

5.3.2 Filters, Humidifiers, and Nebulizers

The application of filters is mandatory during ventilation. There are many types of filters whose action is based on direct interception, diffusional interception, inertial impaction, or electrostatic deposition—depending on the type of contamination, different types of filters are used on different elements of the respirator. During noninvasive ventilation, patients are at particular risk of upper airway dryness. This can lead to edema, increasing respiratory resistance by up to a third, contributing to discomfort and intolerance of ventilation. Factors predisposing to this phenomenon include prolonged ventilation time, restricted fluid intake, respiratory leaks, and high flow rates with increased patient respiratory effort [1]. HME (heat and moisture exchangers) are used in circle systems to retain heat and water vapor and maintain adequate humidity. HMEs can also be merged with antimicrobial filters (HME filters, HMEF). HMEF should be installed proximally to the patient, above the exhalation port, and therefore may carry the risk of impeding exhalation. Alternatives include active humidifiers and heat exchangers mounted on the inhalation arm. It is necessary to pay close attention to additional equipment used, while each has its volume, resistance, and potential leakage points—the use of parts not authorized by the manufacturer can disrupt ventilator operation and pose a danger to the patient. A similar issue arises when using nebulizers. There are several types of nebulizers, but gas-powered and ultrasonic nebulizers are the most commonly used. In a gas-powered nebulizer, a high-velocity stream of gas flows through the end of a tube placed in the reservoir with the administered water solution. The working principle is based on the Venturi effect—the moving gas creates negative pressure, drawing water into the tube and additionally breaking the water into tiny droplets. Ultrasonic nebulizers use vibration of a plate placed in the administered solution. The vibration is transmitted to the water surface and can generate water droplets entrained with fresh gas flowing through the nebulizer chamber. The advantage of ultrasonic nebulizers is the generation of smaller droplets (up to 1 um) than with classic nebulizers and potentially better distribution of the administered solution.

5.3.3 Battery

Each ventilator must have a power source and a battery. ICU ventilators are often equipped with several batteries, allowing uninterrupted operation for hours in case of loss of electrical supply. Manufacturers usually equip portable ventilators with one or more internal batteries. Some types have only an external battery to which the respirator can be connected when needed.

5.4 Special Considerations

During NIV, the patient is at risk of both hypo- and hyperventilation, so the alarm settings, including the leakage limits, should be carefully checked each time. For patients with significant airway secretions, there is a risk of bronchial tree obstruction, especially when using active humidification. In patients ventilated noninvasively for acute conditions such as pulmonary edema, there is a risk of gastric insufflation and aspiration of gastric contents. Additionally, the risk of hemodynamic instability due to positive intrathoracic pressure must be considered in these patients [4]. Finally, contraindications to noninvasive ventilation include severe craniofacial trauma, upper respiratory and gastrointestinal hemorrhage, severe consciousness impairment, and others [1, 2]. Do not use equipment in the presence of flammable gases and in oxygen-enriched atmospheres (high oxygen concentration poses a risk of ignition in electrical equipment). Do not independently modify (e.g., seal) leakage parts of the ventilator and use noncertified/incompatible respiratory components.

5.5 Conclusion

Ventilation modes have improved patient synchronization, and NIV has become an option for managing both acute and chronic respiratory insufficiency. Understanding unintentional leakage, humidification, oxygen delivery, and hemodynamic effects of NIV allows clinicians to select the most appropriate device and ventilation mode tailored to the patient's condition, minimizing complication risk.

References

1. Hasan A. Understanding mechanical ventilation: a practical handbook. 2nd ed. London, New York: Springer; 2010.
2. Carlucci A, Richard JC, Wysocki M, Lepage E, Brochard L, SRLF Collaborative Group on Mechanical Ventilation. Noninvasive versus conventional mechanical ventilation. An epidemiologic survey. Am J Respir Crit Care Med. 2001;163(4):874–80.
3. Majorski DS, Magnet FS, Thilemann S, et al. Portable NIV for patients with moderate to severe COPD: two randomized crossover trials. Respir Res. 2021;22:123.
4. Corp A, Thomas C, Adlam M. The cardiovascular effects of positive pressure ventilation. BJA Educ. 2021;21(6):202–9.

6 Portable Noninvasive Ventilation Devices

Tomasz Cyzowski and Konrad Mendrala

6.1 Introduction

Recent studies show that noninvasive ventilation (NIV) significantly improves numerous outcomes, such as dyspnea, patients' physical activity, and health-related quality of life, compared to standard oxygen therapy [1]. Additionally, the use of portable NIV is well-tolerated by the patients and results in a lower rate of hospital admissions for exacerbations of chronic obturative pulmonary disease (COPD) [2]. Nevertheless, NIV therapy is used mainly in rest and nocturnal settings, especially in COPD and obstructive sleep apnea (OSA) patients. It is primarily due to the inconvenience of carrying the device. Nowadays, manufacturers are making smaller devices with dimensions of bedside alarm clocks. Ventilators have internal batteries, some of them replaceable backup batteries, which enable use without connecting to the power supply. This facilitates using the devices and receiving breathing support during daily activities, outside patients' houses, going out, or traveling.

Most commonly used portable NIV devices are as follows: Philips Respironics Trilogy Evo (4.5 kg, 10 lbs.) and REMstar (1.5 kg, 3.3 lbs.), ResMed Astral 100 (3.2 kg, 7 lbs.) and Lumis 100 (1.1 kg, 2.4 lbs.), Ventec Life Systems VOCSN (7.3 kg, 16 lbs.), Medtronic Puritan Bennett 560 (8.6 kg, 19 lbs.), and Breas Vivo 65 (4.5 kg, 10 lbs.). They can be used with a stroller, backpack, or hook onto the backs of wheelchairs but with restriction of the patient's motion.

T. Cyzowski (✉)
Department of Anaesthesiology and Intensive Care, Faculty of Medical Sciences in Katowice, Medical University of Silesia, Katowice, Poland

Medical University of Silesia, Katowice, Poland

K. Mendrala
Department of Anaesthesiology and Intensive Care, Faculty of Medical Sciences in Katowice, Medical University of Silesia, Katowice, Poland

© The Author(s), under exclusive license to Springer Nature Switzerland AG 2025

K. Panda et al. (eds.), *Noninvasive Ventilatory Approaches in Interventional Procedures*, Noninvasive Ventilation. The Essentials,
https://doi.org/10.1007/978-3-032-05328-2_6

6.2 VitaBreath: Ultraportable NIV Device

The ultraportable device that can provide positive pressure ventilation is VitaBreath Philips Respironics [3] (Fig. 6.1). It is marketed as a lightweight, handheld, battery-operated, easy-to-use device for home or hospital use. The device has a mouthpiece and can be worn on a belt or carried in a bag. It is designed for COPD patients suffering from activity-related shortness of breath. The modes of noninvasive ventilation include continuous positive airway pressure (CPAP) mode and pressure support ventilation (PSV). Auto-titrating mode adjusts the pressure level automatically based on the patient's breathing patterns and needs, which can help optimize therapy and improve patient comfort [4]. The additional feature is the ramp function which gradually increases pressure to the prescribed level over time to help patients adapt to therapy. Scientific research results indicate that the use of portable NIV device VitaBreath increased exercise tolerance by reducing dynamic hyperinflation and breathlessness, may alleviate disease-related anxiety and depression [5], and can improve walking distance and dyspnea during exercise testing [6] in COPD patients (particularly in more severe cases of COPD).

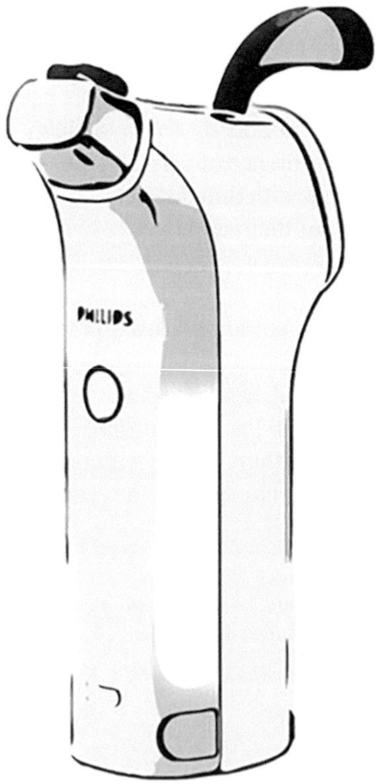

Fig. 6.1 Philips VitaBreath. (Figure source—own material)

6.3 Negative-Pressure Ventilation

A different approach to noninvasive mechanical ventilation represents negative-pressure ventilation (NPV). The principle of NPV devices is based on imitating the physiological way of breathing. The patient's body (or just the chest) is placed in a sealed chamber, while the head and upper respiratory tract remain outside (Fig. 6.2). Inspiration occurs through the periodic negative pressure generation in the chamber, expanding the chest and the lungs. Exhalation can be either passive (by the lungs and chest retraction forces) or assisted with positive pressure.

NPV devices were the most widely used during the polio pandemic, and their popularity has reappeared during the SARS-CoV2 pandemic. Although negative-pressure ventilation has no advantage over modern positive pressure ventilation modes, it remains an interesting option, mainly in neuromuscular diseases and children who do not tolerate interfaces placed on the face. The following represent a few noticeable NPV devices: iron lung, Exovent, jacket (bodysuit) ventilator, cuirass ventilator, and intermittent abdominal pressure ventilator (IAPV). A summary of the advantages and disadvantages of NPV use is presented in Table 6.1.

6.3.1 Iron Lungs

With the widespread use of positive-pressure mechanical ventilation, the iron lung gives a historical viewpoint on mechanical ventilation. Iron lungs, often known as tank ventilators, were among the first NPV devices used to treat respiratory insufficiency during the poliomyelitis epidemic in the mid-twentieth century. They were developed by Drinker and Shaw at Harvard University in 1928 and introduced by John Haven Emerson in 1931. Originally, the chamber made of aluminum (or plastic in later versions) seals the whole body except the head. The patient was lying on a contoured mattress with neck support that ensured proper positioning. The rotary

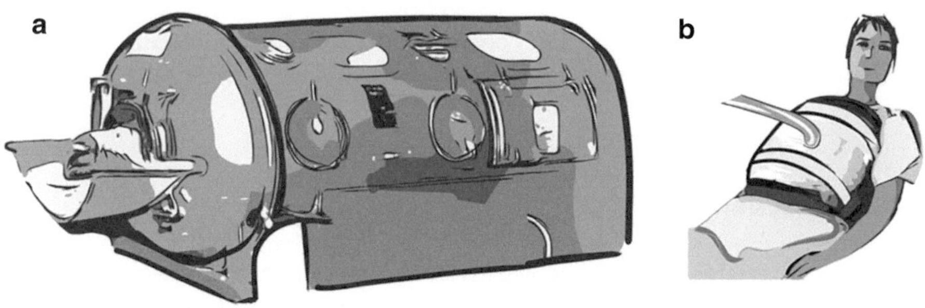

Fig. 6.2 Negative-pressure ventilators. (**a**) Iron lung, an aluminum chamber seals the whole body except the head. (**b**) Chest cuirass, a rigid shell attached tightly to the chest and connected to the ventilator with wide-bore tubing. (Figure source—own material)

Table 6.1 Advantages and disadvantages of negative-pressure ventilation

Advantages	Disadvantages
The most physiological type of ventilation No need for interfaces placed on/in the patient's airway Reduced prevalence of facial pressure injuries Lower risk of ventilator-related events such as ventilator-associated pneumonia and barotrauma Hemodynamic stability Effective in weaning from mechanical ventilation Dependability and simplicity	Higher risk of airway obstruction (especially in flaccid airways) Exacerbate obstructive sleep apnea Less mobility of the device Limited in patients with low thoracic/lungs compliance

pumps eliminated the air within the chamber, allowing the chest to extend and providing a breath. Side openings allowed hygienic activities, patient examination, or physiotherapy [7].

Although current research showed that iron lung ventilation (ILV) can be as effective as positive-pressure mechanical ventilation in improving gas exchange with a tendency toward a lower rate of complications, these are not widely used [8]. Interest in iron lungs has revived during the COVID-19 pandemic. Due to the lack of modern ventilators, some prototypes of new, easy-to-manufactured versions of the iron lung have been developed.

6.3.2 Exovent

A "modern version of the iron lung" was developed by a team of engineers, doctors, and researchers from the Indian Institute of Technology Bombay in April 2020 during the first wave of COVID-19 in India. Unlike a "classic" iron lung, the device encloses only the torso area [9]. The Exovent device provides two modes—negative-pressure ventilation (NPV) and high-frequency oscillatory ventilation (HFOV). NPV mode works similarly to classic iron lungs. In HFOV mode, the device uses high-frequency oscillations to provide mechanical ventilation. This mode is designed for patients who require more advanced respiratory support, such as those with acute respiratory distress syndrome (ARDS) on severe COVID-19 pneumonia. The Food and Drug Administration (FDA) granted the device Emergency Use Authorization (EUA) during the COVID-19 pandemic [9].

6.3.3 Vest Ventilator

Unlike large metal iron lungs, the negative-pressure chamber of vest ventilators is made of airtight synthetic clothing and forms a poncho, jacket, or suit. An inner framework and back plate allow the creation of negative pressure. The usability of the jacket ventilator is mainly limited to out-of-hospital applications due to its lower effectiveness compared to other methods of noninvasive ventilation. Certified negative-pressure ventilation devices include Negavent—Pegaso Vent Dimi Italia, Lifecare Pulmo-wrap, Poncho Wrap, Nu Mo suit, Pneumo Wrap, Pneumo suits, and Zip Suits. Some of the ventilation vests (such as the Gore-Tex® Poncho) come in a variety of sizes. The devices can also support exhalation with positive pressure. The vest ventilators are lightweight, but must be connected to negative-pressure generators, which weigh 15–30 kg.

6.3.4 Cuirass Ventilator

A chest cuirass is a rigid shell attached tightly to the chest and connected to the ventilator with wide-bore tubing. The pressure inside the cuirass affects the dimensions of the thoracic cavity, thus allowing respiration. Inhalation occurs when the device creates negative pressure. During expiration, the ventilator generates positive pressure, thus creating a compression effect on the thorax and facilitating expiration. Cuirass ventilation with both the inhalation and exhalation phases control is called biphasic cuirass ventilation (BCV) [10].

6.3.5 Intermittent Abdominal Pressure Ventilator

This method uses an inflatable belt placed around the patient's abdomen. During the exhalation, the belt inflates, causing an upward displacement of the diaphragm. After this phase, the pressure is removed from the belt, and internal organs and the diaphragm move downward, facilitating inspiration [11].

6.4 Summary

Noninvasive ventilation (NIV) is an effective respiratory support method that offers significant benefits for patients with COPD and other respiratory disorders compared to standard oxygen therapy. Portable NIV devices improve patients' quality of life, reduce hospital admissions, and are well-tolerated. However, patient mobility remains limited due to the size of the devices, although models like VitaBreath provide greater ease of use.

Negative-pressure ventilation (NPV), although less commonly used today, remains an interesting alternative, particularly for patients with neuromuscular diseases and children. Modern devices such as Exovent and vest ventilators are built on the concept of the classic "iron lung." Even new NPV devices like cuirass or vest ventilator are less portable than NIV devices.

References

1. Hasan A. Understanding mechanical ventilation: a practical handbook. 2nd ed. London, New York: Springer; 2010. https://doi.org/10.1007/978-1-84882-869-8.
2. Corp A, Thomas C, Adlam M. The cardiovascular effects of positive pressure ventilation. BJA Educ. 2021;21(6):202–9. https://doi.org/10.1016/j.bjae.2021.01.002.
3. Philips Respironics. VitaBreath: user guide and specifications. Philips Healthcare; 2020.
4. Vogiatzis I, Chynkiamis N, Armstrong M, Lane ND, Hartley T, Gray WK, Bourke SC. Intermittent use of portable NIV increases exercise tolerance in COPD: a randomised, cross-over trial. J Clin Med. 2019;8(1):94. https://doi.org/10.3390/jcm8010094.
5. De Giacomi F, Bonaiti G, Montanelli F, Della Zoppa M, Messinesi G, Carlucci A, Luppi F, Pesci A, Faverio P. Feasibility and clinical impact of a portable bi-level ventilation device in patients with severe chronic obstructive pulmonary disease and exertional dyspnea: preliminary results from a clinical series. Physiother Theory Pract. 2022;38(13):2526–30. https://doi.org/10.1080/09593985.2021.1938309.
6. Majorski DS, Magnet FS, Thilemann S, et al. Portable NIV for patients with moderate to severe COPD: two randomized crossover trials. Respir Res. 2021;22:123.
7. Meyer JA. A practical mechanical respirator, 1929: the "iron lung". Ann Thorac Surg. 1990;50(3):490–3. https://doi.org/10.1016/0003-4975(90)90508-4.
8. Corrado A, Ginanni R, Villella G, Gorini M, Augustynen A, Tozzi D, Peris A, Grifoni S, Messori A, Nozzoli C, Berni G. Iron lung versus conventional mechanical ventilation in acute exacerbation of COPD. Eur Respir J. 2004;23(3):419–24. https://doi.org/10.1183/09031936.04.00029304.
9. Exovent Development Group. Exovent: a study of a new negative pressure ventilatory support device in healthy adults. Anaesthesia. 2021;76(5):623–8. https://doi.org/10.1111/anae.15350.
10. Linton DM. Cuirass ventilation: a review and update. Crit Care Resusc. 2005;7(1):22–8. PMID: 16548815.
11. Volpi V, Volpato E, Compalati E, Pierucci P, Nicolini A, Lax A, Fagetti L, Annunziata A, Cauteruccio R, Fiorentino G, et al. Is intermittent abdominal pressure ventilation still relevant? A multicenter retrospective pilot study. J Clin Med. 2023;12:2453. https://doi.org/10.3390/jcm12072453.

Part III

Interfaces for Noninvasive Ventilation Support: Designs and Options

High-Flow Nasal Cannula

7

Adriana Dias and Pedro Nogueira Costa

7.1 Introduction

Supplemental oxygen therapy is commonly administered to patients experiencing hypoxemia. The purpose of respiratory support is to secure adequate ventilation and oxygenation, enhancing the availability of oxygen to tissues and organs, thereby improving physiological function and patient outcomes.

Traditional methods of delivering supplemental oxygen include devices such as low-flow nasal cannulas (LFNC), simple face masks, and non-rebreather masks. Despite its widespread use, LFNC has several limitations, such as its limitation to deliver between 4 and 6 L of oxygen per minute, which translates to a fraction of inspired oxygen (FiO_2) between 0.37 and 0.45. At higher flow rates, patients may experience nasal mucosal irritation and dryness, which can increase the risk of bleeding over time. FiO_2 is directly dependent on the flow rate, which, in these devices, is limited to no more than 15 L/min. The inspiratory flow of patients with respiratory failure ranges from 30 to over 100 L/min, providing a large difference between the patient inspiratory flow and delivered flow, resulting in an inconstant FiO_2.

Advancements in oxygen therapy have led to the development of high-flow nasal cannula (HFNC) therapy, which can provide up to 100% humidified and heated oxygen at flow rates reaching up to 80 L/min. This system addresses many of the limitations associated with traditional oxygen devices by ensuring higher and more

A. Dias (✉)
Pulmonology Department, Unidade Local de Saúde de Coimbra, Coimbra, Portugal
e-mail: 11897@ulscoimbra.min-saude.pt

P. N. Costa
Pulmonology Department, Unidade Local de Saúde de Braga, Braga, Portugal
e-mail: pedro.mn.costa@ulsb.min-saude.pt

© The Author(s), under exclusive license to Springer Nature Switzerland AG 2025

K. Panda et al. (eds.), *Noninvasive Ventilatory Approaches in Interventional Procedures*, Noninvasive Ventilation. The Essentials,
https://doi.org/10.1007/978-3-032-05328-2_7

consistent levels of oxygen delivery while maintaining patient comfort and reducing the risk of nasal mucosal irritation.

7.2 Components

The basic components of an HFNC system include an air/oxygen blender that generates up to 60–80 L/min flow (depending on the device model and or producing company), active heated humidifier, single heated circuit, and nasal cannula. The air/oxygen is set to a FiO_2 up to 1.0 and 80 L/min, consecutively heated and humidified [1]. The gas is delivered through the heated circuit and administered at high flow to the patient via the large nasal cannula.

The nasal cannula interface is an essential component for the delivery of high-flow therapy. To maintain an effective flush of CO_2, it is important that the cannula should occlude approximately 50% of the nares area.

An adequate interface is crucial to ensure good results. Oronasal masks, nasal masks, facial masks, and helmets have been used in noninvasive mechanical ventilation (NIV) but are frequently not tolerated by the patient. The discomfort, the skin trauma, and the high incidence of air leakage are some of the frequently reported obstacles. Patients with HFNC reported less skin damage and more comfort than with NIV.

Various methods have been investigated to enhance the effectiveness of high-flow nasal cannula (HFNC) support in order to prevent failure and reduce the need for ICU admission. Flows exceeding 60 L/min have been linked to discomfort in patients, with sedation potentially necessary to facilitate this approach [2]. Prone positioning while awake during HFNC support may improve oxygenation, optimize lung protection, and reduce the work of breathing [3]. However, this technique necessitates patient cooperation and may not be appropriate for individuals with postoperative respiratory failure or those who are severely obese.

A new HFNC interface featuring an asymmetrical cannula design has been approved for clinical use. This asymmetrical cannula includes one prong with a smaller diameter and another with a larger diameter, leading to an overall 30%–40% increase in the total cross-sectional area compared to a conventional interface of equal size [4]. The hypothesis is that an increase in asymmetrical occlusion of the nares leads to an improvement in dead-space clearance that resulted in a reduction in rebreathing, as schemed in Fig. 7.1.

7.3 Physiology

The physiological effects of HFNC therapy include the washout of carbon dioxide, the provision of low-level PEEP effect, the constant delivery of FiO_2, and the preservation of mucociliary function.

Studies showed that thoracoabdominal synchrony is better with HFNC than with face mask delivery, leading to a lower breathing frequency. Because PCO_2 and tidal

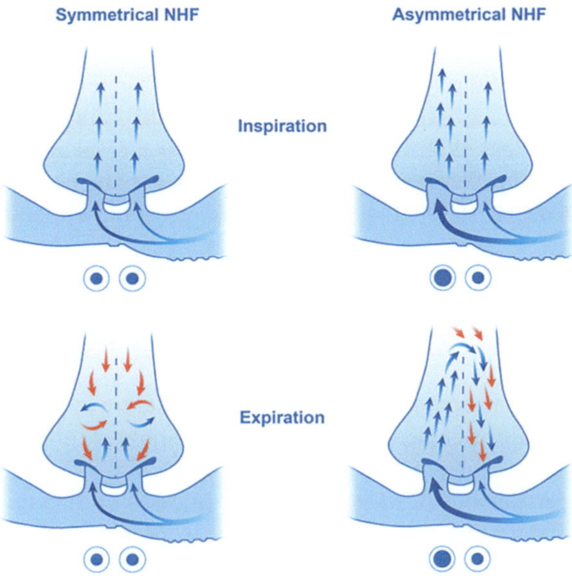

Fig. 7.1 Schematic representation of the flow direction in cannulas and the upper airways during inspiration (top) and expiration (bottom) in a symmetrical interface (SI) (left) and an asymmetrical interface (AI) (right). Blue arrows indicate nasal high flow (NHF), which is equally split between the prongs in the SI. In the AI, NHF is biased toward the larger prong due to its lower resistance and the streamline of gas velocity within the cannula. Expired gas flow is indicated by red arrows. (From Tatkov et al. [4], licensed under CC-BY 4.0)

volume (Vt) remain constant, but breathing frequency is reduced, the minute ventilation is lower. In animal studies, PCO_2 decreased as the HFNC flow increased, suggesting an effective carbon dioxide washout [5, 6].

Although HFNC is an open system, the flow from the cannulas prevails against some resistance of expiratory flow, increasing the airway pressure, as reported in several studies. This effect creates a positive end-expiratory pressure to lower airways, keeping the alveoli from collapsing during exhalation, improving alveolar recruitment, and enhancing the surface for gaseous diffusion.

FiO_2 is not stable with low-flow oxygen delivery given the difference between the patient inspiratory flow and the oxygen delivery system. HFNC provides stable FiO_2 by maintaining a high-flow delivery, supporting the patient's needs.

Conventional oxygen devices deliver dry and cold gas, leading to oral and nasal dryness and mucosal irritation. By contrast, warmed and humidified gas delivered by HFNC minimizes airway constriction, reduces work of breathing, and improves mucociliary function and clearance of secretions and is associated with less atelectasis.

7.4 Limitations

There are some limitations regarding the use of HFNC, in comparison to low-flow devices, starting on the expense for care, increased complexity and training, decreased mobility, loss of positive airway pressure by air leakage, and the potential delay to intubation. Furthermore, there are limitations to the use of nasal cannulas, such as altered mental status, facial injury, risk of aspiration, and hemodynamic instability.

7.5 Indications

Currently, the main indications for HFNC treatment are as follows: acute hypoxemic respiratory failure, hypercapnic respiratory failure, postsurgical respiratory failure, and post-extubation respiratory failure [7, 8].

HFNC has been demonstrated to be effective in cases of mild to moderate acute hypoxemic respiratory failure [9]. It helps reduce work of breathing, heart rate, and dyspnea and enhances thoracoabdominal synchrony and gas exchange, leading to better oxygen saturation. These clinical and physiological advantages provide a solid basis for the early implementation of HFNC to avoid the necessity for noninvasive and invasive positive-pressure ventilation, thereby lowering the mortality risk associated with ventilator-related complications. Compared to NIV, HFNC may be more suitable for patients who have excessive secretions, air leaks due to facial structure, or poor compliance.

HFNC has a physiological basis (such as improving oxygenation, providing positive pressure, and reducing dead space) for use in hypercapnic exacerbations of chronic obstructive pulmonary disease (COPD). Combined with its user-friendliness and patient comfort, HFNC can serve as an alternative to NIV for managing mild to moderate acute-on-chronic hypercapnic respiratory failure with respiratory acidosis. Nevertheless, duc to strong evidence supporting the use of NIV in COPD, current guidelines recommend that NIV should be attempted before considering HFNC.

In postoperative high-risk patients, HFNC has shown a lower re-intubation rate and a reduction in the escalation of respiratory support in comparison to conventional oxygen therapy. Similarly, HFNC reduces post-extubation respiratory failure and lower reintubation rates when compared to conventional oxygen therapy.

Endoscopic procedures such as bronchoscopy and gastrointestinal endoscopies are now widely performed for the diagnosis and treatment of many diseases in clinical practice. Patient discomfort and intolerance may interrupt the procedures; therefore, sedation has been used to increase patient satisfaction and facilitate clinical manipulation.

However, sedation may decrease the patient consciousness, increasing the risk of hypoxemia and other cardiopulmonary complications.

Conventional oxygen therapy (COT) is widely used but can only provide oxygen flow up to 15 L/min and a limited oxygen concentration of 30%–50%, on account of the air mixing and dilution from dead space. Noninvasive ventilation (NIV) has been used in attempt to minimize desaturation; however, patient discomfort and the difficulty of manipulating the endoscopy through the mask disqualify its widespread application. HFNC interface allows better oxygen delivery when compared to COT without the complex setting of NIV. A systematic review found that the use of HFNC was associated with improved oxygenation, decreased need for airway intervention, and reduced procedure interruption in patients undergoing endoscopic procedures [10, 11].

7.6 Conclusion

HFNC has emerged as a promising advancement in supplemental oxygen delivery, addressing many limitations associated with traditional low-flow oxygen devices. Its ability to deliver humidified, heated oxygen at high flow rates offers more consistent oxygenation, improved patient comfort, and reduced risks like nasal mucosal irritation. HFNC's physiological benefits, including carbon dioxide washout, the provision of low-level positive end-expiratory pressure, and preservation of mucociliary function, make it particularly effective for patients with acute hypoxemic and hypercapnic respiratory failure. While HFNC presents certain limitations, such as increased complexity and cost, it serves as a valuable tool in reducing the need for invasive ventilation, improving patient outcomes, and reducing re-intubation rates in postsurgical and post-extubation patients. Its ease of use and comfort make it a suitable alternative to noninvasive ventilation (NIV) in some cases, particularly in managing mild to moderate respiratory failure.

References

1. Nishimura M. High-flow nasal cannula oxygen therapy in adults: physiological benefits, indication, clinical benefits, and adverse effects. Respir Care. 2016;61(4):529–41.
2. Basile MC, Mauri T, Spinelli E, Dalla Corte F, Montanari G, Marongiu I, et al. Nasal high flow higher than 60 L/min in patients with acute hypoxemic respiratory failure: a physiological study. Crit Care. 2020;24(1):654.
3. Ding L, Wang L, Ma W, He H. Efficacy and safety of early prone positioning combined with HFNC or NIV in moderate to severe ARDS: a multi-center prospective cohort study. Crit Care. 2020;24(1):28.
4. Tatkov S, Rees M, Gulley A, van den Heuij LGT, Nilius G. Asymmetrical nasal high flow ventilation improves clearance of CO2 from the anatomical dead space and increases positive airway pressure. J Appl Physiol (1985). 2023;134(2):365–77.
5. Ricard JD, Roca O, Lemiale V, Corley A, Braunlich J, Jones P, et al. Use of nasal high flow oxygen during acute respiratory failure. Intensive Care Med. 2020;46(12):2238–47.
6. Ischaki E, Pantazopoulos I, Zakynthinos S. Nasal high flow therapy: a novel treatment rather than a more expensive oxygen device. Eur Respir Rev. 2017;26(145):170028.
7. Oczkowski S, Ergan B, Bos L, Chatwin M, Ferrer M, Gregoretti C, et al. ERS clinical practice guidelines: high-flow nasal cannula in acute respiratory failure. Eur Respir J. 2022;59(4):2101574.
8. Thille AW, Muller G, Gacouin A, Coudroy R, Decavèle M, Sonneville R, et al. Effect of postextubation high-flow nasal oxygen with noninvasive ventilation vs high-flow nasal oxygen

alone on reintubation among patients at high risk of extubation failure: a randomized clinical trial. JAMA. 2019;322(15):1465–75.
9. Rochwerg B, Einav S, Chaudhuri D, Mancebo J, Mauri T, Helviz Y, et al. The role for high flow nasal cannula as a respiratory support strategy in adults: a clinical practice guideline. Intensive Care Med. 2020;46(12):2226–37.
10. Tao Y, Sun M, Miao M, Han Y, Yang Y, Cong X, et al. High flow nasal cannula for patients undergoing bronchoscopy and gastrointestinal endoscopy: a systematic review and meta-analysis. Front Surg. 2022;9:949614.
11. La Combe B, Messika J, Labbé V, Razazi K, Maitre B, Sztrymf B, et al. High-flow nasal oxygen for bronchoalveolar lavage in acute respiratory failure patients. Eur Respir J. 2016;47(4):1283–6.

8 Full-Face Mask

Raquel Santos Silva, Joana Marques Simões, and Patrícia Trindade

The use of continuous positive airway pressure (CPAP) and noninvasive ventilation (NIV) has been identified as a good alternative in interventional endoscopic procedures [1].

CPAP provides a positive pressure throughout the entire breathing cycle, recruiting lung atelectatic regions, reducing venous admixture, maintaining upper airway patency, and decreasing the patient's inspiratory effort. NIV can also ameliorate gas exchange, thus diminishing the respiratory effort [2].

In a review of oxygenation strategies during flexible bronchoscopy procedures, CPAP, in comparison to conventional oxygen therapy, guaranteed higher SpO_2 during and after the procedure and lowered the number of patients requiring invasive ventilatory assistance within 6 hours following the endoscopic procedure. NIV also provided optimal gas exchange during and after the procedure, causing less hemodynamic impairment compared to invasive ventilation, and was also associated with a low incidence of minor complications and with a small percentage of patients requiring intubation during the first 8 hours after the procedure. Compared to high-flow nasal cannula (HFNC), in mild-to-moderate hypoxemic acute respiratory failure patients, NIV improved oxygenation before, during, and after flexible bronchoscopy, decreasing desaturation ($SpO_2 < 90\%$), without any differences in mortality or in the rate of patients requiring intubation and invasive mechanical ventilation. Also, some bronchoscopy procedures (such as transbronchial biopsies) may require deep sedation and analgesia, which can induce collapse of the airways, affecting the breathing pattern and the respiratory drive. Therefore, NIV may be an option to consider [3].

R. S. Silva (✉) · J. M. Simões · P. Trindade
Pulmonology Service, Thorax Department, Unidade Local de Saúde Santa Maria (ULSSM), Lisbon, Portugal
e-mail: 28864@chln.min-saude.pt; 28844@chln.min-saude.pt; 28813@chln.min-saude.pt

© The Author(s), under exclusive license to Springer Nature Switzerland AG 2025

K. Panda et al. (eds.), *Noninvasive Ventilatory Approaches in Interventional Procedures*, Noninvasive Ventilation. The Essentials,
https://doi.org/10.1007/978-3-032-05328-2_8

In endoscopic procedures, the use of NIV/CPAP is of particular interest and has been used in transesophageal echocardiogram, flexible bronchoscopy, and gastrointestinal procedures which range from esophagogastroduodenoscopy to endoscopic retrograde cholangiopancreatography to percutaneous endoscopic gastrostomy [4, 5]. Standard routine monitoring of patients under sedation and NIV during endoscopic procedures includes continuous electrocardiography, noninvasive arterial pressure measure, pulse oximetry, and transcutaneous capnography (whenever available) [6].

The use of CPAP and NIV in interventional procedures can be accomplished using several interfaces. Interfaces in CPAP/NIV are a potential source of pain and claustrophobia and need to be carefully chosen. In recent years, device manufacturers have developed different types of interfaces with various technologies and materials. There are six main classes of interfaces available: mouthpiece, nasal prongs, nasal mask, oronasal mask, full-face mask, and the helmet [7]. In this chapter, we will focus on the use of full-face masks.

A full-face mask, also named total face, cephalic, or integral mask, is defined as covering the eyes, nose, and mouth, sealing around the perimeter of the face and reducing the leaks. Compared to other interfaces, it is adequate for prominent facial anatomy, makes no pressure on nasal bridge, and lowers the air leaks. However, it is more claustrophobic, has higher costs, and needs to be applied by experienced staff [7, 8].

There are several types of full-face masks commercially available: BiTrac MaxShield Select® [Pulmodyne®, USA], BiTrac SE MaxShield Select® [Pulmodyne®, USA], BiTrac MaxShield VAA® [Pulmodyne®, USA], FitLife® [Phillips Respironics®, USA], FitLife SE® [Phillips Respironics®, USA] (Fig. 8.1), Dimax®, [Dimar®, Italy], Janus Mask® [Biomedical®, Italy], and pediatrics types.

On cardiovascular procedures, in 2010 and 2011, there were reported cases using full-face mask with a self-made hole to allow periprocedural transesophageal echocardiogram guidance [9].

Periprocedural NIV can be provided either by adapting the existing device or using the new technology adaptors available. The disadvantage of using the former is the difficulty in providing an effective positive end-expiratory pressure and positive pressure support due to the opening of the circuit to insert the probe, resulting in increased air leak outside the circuit and suboptimal ventilation.

Some interfaces (helmet and specific face masks) have been specifically designed to be used during endoscopic procedures, allowing both oral and nasal routes for bronchoscope insertion. The first developed device was Patil-Syracuse mask which is an oronasal mask that has an additional port (that can be closed with a plastic cap) and a soft silicone membrane to accommodate different endoscopic devices, and its use was described in flexible bronchoscopy [1, 10].

After Patil-Syracuse mask, full-face masks were the most studied interfaces. The first one created was a full-face mask with a Boussignac valve. Its use was described specially in flexible bronchoscopy. The wall of the device contains four funnel-shaped microchannels able to generate pressure (creating a constant positive pressure), connected to an external opening that is linked to the oxygen source, and

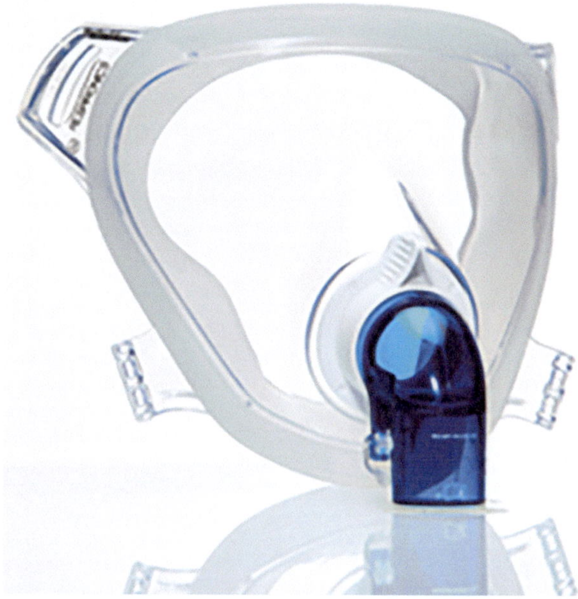

Fig. 8.1 FitLife SE® mask. (Reproduced with permission from Koninklijke Philips N.V.)

remains open to the atmosphere, which allows flexible bronchoscopy to be performed without modifying the jet flow or the resulting pressure, resulting in less leaks and disconnection [1, 11].

Later, it was created with a plastic cylinder secured in the mask to allow for the introduction of the bronchoscope through the mouth and endowed with a disposable cap from a swivel connector that was able to seal the cylinder and prevent air leakage during endoscopic procedures [12].

Another interface, the full-face Janus mask, has a hole covered by a membrane in front of the patient's mouth to allow the insertion of the endoscopic probe. This mask is made of two separable halves with a midline port that allows the insertion of the endoscopic probes into the patient's mouth or nose for diagnostic and/or therapeutic aims without interrupting positive airway pressure support. For this reason, it can be placed on and/or removed from the patient's face even during the endoscopic examination, which becomes relevant in cases of unexpected sudden respiratory deterioration during procedures, thus reducing the risk of intubation. This mask has been applied in transesophageal echocardiogram and flexible bronchoscopy [13].

There are other alternatives such as the use of full-face mask connectors (also denominated as elbows) that have a small hole and a silicone membrane with a sealed hole that allow the entry of the endoscopic device and can be easily adapted to the circuit without increasing air leak and reducing pressurization (Fig. 8.2).

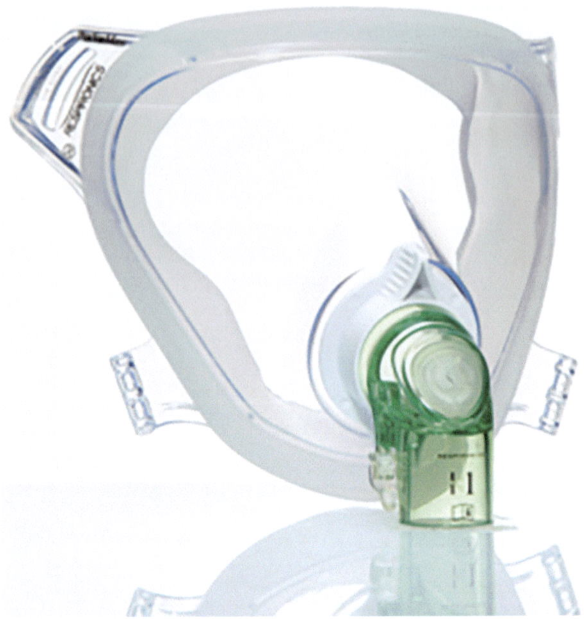

Fig. 8.2 Full-face mask FitLife SE® mask with endoscopic elbow. (Reproduced with permission from Koninklijke Philips N.V.)

However, even with these alternatives, air leaks may occur around the interface or through the dedicated holes, leading to patient-ventilator asynchronies, which can be difficult to manage.

Unfortunately, there is not an available comparative study between the different interfaces previously discussed.

Besides the use of full-face masks, there are some cases reported in literature using nasal masks. There is the case of a woman with cystic fibrosis and on home NIV with a nasal interface (Mirage FX®) with a high ventilatory dependency (>18 h/day) that was submitted to a transesophageal echocardiogram using her own interface and a mouthpiece, with an initial decreased of oxygen to SpO_2 88% during the procedure, but after adjustment of NIV parameters, it was possible to achieve SpO_2 100%, and the procedure occurred without complications [14].

Even though scientific evidence supporting the use of CPAP/NIV during endoscopic procedures is growing, it should be kept in mind that NIV is not 100% successful and not completely free from complications. The most common causes of NIV failure, potentially requiring endotracheal intubation, are respiratory failure, patient intolerance (agitation, delirium, claustrophobia), and facial lesions [15].

In conclusion, the use of full-face masks has been increasing in recent years. It has been used in several endoscopic procedures with evidence of benefits, especially in moderate to severe hypoxemic patients (acute or chronic). However, there is not a comparative study between the interfaces available, suggesting an eventual best choice.

References

1. Pieri M, Landoni G, Cabrini L. Noninvasive ventilation during endoscopic procedures: rationale, clinical use and devices. J Cardiothorac Vasc Anesth. 2018;32(2):928–34.
2. MacIntyre NR. Physiologic effects of noninvasive ventilation. Respir Care. 2019;64(6):617–28.
3. Pelaia C, Bruni A, Garofalo E, et al. Oxygenation strategies during flexible bronchoscopy: a review of the literature. Respir Res. 2021;22(1):253.
4. Folgado MA, De la Serna C, Llorente A, et al. Utility of noninvasive ventilation in high-risk patients during endoscopic retrograde cholangiopancreatography. Lung India. 2014;31(4):331–5.
5. Esquinas A, Zuil M, Scala R, Chiner E. Bronchoscopy during non-invasive mechanical ventilation: a review of techniques and procedures. Arch Bronconeumol. 2013;49(3):105–12.
6. Ergan B, Nasiłowski J, Winck JC. How should we monitor patients with acute respiratory failure treated with noninvasive ventilation? Eur Respir Rev. 2018;27(148):170101.
7. Elliott MW. The interface: crucial for successful noninvasive ventilation. Eur Respir J. 2004;23(1):7–8.
8. Cammarota G, Simonte R, De Robertis E. Comfort during non-invasive ventilation. Front Med (Lausanne). 2022;24(9):874250.
9. Guarracino F, Cabrini L, Baldassarri R, et al. Non-invasive ventilation-aided transoesophageal echocardiography in high-risk patients: a pilot study. Eur J Echocardiogr. 2010;11(6):554–6.
10. Aoyama K, Takenaka I. Patil-Syracuse mask for fiberoptic intubation. Masui. 1999;48(11):1262–6.
11. Maitre B, Jaber S, Maggiore SM, et al. Continuous positive airway pressure during fiberoptic bronchoscopy in hypoxemic patients. A randomized double-blind study using a new device. Am J Respir Crit Care Med. 2000;162(3 Pt 1):1063–7.
12. Heunks LM, de Bruin CJ, van der Hoeven JG, van der Heijden HF. Non-invasive mechanical ventilation for diagnostic bronchoscopy using a new face mask: an observational feasibility study. Intensive Care Med. 2010;36(1):143–7.
13. Beccaria P, Votta CD, Lucchetta L, Silvetti S, Agostoni M, Zangrillo A. Two different endoscopic procedures made feasible by the Janus mask in a high-risk patient. Indian J Crit Care Med. 2017;21(9):613–5.
14. Gomes RE, Redondo MT, Gonçalves MR. Non-invasive ventilation through a nasal interface during transoesophageal echocardiogram in a high-risk chronic patient. Pulmonology. 2021;27(5):455–7.
15. Ozyilmaz E, Ugurlu AO, Nava S. Timing of noninvasive ventilation failure: causes, risk factors, and potential remedies. BMC Pulm Med. 2014;14:19.

9 Helmet Interface for Procedures

Andrzej Swinarew and Szymon Skoczyński

9.1 Introduction

The use of helmets in mechanical ventilation is becoming increasingly common. Initially, this device was developed for use in intensive care unit (ICU) settings. However, over time, the number of procedures utilizing helmets has increased, and they are now being employed in a broader range of cases. Helmets are most frequently used in Italy, but other countries are beginning to recognize their benefits, which has contributed to their growing popularity. One of the key advantages of the helmet device is that it completely covers the patient's face, with none of its components coming into direct contact with the skin, while the neck and shoulders are surrounded by a soft shell gasket.

The helmets used for interventional procedures may differ from those most frequently used in hospitals. While the primary role of the helmet is to provide ventilation, specialized devices can also be utilized for specific medical procedures. Recent developments in helmet technology for these applications are outlined below.

Noninvasive ventilation (NIV) is an increasingly popular method of applying positive pressure to facilitate patient ventilation, aimed at reducing the need for invasive endotracheal intubation. This method requires a secure connection to the patient through interfaces such as various types of masks or helmets. Selecting the

A. Swinarew (✉)
Faculty of Science and Technology, University of Silesia, Katowice, Silesia, Poland

Institute of Sport Science, The Jerzy Kukuczka Academy of Physical Education in Katowice, Katowice, Poland
e-mail: andrzej.swinarew@us.edu.pl

S. Skoczyński
Department of Lung Diseases and Tuberculosis, Faculty of Medical Sciences in Zabrze, Medical University of Silesia in Katowice, Zabrze, Poland

© The Author(s), under exclusive license to Springer Nature Switzerland AG 2025
K. Panda et al. (eds.), *Noninvasive Ventilatory Approaches in Interventional Procedures*, Noninvasive Ventilation. The Essentials,
https://doi.org/10.1007/978-3-032-05328-2_9

appropriate interface is crucial for the effectiveness of the treatment, especially when additional interventions are necessary. The key advantages of NIV include providing noninvasive support for patient ventilation in acute and/or chronic respiratory failure (ARF), preserving airway defense mechanisms, enabling speech and swallowing, and reducing the incidence of ventilator-associated pneumonia, ICU admissions, intubation, and mortality [1].

However, NIV is associated with a significant risk of failure. The likelihood of success or failure depends on the method's ability to reverse hypoxia and/or hypercapnia. Another critical factor impacting NIV's success is patient comfort. Selecting the appropriate interface is particularly important for two patient groups: those with acute respiratory failure, who may require procedures to facilitate ventilation—such as the clearance of pus, mucus, or foreign bodies—and those undergoing chronic or prolonged hospital treatment, where comfort and the potential for complications, such as skin breakdown or pressure ulcers, are significant concerns [1].

NIV-induced complications are primarily observed when masks are used in cases of acute respiratory failure. The pressure applied by the interface on the patient's skin often exceeds capillary pressure, leading to a high chance of skin breakdown, which can ultimately result in NIV discontinuation due to pain and treatment intolerance. The probability of facial pressure ulcers can be as high as 31% and largely depends on the type of mask used, the duration of treatment, ventilator settings, humidification, nutritional status, and skin fragility. Preventative measures, including proper interface fitting, interrupted ventilation, wound dressings, or interface changes, can significantly reduce this risk. From a pathophysiological standpoint, a particularly effective approach is to use an interface that avoids direct contact with the skin, such as ventilation helmets.

The COVID-19 pandemic highlighted that NIV/CPAP might offer better prognoses compared to high-flow nasal cannula (HFNC) treatment. It also underscored the importance of selecting interfaces based on patient preferences as well as healthcare worker safety, particularly in preventing aerosol spread. These factors, along with the frequent need for prolonged NIV, have led to the worldwide popularity of helmets. Their role has expanded from primarily providing ventilation to encompassing procedural support and protection for medical personnel [2, 3].

In addition to helmets, barrier tents offer another effective solution for managing respiratory care in clinical settings. They are designed to protect healthcare workers, facilitate prolonged passive oxygen therapy, and, most importantly, support the safe performance of aerosol-generating procedures for patients with respiratory failure. The barrier tent, as illustrated in Fig. 9.1, incorporates a structure and materials similar to those used in ventilation helmets [4, 5].

The barrier tent was found effective for procedures such as FOB stands for Flexible (Fiberoptic) Bronchoscopy (FOB) in hypoxemic patient. However, taking into account large dead space, the barrier tent (Fig. 9.1) is not feasible for ventilation. The tent facilitates only passive oxygen therapy where oxygen is administered through gas ports, whereas used air is being removed via HEPA filter to protect healthcare workers. As presented in Fig. 9.1, patients were experiencing severe type 2 respiratory failure; therefore, to safely perform FOB, NIV was added, and the

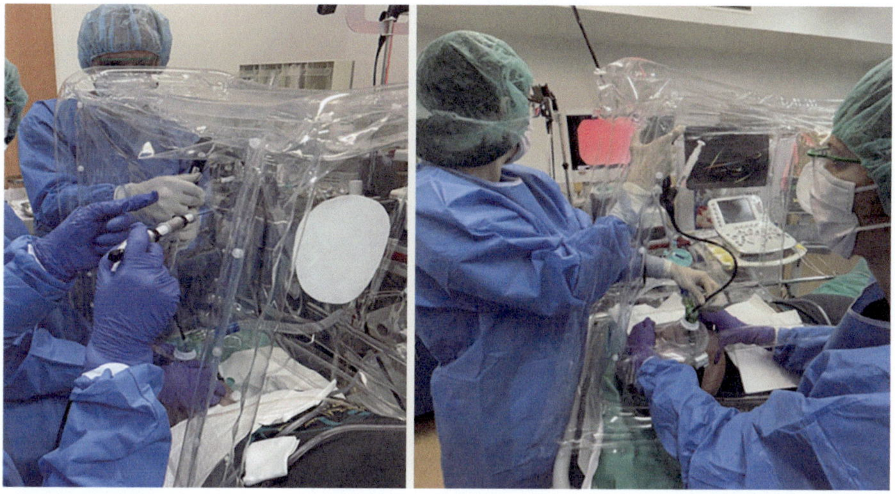

Fig. 9.1 Automatic, pneumatic barrier tent in a clinical setting. (Patent application to The Polish Patent Office: P.440079 [WIPO ST 10/C PL440079])

barrier tent served as the only protective device for the healthcare providers. Several years ago, helmet was found to be an effective interface to facilitate safe diagnostic FOB in patients with acute hypoxemic respiratory failure. In this scenario, helmet prevented gas exchange deterioration. The patients on NIV provided by helmet were stable in terms of cardiovascular function and were free from endotracheal intubation. This should support for further development of new tents with smaller than barrier tent dead space and well-adjusted procedure ports for endoscopic procedures. Large volume may be considered problematic in helmet ventilation; therefore, the interface is used more frequently with CPAP settings. Another possible NIV adjustment is based on the neural signaling on the inspiratory phase. It was found that the neural signaling improves patient ventilator asynchrony and shortens inspiratory delay compared to PSV. This has not been checked on patients requiring medical procedures such as FOB. However, promising neural signaling seems to generate excessive costs in the case of patients requiring only short procedures. Therefore, current efforts are focused on developing a specialized helmets suitable both for NIV and CPAP.

Helmet ventilation seems to be especially promising in children and infants, as it improves respiratory rate and ventilation comfort in comparison with face mask. The helmet ventilation decreases air leaks and skin redness over contact points and is therefore especially promising in infants since facial ossification is ongoing [6–8].

Helmet CPAP was also found effective in pediatric liver transplant patient as a post-extubation respiratory support tool.

Moreover, a helmet can be broadly used in patients with facial trauma or congenital facial deformity or even for otorhinolaryngological surgery.

The new development will incorporate functionality insights gained from the barrier tent, with adjustments required for whole range of procedures, as well as for patients anthropometric features and age.

9.2 General Helmet Design and Functionality

Main components

- Transparent shell.
- Sealing gasket.
- Oxygen/ventilation supply system.
- Integrated humidifiers.
- Exhaust system.

9.2.1 Materials

The proper selection of materials is crucial for creating a transparent, lightweight, and airtight barrier while maintaining the necessary structural integrity.

The *transparent shell* of the helmet is made from high-density polycarbonate or medical-grade polyurethane. Both materials provide excellent clarity, ensuring that medical staff can freely observe the patient. Polycarbonate and polyurethane are highly durable and resistant to impact, providing protection against physical damage, which is essential when carrying out procedures such as bronchofiberoscopy. These materials are also resistant to chemicals and disinfectants, allowing for easy cleaning in terms of prolonged usage. Additionally, their lightweight quality makes the helmet comfortable for extended wear.

The *sealing gasket* is made from medical-grade silicone, providing a flexible and comfortable seal around the neck and shoulder girdle for an airtight fit. Medical-grade silicon is hypoallergenic, minimizing the risk of allergic reactions, and is durable enough to withstand repeated sterilization cycles.

The *oxygen and exhaust channels* consist of medical-grade silicone tubing, known for its flexibility, wear resistance, and chemical durability, making it suitable for medical environments with frequent disinfectant exposure.

Altogether, the materials used in the construction of the individual isolation helmet are selected to provide a balance of transparency, durability, flexibility, and chemical resistance, ensuring the safety and comfort of both the patient and medical personnel.

9.2.2 Design Features

The individual isolation helmet is a protective device designed to isolate the patient's head, providing a protective barrier between the patient and medical staff. It is particularly useful for patients with respiratory viral or bacterial infections, ensuring healthcare workers' safety while allowing for full interaction with the patient.

The transparent shell provides a clear view of the patient's face and is sealed around the neck and shoulders with a flexible, airtight gasket for a secure and comfortable fit. The helmet is lightweight and portable, making it easy to put on and take off, and suitable for both hospital and transport scenarios.

The oxygen supply and exhaust systems are designed to ensure that the patient can breathe comfortably while maintaining a sterile environment. The system provides a continuous flow of fresh air and oxygen mixture and safely removes exhaled gases, preventing the spread of infectious pathogens. Integrated humidifiers maintain adequate humidity in the oxygen supply, preventing dryness and irritation of the respiratory tract.

Helmets are lightweight and are produced to fit various head and neck sizes comfortably.

9.2.3 Advantages

The individual isolation helmet offers numerous advantages from both medical and technical perspectives, making it an effective and essential tool in healthcare settings. It provides a complete barrier around the patient's head, significantly reducing the risk of airborne transmission of infectious agents to medical staff. The airtight seal around the neck and shoulders ensures that no pathogens escape the isolated environment.

The use of lightweight and transparent materials enhances patient comfort, reducing the risk of claustrophobia. The integrated humidification system maintains appropriate moisture levels in the air supply, preventing dryness and irritation of the respiratory tract. The transparent shell allows healthcare providers to continuously monitor the patient's condition without the need for physical contact. The design facilitates full interaction between medical staff and the patient, allowing necessary procedures to be performed without removing the helmet.

The high-density polycarbonate or medical-grade polyurethane helmet provides excellent clarity and durability, guaranteeing long-term use and resistance to physical damage. The medical-grade silicone gasket creates a flexible, airtight, and hypoallergenic seal, enhancing both patient comfort and safety. The flexible and durable medical-grade silicone tubing used for oxygen and exhaust channels allows for easy adjustment and long-lasting performance.

The helmet's lightweight construction makes it easy to transport and use in various healthcare settings, including hospitals and emergency response scenarios. The device is easy to clean and sterilize and can be reused safely and efficiently.

Overall, the individual isolation helmet combines advanced materials and design features to provide high levels of protection, comfort, and ease of use, benefiting both patients and healthcare providers.

9.3 Specialized Helmet Designs

9.3.1 Anesthesia Helmet

In recent years, a helmet designed for outdoor anesthesiological procedures has been developed to address the need for effective battlefield first aid. The invention consists of a helmet, a breathing mask, an anesthetic rod, a cover plate, a ventilation hole, and disc hinges. The top of the helmet features venting holes. Disc hinges are mounted on both sides of the helmet, with the ends of the anesthetic rod, which includes a honeycomb hole, attached to these hinges. A breathing mask is positioned on one side of the helmet, while the front opening is covered by the cover plate [9].

The concept behind this development is to use a standard helmet with an anesthetic rod mounted on the cover plate to facilitate anesthesia procedures in environments where accidents are likely to occur, such as in the field. The design employs a lightweight helmet as the base, which not only protects the patient's head but also functions as a closed container. This allows the anesthesiologist to administer anesthetic gas, making it convenient for field use and enabling the doctor to perform surgery [10].

The principle of this invention is to use the helmet both as a protective device and as a container for administering anesthetic gas. The helmet includes ventilation holes that facilitate airflow and help expel anesthetic gas after the procedure, allowing the patient to wake up more easily.

9.3.2 Infectious Disease Gastroscopy Helmet

The main idea behind the design was to provide a helmet suitable for both ventilation and performance of gastroscopic procedures. This invention enhances the ability to perform gastrointestinal procedures while ensuring the safety of healthcare providers [9].

The device includes a mouthpiece tube that extends into the helmet body near the patient's face, serving as a conduit for the patient's mouth. One end of the tube enters the helmet body and is used for oxygen intake, connecting to an oxygen delivery device. Another tube, positioned above the first, allows for the removal of exhaled gases. The helmet is equipped with an additional through hole on one side of the mouthpiece tube, which has a rotatable cover. This cover, mounted on a shaft, can rotate to either close or open the through hole as needed [9].

The helmet body is molded from silicone or polyolefin material, and the flexible connecting belt is also made of silicone. The mouthpiece tube, along with the exhaust tube, is integrally formed with the helmet body.

9.4 Key Insights and Implications

- The use of helmets in medical procedures is expanding rapidly, with notable benefits in anesthesiology and respiratory care.
- The specialized helmets offer significant benefits, including improved safety, patient comfort, and effective ventilation with advanced features like swirling airflow designs.
- The clinical and physiological rationale supports increasing helmet use for safer and more efficient patient care.
- Many specialized helmet designs have emerged for specific procedures, reflecting ongoing innovation.
- Although current helmets are not universally adaptable for all procedures, efforts are underway to improve their functionality.

9.5 Conclusions

The increasing use of helmet-based interfaces in noninvasive ventilation (NIV) and interventional procedures underscores their clinical value in improving patient outcomes and healthcare worker safety. Compared to traditional mask-based interfaces, helmets provide superior patient comfort, reduce complications such as pressure ulcers, and enable safer execution of procedures requiring prolonged respiratory support.

Key advancements in helmet technology, including the integration of specialized procedural ports and barrier tents, have expanded their applications beyond ICU settings. Helmets have demonstrated particular efficacy in facilitating bronchoscopy, pediatric ventilation, and anesthesia in challenging environments, such as field conditions and infectious disease management.

Despite these advantages, challenges remain in optimizing helmet designs to minimize dead space, enhance ventilation efficiency, and ensure compatibility with different medical procedures. Emerging technologies, such as neural signaling for ventilatory synchronization, offer promising improvements but require further investigation to justify their cost-effectiveness.

Future developments should focus on refining helmet structures to accommodate various clinical scenarios, improve patient adherence, and enhance procedural safety. By continuing to innovate and adapt helmet-based interfaces, healthcare providers can maximize the benefits of noninvasive ventilation while maintaining high standards of care in interventional medicine.

References

1. Vaschetto R, Gregoretti C, Scotti L, et al. A pragmatic, open-label, multi-center, randomized controlled clinical trial on the rotational use of interfaces vs standard of care in patients treated with noninvasive positive pressure ventilation for acute hypercapnic respiratory failure: the

ROTAtional-USE of interface STUDY (ROTA-USE STUDY). Trials. 2023;24(1):527. https://doi.org/10.1186/s13063-023-07560-1.
2. Grasselli G, Calfee CS, Camporota L, European Society of Intensive Care Medicine Taskforce on ARDS, et al. ESICM guidelines on acute respiratory distress syndrome: definition, phenotyping and respiratory support strategies. Intensive Care Med. 2023;49(7):727–59. https://doi.org/10.1007/s00134-023-07050-7.
3. Antonelli M, Pennisi MA, Conti G, et al. Fiberoptic bronchoscopy during noninvasive positive pressure ventilation delivered by helmet. Intensive Care Med. 2003;29(1):126–9. https://doi.org/10.1007/s00134-002-1554-5.
4. Costa A, Merlo F, Pagni A, et al. The new neural pressure support (NPS) mode and the helmet: did we find the dynamic duo? J Anesth Analg Crit Care. 2024;4(1):35. https://doi.org/10.1186/s44158-024-00170-6.
5. Chiusolo F, Fanelli V, Ciofi Degli Atti ML, et al. CPAP by helmet for treatment of acute respiratory failure after pediatric liver transplantation. Pediatr Transplant. 2018;22(1) https://doi.org/10.1111/petr.13088.
6. Frassoni E, Shankar-Aguilera S, Yousef N, De Luca D. Helmet-delivered respiratory support in neonate with severe facial malformation. J Paediatr Child Health. 2017;53(8):825. https://doi.org/10.1111/jpc.13635.59.
7. Liu Q, Shan M, Zhu H, Cao J, Chen R. Noninvasive ventilation with a helmet in patients with acute respiratory failure caused by chest trauma: a randomized controlled trial. Sci Rep. 2020;10(1):21489. https://doi.org/10.1038/s41598-020-78607-5.
8. Pelosi P, Severgnini P, Aspesi M, et al. Non-invasive ventilation delivered by conventional interfaces and helmet in the emergency department. Eur J Emerg Med. 2003;10(2):79–86. https://doi.org/10.1097/00063110-200306000-00002.
9. CN212661788U Infectious disease gastroscopy helmet.
10. CN204409718U Anesthesia helmet for outdoor emergency.

Supraglottic Airways 10

Daniel Raboin and Shaun L. Thompson

10.1 Types of Supraglottic Airways

Supraglottic airways (SGAs) are commonly used to support noninvasive ventilation in procedural settings. Patient comorbidities and/or procedural sedation/anesthesia may lead to a loss of airway patency above the glottis. Any device that improves airway patency above the level of the glottis performs the function of an SGA; therefore, airway adjuncts such as the nasopharyngeal and oropharyngeal airways warrant discussion (Fig. 10.1).

Nasopharyngeal airways (NPAs) form a conduit from the anterior nare to the supraglottic space by stenting open soft tissue. They are manufactured from a wide variety of materials with differing levels of rigidity and come in many designs and sizes. Patients with minimal or no sedation generally tolerate NPAs well [1]. For this reason, NPAs are particularly useful to treat airway obstruction in patients undergoing minor procedures which may not require sedation up to patients needing moderate sedation. Airway professionals may pair NPAs with oxygen delivery devices such as nasal cannula or a range of other oxygen delivery systems such as non-rebreather devices.

The oropharyngeal airway (OPA) [2] is the next most invasive device. Generally manufactured of rigid plastic, they come in an array of designs and sizes. OPA's stent open the soft tissue of the oropharynx to provide an unobstructed pathway from the oral opening to the supraglottic space. These tend to cause more stimulation than an NPA and are poorly tolerated without some degree of sedation [1]. As

D. Raboin
US Army Institute of Surgical Research, Burn Center Division, San Antonio, TX, USA

S. L. Thompson (✉)
Department of Anesthesiology, University of Nebraska Medical Center, Omaha, NE, USA
e-mail: slthomps@unmc.edu

© The Author(s), under exclusive license to Springer Nature Switzerland AG 2025

K. Panda et al. (eds.), *Noninvasive Ventilatory Approaches in Interventional Procedures*, Noninvasive Ventilation. The Essentials,
https://doi.org/10.1007/978-3-032-05328-2_10

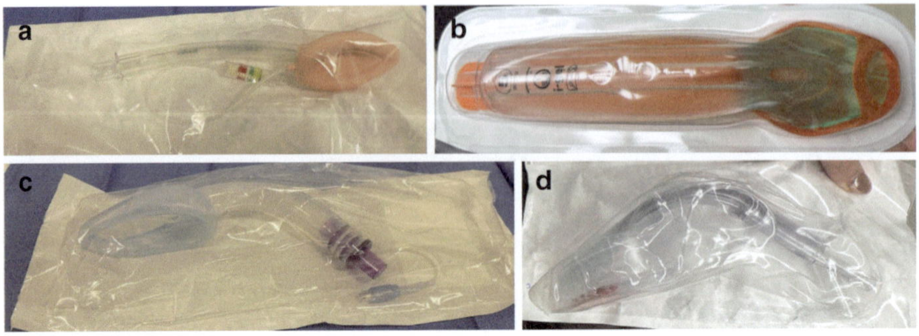

Fig. 10.1 Types and generations of SGAs used in current practice. (**a**) LMA®UniqueTM—1st generation, cuffed perilaryngeal sealer, mask aperture bars. (**b**) Air-Q®—1st generation, cuffed perilaryngeal sealer, without mask aperture bars, integrated bite block. (**c**) i-gel®—2nd generation, cuffless anatomically preshaped sealer, integrated bite block. (**d**) LMA®Supreme™—2nd generation, cuffed perilaryngeal sealer, mask aperture bars

such, the OPA has more of a role in procedures requiring moderate to deep sedation. Like the NPA, OPAs may be paired with oxygen delivery devices.

Both the NPA and OPA serve as bridges to the patient recovering the ability to protect their airway or placement of a more invasive airway. When used to support noninvasive ventilation with procedural sedation, once periprocedural sedation is discontinued, the former is usually the case. In contrast, when used as part of a general anesthetic or in preparation for intubation, they often serve as bridge to and/or from a more invasive airway.

Devices typically referred to as SGAs represent a heterogenous group of airways which provide a means of oxygenation, ventilation, and delivery of volatile anesthetic. The term laryngeal mask airway [3] is commonly used interchangeably with SGAs, but refers to proprietary, trademarked designs. SGAs are generally inserted without guidance into the pharynx. While SGAs are more invasive than OPA/NPAs, they provide more reliable airway patency when properly positioned. In comparison to endotracheal intubation, SGAs are less invasive, but also less secure. Like endotracheal intubation, either spontaneous or positive pressure ventilation may be used. In addition to serving as a primary airway, SGAs are frequently used as rescue devices [4, 5], or as a route for intubation [6, 7].

10.2 Classification

Despite the significant evolution of SGAs and the development additional features since they were originally described in the 1980s [8], no consensus on a universal classification system exists. As such, SGA classification occurs via generation, sealing mechanism, features, or a combination of all the above.

SGAs with only an airway conduit are considered first generation. Second-generation SGAs include an esophageal port to help alleviate the risk of aspiration of gastric contents. Depending on the particular SGA, the esophageal conduit may serve as a pathway for passive venting of the esophagus, a connection point for suction, and/or a conduit for a narrow bore orogastric tube [9]. Van Zundt et al. proposed a third generation of SGA which includes visual guidance [10], to help overcome the common occurrence of sub-optimal placement [11]. The third generation provides verification of the correct placement and a means to visually evaluate manipulations required to improve the placement of the SGA.

Sealing mechanism refers to how the SGA forms a seal with the larynx. Miller proposed three main mechanisms: cuffed perilaryngeal sealers, cuffed pharyngeal sealers, and cuffless anatomically preshaped sealers [12]. Perilaryngeal sealers use a cuff to form a seal around the laryngeal opening. An example of this type of SGA is the LMA® Classic™ or Unique™ (Teleflex, Wayne, PA). In contrast, cuffed pharyngeal sealers create the seal at the base of the tongue in the posterior pharynx. This type of airway includes devices such as the Combitube®; however, these are rarely used outside of the prehospital setting. Finally, many cuffless anatomically preshaped sealers have entered the market. Due to their shape and physical properties, these devices form a perilaryngeal seal without a cuff. The iGel™ (Intersurgical, Berkshire UK) is a commonly encountered example of this sealing mechanism.

A plethora of different modifications have been made to enhance the performance of SGAs. Integrated bite blocks and more rigid conduits have been added to prevent obstruction from external compression. In the past, there was concern that the epiglottis may obstruct the airway conduit. This resulted in development of mask aperture bars and epiglottic elevator bars. These modifications were found to be unnecessary [7] and have largely been abandoned in newer SGAs [10]. Some cuffed perilaryngeal sealers such as the LMA Unique™ (Teleflex, Wayne, PA) include a built-in manometer to assess cuff pressure. Third-generation devices include the use of a camera to accurately guide and confirm optimal placement [11].

SGAs provide a primary airway option for procedures which require general anesthesia, but the risk/benefit profile does not favor endotracheal intubation. The SGA's use in general anesthesia has become common, with 56% of over 111,000 anesthetics performed with an SGA in Great Britain over a 2-week period in 2008 [13]. In the United States where adoption of SGAs has been more conservative [14], a multiyear retrospective study comparing reintubation after general anesthesia administered with a SGA versus an endotracheal intubation found the frequency of SGA use increased over time [15].

Although typically used with general anesthesia, SGAs may be placed with sedation and appropriate localization of the airway to blunt airway reflexes [16–18]. While the described placement was done to facilitate general anesthesia with or without placement of an endotracheal tube, one can think of situations where an SGA could be used to support noninvasive ventilation without general anesthesia. Examples of such would be procedures that require patient participation, wanting to avoid induction doses of sedatives for hemodynamic reasons, or the desire to maintain spontaneous respiration to prevent airway collapse.

Some authors suggest that compared to endotracheal intubation, SGAs may have fewer airway and/or respiratory complications [19–21]. The rate of reintubation may be less with SGAs; however, any conclusion is confounded by neuromuscular blockers used with endotracheal intubation [14, 15]. In many ambulatory practices, SGAs have reduced the need for routine endotracheal intubation and the hemodynamic stresses associated with it [22]. Theoretically, placement and maintenance of an SGA require less anesthetic and less need for neuromuscular blocking agents, which could result in expedited recover and discharge [23].

There are some relative contraindications to SGAs. In patients at high risk for aspiration, the risk/benefit ratio probably leans against using an SGA [24]. A single-center study found that surgical table rotation, male sex, poor dentition, and increased body mass index were independent risk factors for SGA failure [25]. A meta-analysis and numerous studies address failure rates for different SGAs, but the differing definitions make it difficult to compare and draw definitive conclusions.

Length of the planned procedure is another common consideration when deciding whether to use an SGA. While manufacturers of the original SGAs recommended up to 2 h of continuous use, the iGel (Intersurgical, Berkshire, UK) manufacturer allows up to 4 h [9]. The lack of high-quality studies makes it difficult to determine a definitive time cutoff.

10.3 Choice of SGA

The choice of one SGA over another largely depends on provider preference, the procedure, patient factors, and availability at the practicing institution. The Difficult Airway Society recommends using at least a second-generation device [26, 27]. The Fourth National Audit Project of the Royal College of Anaesthetists and Difficult Airway Society (NAP4) reported three issues regarding SGAs: aspiration associated with supraglottic airway devices (SADs) is an important contributor to overall aspiration risk; (>80%) of SGAs used were first-generation devices; and complications were associated with use of first-generation SADs in obese patients [13, 28]. With the benefit of higher sealing pressures and features designed to limit the risk of aspiration, second-generation SGAs potentially mitigate the problems identified in NAP4 [29].

The selection and use of SGAs to support noninvasive ventilation for specific types of procedures will be covered in subsequent chapters.

10.4 Conclusions

1. Many types of supraglottic airways exist and depending upon the situation that the provider finds themselves in will determine the specific type of airway adjunct to be used between a nasopharyngeal airway, oropharyngeal airway, or a laryngeal mask airway. A laryngeal mask airway (LMA) confers a somewhat more secure airway but is not superior in airway security compared to an endotracheal tube.

2. Placement of supraglottic airways is typically easily performed and can be done by practitioners without advanced airway experience. There are some contraindications to placement of a SGA versus and endotracheal tube (ETT), with the possibility of aspiration being a major complication.
3. Choice between the use of SGA and ETT is provider dependent and will be determined based on patient factors, situation that airway is required (rescue airway versus procedural for anesthesia), and provider expertise.
4. SGAs, in particular LMA, can act as a guide for placement of ETT in difficult airway situations.

Disclaimer The identification of specific products or scientific instrumentation is considered an integral part of the scientific endeavor and does not constitute endorsement or implied endorsement on the part of the author(s), DoD, or any component agency. The views expressed in this chapter are those of the author(s) and do not reflect the official policy or position of the U.S. Army Medical Department, Department of the Army, DoD, or the U.S. Government.

References

1. Miller RD, Cohen NH. Miller's anesthesia. 8th ed. Philadelphia: Elsevier Saunders; 2015.
2. Boling B, Dennis DR, Tribble TA, Rajagopalan N, Hoopes CW. Safety of nurse-led ambulation for patients on venovenous extracorporeal membrane oxygenation. Prog Transplant. 2016;26:112–6.
3. Severinghaus JW, Spellman MJ Jr. Pulse oximeter failure thresholds in hypotension and vasoconstriction. Anesthesiology. 1990;73:532–7.
4. Apfelbaum JL, Hagberg CA, Connis RT, Abdelmalak BB, Agarkar M, Dutton RP, et al. 2022 American Society of Anesthesiologists practice guidelines for management of the difficult airway. Anesthesiology. 2022;136:31–81.
5. Rosenblatt WH, Yanez ND. A decision tree approach to airway management pathways in the 2022 difficult airway algorithm of the American Society of Anesthesiologists. Anesth Analg. 2022;134:910–5.
6. Wong DT, Yang JJ, Mak HY, Jagannathan N. Use of intubation introducers through a supraglottic airway to facilitate tracheal intubation: a brief review. Can J Anaesth. 2012;59:704–15.
7. Van Zundert TC, Hendrickx JF, De Witte JL, Wong DT, Cattano D, Brimacombe JR. Do mask aperture bars of extraglottic airway devices prevent prolapse of epiglottis causing airway obstruction? A randomized crossover trial in anesthetized adult patients. J Clin Anesth. 2016;31:231–7.
8. Sorbello M. Evolution of supraglottic airway devices: the Darwinian perspective. Minerva Anestesiol. 2018;84:297–300.
9. Kwanten LE, Madhivathanan P. Supraglottic airway devices: current and future uses. Br J Hosp Med (Lond). 2018;79:31–5.
10. Van Zundert AAJ, Kumar CM, Van Zundert TCRV, Gatt SP, Pandit JJ. The case for a 3rd generation supraglottic airway device facilitating direct vision placement. J Clin Monit Comput. 2021;35:217–24.
11. Van Zundert AAJ, Gatt SP, Van Zundert T, Kumar CM, Pandit JJ. Features of new vision-incorporated third-generation video laryngeal mask airways. J Clin Monit Comput. 2022;36:921–8.
12. Miller D. A proposed classification and scoring system for supraglottic sealing airways: a brief review. Anesth Analg. 2004;99:1553–9.
13. Woodall NM, Cook TM. National census of airway management techniques used for anaesthesia in the UK: first phase of the Fourth National Audit Project at the Royal College of Anaesthetists. Br J Anaesth. 2011;106:266–71.

14. Hunter JM, Aziz MF. Supraglottic airway versus tracheal intubation and the risk of postoperative pulmonary complications. Br J Anaesth. 2021;126:571–4.
15. Hammer M, Santer P, Schaefer MS, Althoff FC, Wongtangman K, Frey UH, et al. Supraglottic airway device versus tracheal intubation and the risk of emergent postoperative intubation after general anaesthesia in adults: a retrospective cohort study. Br J Anaesth. 2021;126:738–45.
16. Lim WY, Wong P. Awake supraglottic airway guided flexible bronchoscopic intubation in patients with anticipated difficult airways: a case series and narrative review. Korean J Anesthesiol. 2019;72:548–57.
17. Matsunami S, Komasawa N, Kuzukawa Y, Fujitate Y, Minami T. Awake insertion of i-gel under dexmedetomidine sedation in a patient with severe obstructive sleep apnea syndrome. Masui. 2014;63:807–9.
18. Ludena JA, Bellas JJA, Alvarez-Rementeria R, Munoz LE. Fiberoptic-guided intubation after awake insertion of the I-gel™ supraglottic device in a patient with predicted difficult airway. J Anaesthesiol Clin Pharmacol. 2017;33:560–1.
19. Yu SH, Beirne OR. Laryngeal mask airways have a lower risk of airway complications compared with endotracheal intubation: a systematic review. J Oral Maxillofac Surg. 2010;68:2359–76.
20. Nicholson A, Cook TM, Smith AF, Lewis SR, Reed SS. Supraglottic airway devices versus tracheal intubation for airway management during general anaesthesia in obese patients. Cochrane Database Syst Rev. 2013;2013:Cd010105.
21. van Esch BF, Stegeman I, Smit AL. Comparison of laryngeal mask airway vs tracheal intubation: a systematic review on airway complications. J Clin Anesth. 2017;36:142–50.
22. Hinkelbein J, Hohn A, Genzwürker H. Airway management for anaesthesia in the ambulatory setting. Curr Opin Anaesthesiol. 2015;28:642–7.
23. Luba K, Cutter TW. Supraglottic airway devices in the ambulatory setting. Anesthesiol Clin. 2010;28:295–314.
24. Kristensen MS, Teoh WH, Asai T. Which supraglottic airway will serve my patient best? Anaesthesia. 2014;69:1189–92.
25. Ramachandran SK, Mathis MR, Tremper KK, Shanks AM, Kheterpal S. Predictors and clinical outcomes from failed Laryngeal Mask Airway Unique™: a study of 15,795 patients. Anesthesiology. 2012;116:1217–26.
26. Higgs A, McGrath BA, Goddard C, Rangasami J, Suntharalingam G, Gale R, et al. DAS guidelines on the airway management of critically ill patients. Anaesthesia. 2018;73:1035–6.
27. Higgs A, McGrath BA, Goddard C, Rangasami J, Suntharalingam G, Gale R, et al. Guidelines for the management of tracheal intubation in critically ill adults. Br J Anaesth. 2018;120:323–52.
28. Cook TM, Woodall N, Harper J, Benger J. Major complications of airway management in the UK: results of the Fourth National Audit Project of the Royal College of Anaesthetists and the Difficult Airway Society. Part 2: intensive care and emergency departments. Br J Anaesth. 2011;106:632–42.
29. Cook TM, Kelly FE. Time to abandon the 'vintage' laryngeal mask airway and adopt second-generation supraglottic airway devices as first choice. Br J Anaesth. 2015;115:497–9.

Part IV

Methodology: Noninvasive Approach For Procedures

11 Patient Selection: Score Discomfort and Airway Evaluation

Efthymia Papadopoulou, Effimia Kamariotou, and Stavros Tryfon

11.1 Introduction

Noninvasive ventilation (NIV) improves alveolar hypoventilation and decreases the work of breathing, preventing endotracheal intubation in appropriately selected cases. Compared to invasive mechanical ventilation, NIV decreases the length of intensive care unit and hospital stay, morbidity, and mortality. However, worse outcomes have been reported in clinical practice than in randomized controlled trials [1]. Available guidelines advocate timely NIV initiation with individualized settings in appropriate patients and close monitoring by an experienced healthcare team to ensure favorable outcomes. In parallel, patient comfort should be optimized during NIV to prevent intolerance and subsequent NIV failure. Evaluation of the airway, namely, the upper airway, serves to identify potential indications for treatment with NIV and to investigate untoward responses during NIV.

11.2 Patient Selection

11.2.1 NIV in the Acute Care

Criteria for NIV in acute disease states include moderate to severe dyspnea, clinical signs of respiratory distress with increased work of breathing (tachypnea, labored breathing with the use of accessory respiratory muscles, paradoxical breathing), hypercapnic respiratory acidosis, and severe hypoxemia unresponsive to conventional oxygen therapy.

E. Papadopoulou · E. Kamariotou · S. Tryfon (✉)
Pulmonology Department, "G. Papanikolaou" General Hospital of Thessaloniki, Exochi, Greece

© The Author(s), under exclusive license to Springer Nature Switzerland AG 2025
K. Panda et al. (eds.), *Noninvasive Ventilatory Approaches in Interventional Procedures*, Noninvasive Ventilation. The Essentials,
https://doi.org/10.1007/978-3-032-05328-2_11

Prior to NIV initiation and during NIV use, a holistic patient assessment should reveal potential contraindications requiring immediate intubation. These include coma, cardiac arrest, respiratory arrest, hemodynamic instability, and inability to protect the upper airway, as in uncontrollable gastrointestinal or respiratory bleeding, intractable emesis, continuous rhinorrhea following fracture of skull base, impaired cough or swallowing predisposing to aspiration, difficulty in expectoration of secretions, lethargy, status epilepticus and upper airway obstruction secondary to angioedema, anaphylaxis, or extensive head and neck lesions. NIV efficacy may be compromised in cases with facial trauma or burns leading to inadequate or painful interface fitting. Consultation by the surgical team should precede NIV initiation in patients with recent upper airway or upper gastrointestinal tract surgery. Finally, pneumothorax drainage prior to NIV is crucial to the prevention of further lung collapse.

Patients with acute respiratory failure and hypercapnia are generally more responsive to NIV than those that have normocapnia, due to the underlying pathophysiological mechanisms, as NIV relieves respiratory muscle workload, but may not suffice in cases of parenchymal disease. NIV recommendations in acute respiratory failure differ depending on the underlying disease [2], as shown in Table 11.1. Patient cooperation, close monitoring, and regular assessment of treatment response are of fundamental importance. Lack of improvement after 1–2 treatment hours signifies NIV failure. Treatment success pivots on the proper therapeutic approach to the underlying disease.

11.2.2 Long-Term NIV

Domiciliary NIV is indicated in chronic respiratory diseases with symptoms and clinical signs of respiratory distress, diurnal hypercapnia or manifestations of sleep-disordered breathing, and findings of nocturnal hypoventilation in polysomnography or nocturnal respiratory monitoring [3]. Patients should be closely followed up at specialized centers, with reassessment and titration of ventilator settings following the disease course and patient needs. Specific indications for long-term NIV are shown in Table 11.1.

11.3 Patient Discomfort

As per the 2012 National Institute for Health and Care Excellence Patient Experience Guideline [4], comfort comprises a major parameter in a patient-centered healthcare framework. Despite the favorable outcomes with NIV use, NIV experience is deemed stressful and disagreeable [5]. Patient discomfort compromises cooperation predisposing to NIV failure, with high intubation and mortality rates [6].

Indeed, up to 30–50% of patients experience discomfort during NIV with subsequent intolerance accounting for 12–33% cases of NIV failure [7]. An observational study in the respiratory intensive care unit (ICU) noted younger age and higher heart

Table 11.1 Indications for NIV

Disease state	Clinical indications	Notes
In the acute care		
COPD exacerbation	Acute or acute-on-chronic respiratory acidosis	Bilevel NIV of choice. HFNC superior to conventional oxygen therapy in compensated hypercapnic respiratory failure
Acute cardiogenic pulmonary edema	Respiratory distress or severe dyspnea and acidosis	CPAP or bilevel NIV in severe hypercapnia; if prolonged, HFNC better tolerated
Immunocompromised patients	Acute respiratory failure secondary to opportunistic infections or drug-induced toxicity	Bilevel NIV or CPAP; HFNC better tolerated
Obesity hypoventilation syndrome	Acute hypercapnic respiratory failure	Bilevel NIV as standard practice, despite the lack of randomized trials
Acute decompensation of neuromuscular diseases, bronchiectasis, cystic fibrosis	Clinical signs of respiratory distress with hypercapnic respiratory failure	Complementary to physiotherapy and airway secretions clearance techniques
Weaning from invasive mechanical ventilation	Hypercapnic respiratory failure	
Terminal conditions	Palliative support for dyspnea, respiratory distress	For example, cancer, COPD or congestive heart failure with no prospect of ICU support
Postoperative setting	Acute respiratory failure	CPAP or bilevel NIV, preferably with lower pressures. HFNC as an alternative
Perioperative use	High-risk cases, such as obstructive sleep apnea	Preoperative initiation of CPAP upon meticulous evaluation of patients at risk
Chest trauma (rib fractures, flail chest, etc.)	Acute respiratory failure without severe hypoxemia	Measures for adequate control of pain
Post-extubation	High-risk patients (e.g., >65 years of age with underlying cardiac or respiratory disease)	Reintubation should not be delayed in cases of post-extubation respiratory failure. HFNC superior to conventional oxygen therapy in low-risk nonsurgical patients
Viral infections	Acute respiratory failure	Appropriate precautions to limit viral spread. Prompt intubation upon NIV failure
ARDS	Increased work of breathing	Risk for lung injury in cases of excessive respiratory demand with high tidal volumes. HFNC better tolerated

(continued)

Table 11.1 (continued)

Disease state	Clinical indications	Notes
Long term		
Neuromuscular disorders, chest wall deformities	Reduced vital capacity, orthopnea, diurnal hypercapnia, or symptomatic nocturnal hypoventilation	Meticulous titration and, ultimately, switch to tracheostomy-delivered mechanical ventilation in deteriorating cases, as in bulbar involvement with inability to protect the airway or 24-h ventilator dependence
Obstructive sleep apnea	Clinical manifestations of sleep-disordered breathing or complications	CPAP or bilevel NIV in significant hypercapnia Weight loss and exercise as treatment cornerstones
Obesity hypoventilation syndrome	Diurnal hypercapnia or complications	CPAP or bilevel NIV in significant hypercapnia. Weight loss and exercise as treatment cornerstones.
COPD	Persistent diurnal hypercapnia following a severe exacerbation with hospitalization; stable very severe COPD; overlap syndrome	
Cystic fibrosis, diffuse bronchiectasis, post-tuberculosis lung disease	Selected cases with hypercapnic respiratory failure or sleep-induced hypoventilation	
Central sleep apnea	Symptoms of sleep-disordered breathing persisting despite optimal treatment of the underlying disorder	

COPD chronic obstructive pulmonary disease, *ARDS* acute respiratory distress syndrome, *NIV* non-invasive ventilation, *CPAP* continuous positive airway pressure, *HFNC* high-flow nasal cannula, *ICU* intensive care unit

rate prior to NIV initiation, as well as higher heart rate and respiratory rate after 1–2 h under NIV, as independent factors for NIV intolerance [8]. Patients complained frequently of distress, dyspnea, and unbearably strong NIV-delivered flow, but also cough, headache, and facial pain. Apart from emotional or physical distress, lack of response to NIV and deterioration of the underlying disorder may cause discomfort dictating prompt escalation to intubation.

Specific parameters should be considered when assessing patient discomfort:

- *Patient-ventilator asynchrony*

  Discordance between the patient's respiratory effort and ventilator-provided support should be promptly recognized [9]. Clinical signs and screen ventilator waveforms may reveal delayed or premature cycling due to inappropriate pressure support or tidal volume level, ineffective triggering (weak inspiratory muscles, intrinsic positive end-expiratory pressure, low respiratory drive), double-triggering, or auto-triggering (random noise, fluid in the circuit, cardiogenic oscillations).

- *The ventilation mode*

  Comfort levels are worse with volume-controlled ventilation [7] than with pressure support, where maximal pressures correspond to lower comfort creating a U-shaped comfort level [10]. NIV initiation at lower pressures and gradual upward titration appears advantageous [5] but may not be appropriate in severe life-threatening cases.

- *NIV interface*

  NIV interface may induce claustrophobia, a feeling of suffocation or confinement to the equipment, compromising eating, drinking, and communication [5]. Selection of the type and size should be individualized depending on the patient's facial features and preference, as well as the duration of NIV support. Healthy individuals rated the total face mask as most uncomfortable [11], but there was no significant difference in comfort levels according to another study [12]. The nasal mask reduces claustrophobia, allows communication, and may be suitable in cases with frequent cough, but mouth respiration causes air loss. The helmet has shown greater tolerability compared to masks, while facilitating oral nutrition and fluid administration [13], and has been associated with more favorable outcomes in a randomized controlled trial of patients with ARDS [14]. NIV interface rotation may improve tolerance and relevant outcomes, as suggested in one study [15]. Excessively tightened interface should be avoided to prevent facial skin erythema and abrasions. High-flow nasal cannula (HFNC) enhances tolerance during breaks from NIV in selected cases, with greater comfort and lower incidence of facial pressure ulcers compared to the NIV face mask [16].

- *Air leaks*

  Major leaks cause patient-ventilator asynchrony and increase respiratory muscles workload or ventilator inspiratory flow, whereas smaller leaks cause eye irritation and noise. Selection of the proper interface minimizes air leaks during NIV.

- *Physical distress*

  Physical distress may result from NIV complications, including skin abrasions or pressure ulcers from the NIV interface, gastric insufflations, or nasal congestion. Flow rates exceeding 4L/min surpass the humidification capacity of the upper airway inducing airway dryness with subsequent swallowing difficulty and throat irritation. More serious complications, such as pneumonia, barotrauma, and hemodynamic effects, should be prevented and monitored [7].

On top of NIV-related discomfort, physical distress arises from insufficient management of symptoms, such as postoperative nausea, fatigue, sleep disorders, constipation, loss of appetite, fluid retention, or palpitations and breathlessness. Amelioration of symptoms, especially pain and dyspnea, is crucial to minimizing discomfort. The Fowler's position is preferable during NIV, but the recumbent position may be more comfortable in obese patients [17]. Physical distress may also ensue from restricted mobility due to surgery or underlying disorders, as well as noise and lights disturbing sleep.

- *Emotional discomfort*

  Patients experience emotional discomfort [18] as a result from the uncertainty surrounding treatment procedures and expectations, the sense of dependency and weakness due to a limited functional status, or the perceived loss of privacy and dignity [19]. Patients who had been treated in the ICU due to acute respiratory failure reported similar symptoms as in post-traumatic stress disorder [20]. Adequate nursing care, physician surveillance, and establishment of a patient-physician trust relationship with informative discussions may inspire confidence, provide a sense of involvement in care decisions, and increase patient cooperation [21]. Well-equipped facilities and encouragement of interaction with family may promote resilience in the unfamiliar environment.

11.3.1 Comfort Scores

Standardized tools for emotional discomfort, like the Faces Anxiety Scale [22] and the State-Trait Anxiety Inventory [23], are available in clinical practice. However, there is a lack of tools addressing the overall patient comfort during NIV. Previous studies have utilized mostly *non-validated scores*, including Likert scales [24–28] and visual analog scales [29–32]. There was no association between the subjective discomfort captured in a Likert scale and physiological parameters related to stress, including heart and respiratory rate, heart rate variability, and electrodermal activity, in healthy individuals receiving NIV for 10 min [11]. Two studies developed a questionnaire with specific parameters regarding interface-related discomfort [12, 33].

Figure 11.1 illustrates a proposed clinical algorithm for the systematic approach to patient discomfort during NIV.

Optimizing patient comfort merits an individualized and holistic approach. Close patient monitoring should include routine assessment of symptoms and vital signs, adjustment of NIV settings and interface, correction of air leakage and patient-ventilator asynchrony, and prevention of NIV-related complications, in parallel with a meticulous therapeutic approach to the underlying disorders within a patient-physician trust relationship. Ultimately, sedation potentially improves tolerance, preventing intubation in some cases [34], but a false outward appearance of comfort in patients who may actually suffer has been reported [35]. Analgesic and sedative agents should be cautiously administered by experienced ICU physicians only in selected cases. Importantly, persistent patient discomfort may signify lack of response to NIV or even deterioration of underlying disorders, dictating timely escalation to invasive mechanical ventilation.

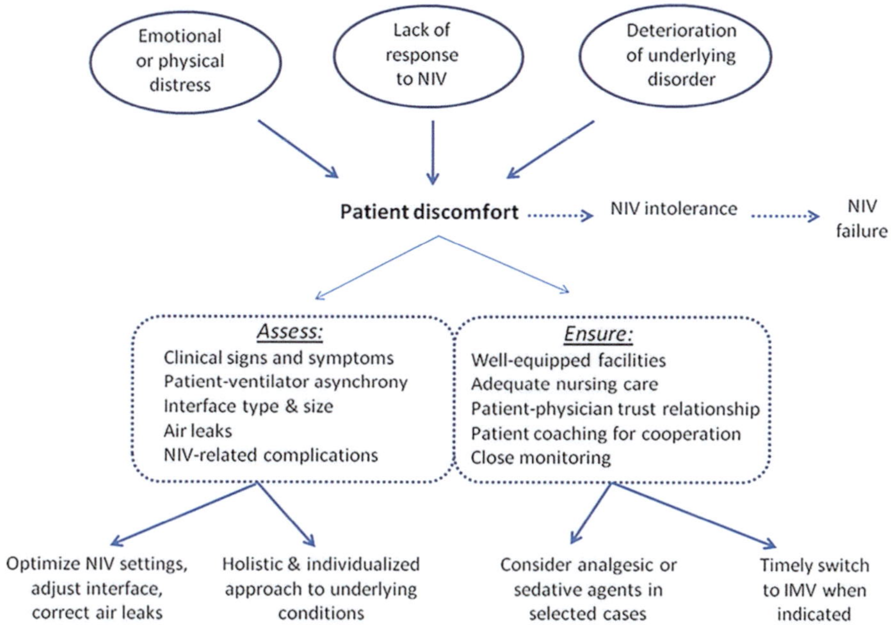

Fig. 11.1 Clinical algorithm for the systematic approach to patient discomfort during noninvasive ventilation

11.4 Upper Airway Evaluation

The upper airway, comprising the nose, oral cavity, pharynx, and larynx, facilitates airflow passage to the tracheobronchial tree while humidifying, warming, and filtering the delivered air. Complementary functions include speech and phonation, swallowing, and cough. The upper airway patency impacts airflow resistance and, consequently, may pose an indication for treatment with NIV or affect the NIV-delivered volume or pressure to the lungs [36].

A systematic evaluation of the upper airway is essential to identify potential underlying disorders and ensure efficient NIV implementation [37]. *Medical history and physical examination* can reveal abnormalities in the general appearance (obesity, increased neck circumference) and specific facial and cervical features (micrognathia, retrognathia, midfacial hypoplasia, abnormal positioning of the hyoid) as in craniofacial syndromes. The following disorders potentially disrupt the upper airway patency:

- *Nasal cavity*: External nasal valve collapse due to alar rim weakening or wide columella, deflection of the nasal septum in the internal nasal valve, deviations of the nasal septum, allergic rhinitis or sinusitis, nasal polyposis, canal stenosis or atresia [38].

- *Oral cavity*: Tonsillar hypertrophy, dental disorders, tongue tumors, macroglossia, long or flaccid palate velum, soft palate elongation. A high arched palate and hypertrophic gums may imply chronic mouth respiration due to nasal obstruction [39].
- *Palate position*, *tonsil size*, and *body mass index* determine clinical stages in obstructive sleep apnea, as per the *Friedman staging system* [40].
- Depending on the visibility of the *soft palate*, *faucial pillars*, and *uvula base* upon tongue protrusion, the modified *Mallampati score* [41] is estimated to predict difficulty in airway management during intubation and has been associated with obstructive sleep apnea [42].
- *Pharynx and larynx*: decreased pharyngeal muscle tone, adenoid hypertrophy in nasopharynx, retroflex movement of epiglottis (prolapse during inspiration), redundant mucosa in the arytenoid-aryepiglottic folds.

The pharynx and larynx are muscular structures affecting the upper airway *patency* [43]. The *larynx* has been reported to exert approximately 25% of the total airflow resistance during quiet mouth respiration [44]. Laryngeal abduction is induced by the posterior cricoarytenoid muscle immediately prior to diaphragmatic contraction to allow inspiration [45]. Increased activity of the intrinsic laryngeal adductor muscles leads to glottis narrowing during inspiration and increases airflow resistance [46]. Receptors are sensitive to mechanical, chemical, or thermic stimuli [47]. Among them, C-fiber receptors have been found to exert inhibitory effects related to intermittent upper airway obstruction, namely, apnea, bradypnea, and glottis adduction [36].

Additionally, NIV settings may affect the upper airway patency [48]. A laryngeal closure reflex is potentially triggered by positive air pressure to the laryngeal vestibular mucosa [49]. Genioglossus muscle activity prior to the onset of inspiratory flow differs during quiet and forced inspiration [50]. Posterior cricoarytenoid muscle activity increases with negative pressure and inspiratory flow, whereas thyroarytenoid muscle activity increases with positive pressure and expiratory flow [48]. Healthy individuals undergoing NIV at higher pressures presented adduction of the vocal chords and significantly narrow glottic aperture with subsequent higher airflow resistance and decreased NIV-delivered tidal volume [51–53]. Patient-ventilator asynchrony may also increase the phasic activity of intrinsic laryngeal muscles [54, 55].

Various underlying disorders may cause upper airway dysfunction or collapsibility and intermittent obstruction, potentially leading to *untoward responses during NIV* [36]. Close monitoring and regular reassessments of efficacy are required in:

- Vocal cord dysfunction [56–58] or laryngeal injury secondary to prolonged NIV implementation [59].
- Obstructive sleep apnea and obesity hypoventilation syndrome, where increased adiposity or tongue enlargement lead to soft tissue collapse decreasing airway

diameter and increasing resistance, especially in the supine position [60, 61]; upper airway muscles may also respond poorly during sleep.

- COPD, where dynamic laryngeal narrowing may occur during expiration, depending on disease severity as reflected by exercise capacity [62]. However, NIV high pressures during COPD exacerbations were not related with obstructive events, but rather increased tidal volume [62]; chronic hypercapnia has been postulated to modulate a different C-fiber receptors response accounting for this phenomenon [63].
- Neurodegenerative diseases, especially amyotrophic lateral sclerosis (ALS), where upper motor neuron involvement and bulbar function impairment may cause hyperresponsiveness or dysfunction of the intrinsic laryngeal muscles increasing upper airway resistance [64]. Lower pressures and longer inspiratory times are more efficient; high pressures cause laryngeal adduction in *pseudobulbar ALS* or supraglottic adduction in *bulbar hypotonic ALS* [65].

There is *no specific algorithm* to guide evaluation of the upper airway during NIV. The development of standardized protocols merits attention in specialized centers. In cases of untoward responses during NIV, the following methods may prove useful:

- Endoscopy may reveal the underlying disorder in selected cases with persistent residual obstructive events or signs of bulbar dysfunction [37] and contribute to NIV setting titration [66]. Complementary *dynamic tests*, such as the Mueller's maneuver, create negative pressure allowing functional assessment.
- *Drug-induced sleep endoscopy* [67] under pharmacologic sedation may tailor treatment in cases of sleep-related pathology evading during wakefulness. For instance, positional therapy is potentially indicated in cases with epiglottis collapse, while CPAP is recommended for tongue-related obstruction. The *VOTE classification system* delineates obstruction at the velum, oropharynx lateral walls, tongue base and epiglottis [68].
- The visualization of responses during NIV with *transnasal fiberoptic laryngoscopy (TLF)* may contribute to appropriate titration of settings with fewer obstructive events [69, 70]. However, adduction of aryepiglottic folds or excessive secretions may hinder inspection of the glottis.
- Polygraphic monitoring of cardiorespiratory parameters identifies obstructive events, while polysomnography and capnography serve for NIV titration [71, 72].
- The ultrasound offers an alternative practical approach [73, 74] for cases with contraindications or difficulties to proceed with endoscopy. Although it is already used to evaluate the upper airway, as in vocal cord dysfunction following thyroid surgery or intubation [75–77], its accuracy in depicting laryngeal movements warrants standardization [78].

References

1. Bourke SC, Piraino T, Pisani L, Brochard L, Elliott MW. Beyond the guidelines for noninvasive ventilation in acute respiratory failure: implications for practice. Lancet Respir Med. 2018;6:935–47.
2. Rochwerg B, Brochard L, Elliott MW, Hess D, Hill NS, Nava S, Navalesi P, Members Of The Steering Committee, Antonelli M, Brozek J, Conti G, Ferrer M, Guntupalli K, Jaber S, Keenan S, Mancebo J, Mehta S, Raoof S, Members of the Task Force. Official ERS/ATS clinical practice guidelines: noninvasive ventilation for acute respiratory failure. Eur Respir J. 2017;50:1602426.
3. Simonds AK. Home mechanical ventilation: an overview. Ann Am Thorac Soc. 2016;13:2035–44.
4. National Clinical Guideline Centre (UK). Patient experience in adult NHS services: improving the experience of care for people using adult NHS services: patient experience in generic terms. London: Royal College of Physicians (UK); 2012. https://www.nice.org.uk/guidance/cg138/evidence/full-guideline-pdf-185142637. Accessed 5 May 2023.
5. Beckert L, Wiseman R, Pitama S, Landers A. What can we learn from patients to improve their non-invasive ventilation experience? 'It was unpleasant; if I was offered it again, I would do what I was told'. BMJ Support Palliat Care. 2020;10:e7.
6. Ozyilmaz E, Ugurlu AO, Nava S. Timing of noninvasive ventilation failure: causes, risk factors, and potential remedies. BMC Pulm Med. 2014;14:19.
7. Carron M, Freo U, BaHammam AS, Dellweg D, Guarracino F, Cosentini R, Feltracco P, Vianello A, Ori C, Esquinas A. Complications of non-invasive ventilation techniques: a comprehensive qualitative review of randomized trials. Br J Anaesth. 2013;110:896–914.
8. Liu J, Duan J, Bai L, Zhou L. Noninvasive ventilation intolerance: characteristics, predictors, and outcomes. Respir Care. 2016;61:277–84.
9. Longhini F, Colombo D, Pisani L, Idone F, Chun P, Doorduin J, Ling L, Alemani M, Bruni A, Zhaochen J, Tao Y, Lu W, Garofalo E, Carenzo L, Maggiore SM, Qiu H, Heunks L, Antonelli M, Nava S, Navalesi P. Efficacy of ventilator waveform observation for detection of patient-ventilator asynchrony during NIV: a multicentre study. ERJ Open Res. 2017;3:00075–2017.
10. Chiumello D, Pelosi P, Croci M, Bigatello LM, Gattinoni L. The effects of pressurization rate on breathing pattern, work of breathing, gas exchange and patient comfort in pressure support ventilation. Eur Respir J. 2001;18:107–14.
11. da Cunha-Martins BSM, Motta-Ribeiro GC, Jandre FC. Short-term usage of three non-invasive ventilation interfaces causes progressive discomfort in healthy adults. Res Biomed Eng. 2021;37:289–98. https://doi.org/10.1007/s42600-020-00114-3.
12. Holanda MA, Reis RC, Winkeler GF, Fortaleza SC, Lima JW, Pereira ED. Influence of total face, facial and nasal masks on short-term adverse effects during noninvasive ventilation. J Bras Pneumol. 2009;35:164–73.
13. Hong S, Wang H, Tian Y, Qiao L. The roles of noninvasive mechanical ventilation with helmet in patients with acute respiratory failure: a systematic review and meta-analysis. PLoS One. 2021;16:e0250063.
14. Patel BK, Wolfe KS, Pohlman AS, Hall JB, Kress JP. Effect of noninvasive ventilation delivered by helmet vs face mask on the rate of endotracheal intubation in patients with acute respiratory distress syndrome: a randomized clinical trial. JAMA. 2016;315:2435–41.
15. Roy B, Cordova FC, Travaline JM, D'Alonzo GE Jr, Criner GJ. Full face mask for noninvasive positive-pressure ventilation in patients with acute respiratory failure. J Am Osteopath Assoc. 2007;107:148–56.
16. Tan D, Walline JH, Ling B, Xu Y, Sun J, Wang B, Shan X, Wang Y, Cao P, Zhu Q, Geng P, Xu J. High-flow nasal cannula oxygen therapy versus non-invasive ventilation for chronic obstructive pulmonary disease patients after extubation: a multicenter, randomized controlled trial. Crit Care. 2020;24:489.

17. Sanchez D, Smith G, Piper A, Rolls K. Non–invasive ventilation guidelines for adult patients with acute respiratory failure: a clinical practice guideline. Version 1. Chatswood: Agency for Clinical Innovation NSW Government; 2014.
18. Torheim H, Gjengedal E. How to cope with the mask? Experiences of mask treatment in patients with acute chronic obstructive pulmonary disease-exacerbations. Scand J Caring Sci. 2010;24:499–506.
19. Wensley C, Botti M, McKillop A, Merry AF. Maximising comfort: how do patients describe the care that matters? A two-stage qualitative descriptive study to develop a quality improvement framework for comfort-related care in inpatient settings. BMJ Open. 2020;10:e033336.
20. Teixeira C, Rosa RG, Sganzerla D, Sanchez EC, Robinson CC, Dietrich C, Kochhann R, de Souza D, Rech GS, da Dos Santos R, Schneider D, Boldo R, Sharshar T, Bozza FA, Falavigna M, Friedman G. The burden of mental illness among survivors of critical care-risk factors and impact on quality of life: a multicenter prospective cohort study. Chest. 2021;160:157–64.
21. Barry MJ, Edgman-Levitan S. Shared decision making--pinnacle of patient-centered care. N Engl J Med. 2012;366:780–1.
22. McKinley S, Stein-Parbury J, Chehelnabi A, Lovas J. Assessment of anxiety in intensive care patients by using the faces anxiety scale. Am J Crit Care. 2004;13:146–52.
23. Spielberger CD. State-trait anxiety inventory: bibliography. 2nd ed. Palo Alto, CA: Consulting Psychologists Press; 1989.
24. Corley A, Rickard CM, Aitken LM, Johnston A, Barnett A, Fraser JF, Lewis SR, Smith AF. High-flow nasal cannulae for respiratory support in adult intensive care patients. Cochrane Database Syst Rev. 2017;5:CD010172.
25. Antón A, Tárrega J, Giner J, Güell R, Sanchis J. Acute physiologic effects of nasal and full-face masks during noninvasive positive-pressure ventilation in patients with acute exacerbations of chronic obstructive pulmonary disease. Respir Care. 2003;48:922–5.
26. Navalesi P, Fanfulla F, Frigerio P, Gregoretti C, Nava S. Physiologic evaluation of noninvasive mechanical ventilation delivered with three types of masks in patients with chronic hypercapnic respiratory failure. Crit Care Med. 2000;28:1785–90.
27. Criner GJ, Travaline JM, Brennan KJ, Kreimer DT. Efficacy of a new full face mask for noninvasive positive pressure ventilation. Chest. 1994;106:1109–15.
28. Maggiore SM, Idone FA, Vaschetto R, Festa R, Cataldo A, Antonicelli F, Montini L, De Gaetano A, Navalesi P, Antonelli M. Nasal high-flow versus Venturi mask oxygen therapy after extubation. Effects on oxygenation, comfort, and clinical outcome. Am J Respir Crit Care Med. 2014;190:282–8.
29. Costa R, Navalesi P, Antonelli M, Cavaliere F, Craba A, Proietti R, Conti G. Physiologic evaluation of different levels of assistance during noninvasive ventilation delivered through a helmet. Chest. 2005;128:2984–90.
30. Vaschetto R, De Jong A, Conseil M, Galia F, Mahul M, Coisel Y, Prades A, Navalesi P, Jaber S. Comparative evaluation of three interfaces for non-invasive ventilation: a randomized crossover design physiologic study on healthy volunteers. Crit Care. 2014;18:R2.
31. Lee CC, Mankodi D, Shaharyar S, Ravindranathan S, Danckers M, Herscovici P, Moor M, Ferrer G. High flow nasal cannula versus conventional oxygen therapy and non-invasive ventilation in adults with acute hypoxemic respiratory failure: A systematic review. Respir Med. 2016;121:100–8.
32. Ozsancak A, Sidhom SS, Liesching TN, Howard W, Hill NS. Evaluation of the total face mask for noninvasive ventilation to treat acute respiratory failure. Chest. 2011;139:1034–41.
33. Massie CA, Hart RW. Clinical outcomes related to interface type in patients with obstructive sleep apnea/hypopnea syndrome who are using continuous positive airway pressure. Chest. 2003;123:1112–8.
34. Clouzeau B, Bui HN, Vargas F, Grenouillet-Delacre M, Guilhon E, Gruson D, Hilbert G. Target-controlled infusion of propofol for sedation in patients with non-invasive ventilation failure due to low tolerance: a preliminary study. Intensive Care Med. 2010;36:1675–80.
35. Frölich MA, Zhang K, Ness TJ. Effect of sedation on pain perception. Anesthesiology. 2013;118:611–21.

36. Rabec C, Rodenstein D, Leger P, Rouault S, Perrin C, Gonzalez-Bermejo J, SomnoNIV Group. Ventilator modes and settings during non-invasive ventilation: effects on respiratory events and implications for their identification. Thorax. 2011;66:170–8.
37. Georges M, Attali V, Golmard JL, Morélot-Panzini C, Crevier-Buchman L, Collet JM, Tintignac A, Morawiec E, Trosini-Desert V, Salachas F, Similowski T, Gonzalez-Bermejo J. Reduced survival in patients with ALS with upper airway obstructive events on non-invasive ventilation. J Neurol Neurosurg Psychiatry. 2016;87:1045–50.
38. Magliulo G, Iannella G, Ciofalo A, Polimeni A, De Vincentiis M, Pasquariello B, Montevecchi F, Vicini C. Nasal pathologies in patients with obstructive sleep apnoea. Acta Otorhinolaryngol Ital. 2019;39:250–6.
39. Hamans EP, Van Marck EA, De Backer WA, Creten W, Van de Heyning PH. Morphometric analysis of the uvula in patients with sleep-related breathing disorders. Eur Arch Otorrinolaringol. 2000;257:232–6.
40. Friedman M, Ibrahim H, Bass L. Clinical staging for sleep-disordered breathing. Otolaryngol Head Neck Surg. 2002;127:13–21.
41. Samsoon GL, Young JR. Difficult tracheal intubation: a retrospective study. Anaesthesia. 1987;42:487–90.
42. Nuckton TJ, Glidden DV, Browner WS, Claman DM. Physical examination: Mallampati score as an independent predictor of obstructive sleep apnea. Sleep. 2006;29:903–8.
43. Pierce RJ, Worsnop CJ. Upper airway function and dysfunction in respiration. Clin Exp Pharmacol Physiol. 1999;26:1–10.
44. Bartlett D Jr. Respiratory functions of the larynx. Physiol Rev. 1989;69:33–57.
45. England SJ, Bartlett D Jr, Daubenspeck JA. Influence of human vocal cord movements on airflow and resistance during eupnea. J Appl Physiol Respir Environ Exerc Physiol. 1982;52:773–9.
46. Stella MH, England SJ. Modulation of laryngeal and respiratory pump muscle activities with upper airway pressure and flow. J Appl Physiol. 2001;91:897–904.
47. Andersen TM, Hov B, Halvorsen T, Røksund OD, Vollsæter M. Upper airway assessment and responses during mechanically assisted cough. Respir Care. 2021;66:1196–213.
48. Oppersma E, Doorduin J, van der Heijden EH, van der Hoeven JG, Heunks LM. Noninvasive ventilation and the upper airway: should we pay more attention? Crit Care. 2013;17:245.
49. Bhabu P, Poletto C, Mann E, Bielamowicz S, Ludlow CL. Thyroarytenoid muscle responses to air pressure stimulation of the laryngeal mucosa in humans. Ann Otol Rhinol Laryngol. 2003;112:834–40.
50. Cheng S, Butler JE, Gandevia SC, Bilston LE. Movement of the human upper airway during inspiration with and without inspiratory resistive loading. J Appl Physiol. 2011;110:69–75.
51. Jounieaux V, Aubert G, Dury M, Delguste P, Rodenstein DO. Effects of nasal positive-pressure hyperventilation on the glottis in normal sleeping subjects. J Appl Physiol. 1995;79:186–93.
52. Jounieaux V, Aubert G, Dury M, Delguste P, Rodenstein DO. Effects of nasal positive-pressure hyperventilation on the glottis in normal awake subjects. J Appl Physiol. 1995;79:176–85.
53. Delguste P, Aubert-Tulkens G, Rodenstein DO. Upper airway obstruction during nasal intermittent positive-pressure hyperventilation in sleep. Lancet (London, England). 1991;338:1295–7.
54. Hug F, Raux M, Morelot-Panzini C, Similowski T. Surface EMG to assess and quantify upper airway dilators activity during non-invasive ventilation. Respir Physiol Neurobiol. 2011;178:341–5.
55. Schmidt M, Chiti L, Hug F, Demoule A, Similowski T. Surface electromyogram of inspiratory muscles: a possible routine monitoring tool in the intensive care unit. Br J Anaesth. 2011;106:913–4.
56. Heimdal JH, Roksund OD, Halvorsen T, Skadberg BT, Olofsson J. Continuous laryngoscopy exercise test: a method for visualizing laryngeal dysfunction during exercise. Laryngoscope. 2006;116:52–7.
57. Maat RC, Røksund OD, Halvorsen T, Skadberg BT, Olofsson J, Ellingsen TA, Aarstad HJ, Heimdal JH. Audiovisual assessment of exercise-induced laryngeal obstruction: reliability and validity of observations. Eur Arch Otorrinolaringol. 2009;266:1929–36.

58. Røksund OD, Maat RC, Heimdal JH, Olofsson J, Skadberg BT, Halvorsen T. Exercise induced dyspnea in the young. Larynx as the bottleneck of the airways. Respir Med. 2009;103:1911–8.
59. Shinn JR, Kimura KS, Campbell BR, Sun Lowery A, Wootten CT, Garrett CG, Francis DO, Hillel AT, Du L, Casey JD, Ely EW, Gelbard A. Incidence and outcomes of acute laryngeal injury after prolonged mechanical ventilation. Crit Care Med. 2019;47:1699–706.
60. Genta PR, Schorr F, Eckert DJ, Gebrim E, Kayamori F, Moriya HT, Malhotra A, Lorenzi-Filho G. Upper airway collapsibility is associated with obesity and hyoid position. Sleep. 2014;37:1673–8.
61. Marques M, Genta PR, Sands SA, Azarbazin A, de Melo C, Taranto-Montemurro L, White DP, Wellman A. Effect of sleeping position on upper airway patency in obstructive sleep apnea is determined by the pharyngeal structure causing collapse. Sleep. 2017;40:zsx005.
62. Baz M, Haji GS, Menzies-Gow A, Tanner RJ, Hopkinson NS, Polkey MI, Hull JH. Dynamic laryngeal narrowing during exercise: a mechanism for generating intrinsic PEEP in COPD? Thorax. 2015;70:251–7.
63. Oppersma E, Doorduin J, Gooskens PJ, Roesthuis LH, van der Heijden EHFM, van der Hoeven JG, Veltink PH, Heunks LMA. Glottic patency during noninvasive ventilation in patients with chronic obstructive pulmonary disease. Respir Physiol Neurobiol. 2019;259:53–7.
64. Andersen T, Sandnes A, Brekka AK, Hilland M, Clemm H, Fondenes O, Tysnes OB, Heimdal JH, Halvorsen T, Vollsæter M, Røksund OD. Laryngeal response patterns influence the efficacy of mechanical assisted cough in amyotrophic lateral sclerosis. Thorax. 2017;72:221–9.
65. Andersen TM, Sandnes A, Fondenes O, Nilsen RM, Tysnes OB, Heimdal JH, Clemm HH, Halvorsen T, Vollsæter M, Røksund OD. Laryngeal responses to mechanically assisted cough in progressing amyotrophic lateral sclerosis. Respir Care. 2018;63:538–49.
66. Conde B, Martins N, Brandão M, Pimenta AC, Winck JC. Upper airway video endoscopy: assessment of the response to positive pressure ventilation and mechanical in-exsufflation. Pulmonology. 2019;25:299–304.
67. De Vito A, Carrasco Llatas M, Ravesloot MJ, Kotecha B, De Vries N, Hamans E, Maurer J, Bosi M, Blumen M, Heiser C, Herzog M, Montevecchi F, Corso RM, Braghiroli A, Gobbi R, Vroegop A, Vonk PE, Hohenhorst W, Piccin O, Sorrenti G, et al. European position paper on drug-induced sleep endoscopy: 2017 update. Clin Otolaryngol. 2018;43:1541–52.
68. Kezirian EJ, Hohenhorst W, de Vries N. Drug-induced sleep endoscopy: the VOTE classification. Eur Arch Otorrinolaringol. 2011;268:1233–6.
69. Sayas Catalán J, Jiménez Huerta I, Benavides Mañas P, Luján M, López-Padilla D, Arias Arias E, Hernández Voth A, Rabec C. Videolaryngoscopy with noninvasive ventilation in subjects with upper-airway obstruction. Respir Care. 2017;62:222–30.
70. Johnson PE, Belafsky PC, Postma GN. Topical nasal anesthesia for transnasal fiberoptic laryngoscopy: a prospective, double-blind, cross-over study. Otolaryngol Head Neck Surg. 2003;128:452–4.
71. Finder J, Gozal D, Iber C, Kushida CA, Morgenthaler T, et al. Best clinical practices for the sleep center adjustment of noninvasive positive pressure ventilation (NPPV) in stable chronic alveolar hypoventilation syndromes. J Clin Sleep Med. 2010;6:491–509.
72. Gobbi R, Baiardi S, Mondini S, Cerritelli L, Piccin O, Scaramuzzino G, Milano F, Melotti MR, Mordini F, Pirodda A, Cirignotta F, Sorrenti G. Technique and preliminary analysis of drug-induced sleep endoscopy with online polygraphic cardiorespiratory monitoring in patients with obstructive sleep apnea syndrome. JAMA Otolaryngol. 2017;143:459–65.
73. Ruan Z, Ren R, Dong W, Ma J, Xu Z, Mao Y, Jiang L. Assessment of vocal cord movement by ultrasound in the ICU. Intensive Care Med. 2018;44:2145–52.
74. Tsui PH, Wan YL, Chen CK. Ultrasound imaging of the larynx and vocal folds: recent applications and developments. Curr Opin Otolaryngol Head Neck Surg. 2012;20:437–42.
75. Cheng SP, Lee JJ, Liu TP, Lee KS, Liu CL. Preoperative ultrasonography assessment of vocal cord movement during thyroid and parathyroid surgery. World J Surg. 2012;36:2509–15.

76. Fukuhara T, Donishi R, Matsuda E, Koyama S, Fujiwara K, Takeuchi H. A novel lateral approach to the assessment of vocal cord movement by ultrasonography. World J Surg. 2018;42:130–6.
77. Kandil E, Deniwar A, Noureldine SI, Hammad AY, Mohamed H, Al-Qurayshi Z, Tufano RP. Assessment of vocal fold function using transcutaneous laryngeal ultrasonography and flexible laryngoscopy. JAMA Otolaryngol Head Neck Surg. 2016;142:74–8.
78. Brekka AK, Vollsæter M, Ntoumenopoulos G, Clemm HH, Halvorsen T, Røksund OD, Andersen TM. Adjustments of non-invasive ventilation and mechanically assisted cough by combining ultrasound imaging of the larynx with transnasal fibre-optic laryngoscopy: a protocol for an experimental study. BMJ Open. 2022;12:e059234.

Monitoring During Bronchoscopy: Essential Key Recommendations

12

Setu Patolia

12.1 Introduction

Bronchoscopy is a key procedure for the diagnosis and management of various pulmonary diseases. It is mainly performed under moderate sedation as an elective procedure. However, when patient presenting with hypoxic respiratory failure undergoes bronchoscopy, approach and techniques become a dilemma. More and more bronchoscopist and respiratory staff are becoming familiar with the noninvasive ventilation (NIV). They are using NIV for bronchoscopy in hypoxic patients to avoid intubation. In this chapter, we will describe key recommendations for monitoring during bronchoscopy on patients with hypoxic respiratory failure.

12.2 Physiological Changes During Bronchoscopy and Rationale for Monitoring

12.2.1 Respiratory

Some degree of alveolar de-recruitment is expected with sedation and suction during bronchoscopy. This may result in decreased oxygenation [1, 2]. Mohan et al. studied 88 patients before and after bronchoscopy. In their study, mean duration of the bronchoscopy was 15 min. During these 15 min, they noticed a mean decline in Forced Vital Capacity (FVC) and Forced Expiratory Volume in 1 second (FEV1) by 130 and 210 mL, respectively [3].

S. Patolia (✉)
Saint Louis University, Saint Louis, MO, USA
e-mail: Setu.patolia@health.slu.edu

© The Author(s), under exclusive license to Springer Nature Switzerland AG 2025

K. Panda et al. (eds.), *Noninvasive Ventilatory Approaches in Interventional Procedures*, Noninvasive Ventilation. The Essentials,
https://doi.org/10.1007/978-3-032-05328-2_12

Davies et al. studied 45 patients undergoing bronchoscopy. They found that 19 of the 45 (42.2%) patients developed desaturation. Patients with poor lung function were more likely to develop desaturation [4]. Jones et al. studied 1051 bronchoscopies done between 1992 and 1997. In their study, 14.4% patients required oxygen supplementation during the procedure, and additional 9.6% had transient desaturation (<20 s) [5]. Risk of oxygen desaturation was higher with lower FEV_1 [5]. This study showed that patient with $FEV_1 < 1$ L had 35% incidence of hypoxia requiring supplemental oxygen as compared to 14% and 7% for FEV_1 1–1.5 L and > 1.5 L, respectively. Hasan et al. studied 56 patients undergoing bronchoscopy, wherein 21.4% of these patients developed oxygen saturation below 80% and 8.9% of patients had oxygen saturation below 75%. In 67.8% of these patients, oxygen desaturation persisted for more than half an hour [6]. Similar findings were noted by Katz et al. [7] Stanopoulos et al. studied 167 bronchoscopies. They found 87 of the 167 (52%) patients had desaturation <90% despite routing oxygen supplementation. This was more likely to happen in patients with FEV_1 or FVC below the lower limit of normal or patients with lower preprocedure oxygen saturation [8]. Overall, PaO_2 decline of 10–20 mm of Hg is noted during fiberoptic examination, and this can decline up to 40% more with suctioning [9–11].

Bronchoscope also reduces cross-sectional area of tracheobronchial tree and, as a result, increases the work of breathing. Sedation can also reduce ventilatory drive [1]. This can result in carbon dioxide retention [9]. Taher et al. studied 200 patients and found that 59% of patients had a decrease in ET-PCO_2 of equal or greater than 4 mm of Hg, suggestive of airway obstruction by the instrument [12]. Yumrukuz Senel et al. studied 74 patients undergoing bronchoscopy and monitored $TcPCO_2$ and $TcSO_2$. Mean increase in $TcPCO_2$ was 3.25 ± 2.12 mm of Hg [13]. Rise of PCO_2 up to 8 mm of Hg can be seen during bronchoscopy [11].

12.2.2 Cardiovascular

Bronchoscopy is associated with significant hemodynamic changes. Coughing and positive pressure associated with NIV can increase intrathoracic pressure. This will decrease the cardiac preload.

Davies et al. studied cardiovascular consequences of bronchoscopy on 45 patients [4]. In their study, mean heart rate increased from 93 to 134/min during the procedure. Seven patients had significant tachycardia, and their BP increase to >220/110. Four of these patients had ST segment depression, and the other three developed bundle branch block. Mohan et al. had similar finding in their study where Systolic Blood Pressure (SBP), Diastolic Blood Pressure (DBP), and Heart Rate (HR) increased during the procedure and were higher at 5 and 10 min as compared to the baseline [3]. In the study by Hasan et al., 41.07% (23/56) patients developed cardiac arrythmia [6]. Most common arrythmias were sinus (16/26–69.5%). Premature ventricular contraction (PVC) was noted in five (21.7%) patients and paroxysmal supraventricular tachycardia (PSVT) in two (8.6%) patients. In Katz et al. study, 20 patients (40%) developed arrythmia. PVC were seen in 10 and atrial arrythmia in

16. PVCs occurred during passage from the vocal cord [7]. In both studies, arrythmia was common during periods of desaturation.

12.3 Current Guideline Recommendations

British thoracic guidelines (BTS) recommend continuous pulse oximetry monitoring during bronchoscopy [14]. In patients at high risk of arrythmia, BTS guideline recommends continuous ECG monitoring and blood pressure optimization [14].

12.4 Our Practice

Patients undergoing bronchoscopy with noninvasive ventilation are hypoxemic at baseline and likely to develop worsening hypoxemia during the procedure. This also puts them at higher risk of arrythmia during the procedure. We routinely use continuous Electrocardiogram (EKG) and pulse oximetry monitoring for patients undergoing bronchoscopy with noninvasive ventilation. We also set up automated blood pressure recording for every 2–3 min during the procedure. With minimal increase demonstrated in PCO_2, we do not routinely monitor $ETCO_2$ or TCO_2 during the procedure.

12.5 Conclusion

There are significant physiological changes during bronchoscopy. Various phases of bronchoscopy like passing through the vocal cord, suctioning, and bronchoalveolar lavage are associated with exacerbation of those changes. Patients undergoing bronchoscopy under noninvasive ventilation are at high risk of desaturation and arrythmia-related complications. They should be routinely monitored with pulse oximetry and continue EKG monitoring.

References

1. Lindholm CE, Ollman B, Snyder JV, Millen EG, Grenvik A. Cardiorespiratory effects of flexible fiberoptic bronchoscopy in critically ill patients. Chest. 1978;74:362–8.
2. Matsushima Y, Jones RL, King EG, Moysa G, Alton JD. Alterations in pulmonary mechanics and gas exchange during routine fiberoptic bronchoscopy. Chest. 1984;86:184–8. Miller EJ. Hypoxemia during fiberoptic bronchoscopy. Chest. 1979;75:103
3. Mohan A, Ansari A, Uniyal A, Upadhyay AD, Guleria R. Acute changes in physiological cardiopulmonary parameters during and after flexible fiberoptic bronchoscopy. Lung India. 2016;33:111–2.
4. Davies L, Mister R, Spence DP, Calverley PM, Earis JE, Pearson MG. Cardiovascular consequences of fibreoptic bronchoscopy. Eur Respir J. 1997;10:695–8.
5. Jones AM, O'Driscoll R. Do all patients require supplemental oxygen during flexible bronchoscopy? Chest. 2001;119:1906–9. https://doi.org/10.1378/chest.119.6.1906.

6. Hassan G, Khan GQ, Yaseen M, Masood T, Qureshi W. Cardiac arrhythmias during fiberoptic bronchoscopy and relation with oxygen saturation. Lung India. 2005;22:54–9.
7. Katz AS, Michelson EL, Stawicki J, Holford FD. Cardiac arrhythmias. Frequency during fiberoptic bronchoscopy and correlation with hypoxemia. Arch Intern Med. 1981;141:603–6.
8. Stanopoulos IT, Pickering R, Beamis JF, Martinez FJ. Oximetric monitoring during routine, oxygen-supplemented flexible bronchoscopy: what role does it have? J Bronchol. 1995;2:5–11.
9. Antonelli M, Conti G, Rocco M, et al. Noninvasive positive-pressure ventilation versus conventional oxygen supplementation in hypoxemic patients undergoing diagnostic fiberoptic bronchoscopy. Chest. 2002;121:1149–54.
10. Maitre B, Jaber S, Maggiore SM, et al. Continuous positive airway pressure during fiberoptic bronchoscopy in hypoxemic patients: a randomized double blind study using a new device. Am J Respir Crit Care Med. 2000;162:1063–7.
11. Tai DYH. Bronchoscopy in the intensive care unit (ICU). Ann Acad Med Singap. 1998;27:552–9.
12. Taher MA, Kamash FA, Al-Momani JA. End-tidal carbon dioxide monitoring during flexible fiberoptic bronchoscopy. Pak J Med Sci. 2006;22:149–53.
13. Yumrukuz Şenel M, Fırat H, Kurt EB. Evaluation of transcutaneous carbon dioxide and saturation monitoring during fiberoptic bronchoscopy. Tuberk Toraks. 2020;68:379–87.
14. Du Rand IA, Blaikley J, Booton R, Chaudhuri N, Gupta V, Khalid S, Mandal S, Martin J, Mills J, Navani N, Rahman NM, Wrightson JM, Munavvar M, British Thoracic Society Bronchoscopy Guideline Group. British Thoracic Society guideline for diagnostic flexible bronchoscopy in adults: accredited by NICE. Thorax. 2013;68:i1–i44.

13 Patient-Ventilator Asynchronies: Leak Prevention

Raffaele Merola and Maria Vargas

13.1 Introduction

In patients with acute respiratory failure, mechanical ventilation is a life-saving treatment. The effects of mechanical ventilation on gas exchange, respiratory muscle load, and dyspnea depend on the matching between the ventilator settings and the patient's respiratory physiology. However, mechanical ventilation is rarely optimized, which would require ventilator settings based on accurate and reproducible measurements of the patient's respiratory mechanics [1–4].

Patient-ventilator asynchrony (PVA) is defined as a mismatch between the breathing efforts of a patient and breath delivery by a ventilator [5]. It is a common problem in mechanically ventilated patients and has an incidence of up to 80% [6]. PVA may cause ventilator-induced lung injury (VILI) due to excessive tidal volume [7, 8] and diaphragm injury from eccentric contractions [9], both of which can affect clinical outcomes.

13.2 Respiratory Physiology

The goal of the intrinsic ventilatory control system is to integrate the timing and intensity of the phrenic nerve signal, inputs from chemoreceptors and pulmonary stretch receptors, and changes in metabolic demands. Contraction of the respiratory muscles generates flow and volume to provide adequate alveolar ventilation with a tolerable work of breathing [10]. During spontaneous breathing, the respiratory

R. Merola (✉) · M. Vargas
Anesthesia and Intensive Care Medicine, Department of Neurosciences, Reproductive and Odontostomatological Sciences, University of Naples Federico II, Naples, Italy
e-mail: raffaele.merola@unina.it; maria.vargas@unina.it

© The Author(s), under exclusive license to Springer Nature Switzerland AG 2025

K. Panda et al. (eds.), *Noninvasive Ventilatory Approaches in Interventional Procedures*, Noninvasive Ventilation. The Essentials,
https://doi.org/10.1007/978-3-032-05328-2_13

muscles generate pressure (P_{mus}) to produce flow against the resistive properties (R_{RS}), deliver volume against the elastic properties (E_{RS}) of the respiratory system, and overcome any intrinsic positive end-expiratory pressure (PEEPi, known better clinically as auto-PEEP) [11]. Therefore, the act of spontaneous breathing can be described as follows:

$$P_{mus} = P_{res} + P_{el} + \text{PEEPi}$$

where P_{res} represents the resistive pressure and is a function of flow ($P_{res} = \text{Flow} \times R_{RS}$) and P_{el} represents the elastic recoil pressure generated by lung expansion and is a function of volume ($P_{el} = \text{Volume} \times E_{RS}$). So, the equation becomes:

$$P_{mus} = \left(\text{Flow} \times R_{RS}\right) + \left(\text{Volume} \times E_{RS}\right) + \text{PEEPi}$$

In patients with acute respiratory failure requiring ventilatory support, pressure generated by the ventilator (P_{appl}) is added to the pressure generated by the contraction of the respiratory muscles according to the following equation:

$$P_{mus} + P_{appl} = \left(\text{Flow} \times R_{RS}\right) + \left(\text{Volume} \times E_{RS}\right) + \text{PEEPi}$$

The patient interacts with the ventilator based on three physiologic variables:

- Respiratory drive [12]
- Ventilatory requirements [4]
- Timing of the breathing pattern [13]

The ventilator interfaces with the patient's physiology based on three technologic variables:

- Inspiratory trigger (phase trigger variable), that is, what triggers the breath delivered by the ventilator [14, 15]
- Delivery mechanism (control variable), that is, what governs the way in which the air flow is delivered [16–20]
- Cycle-off criterion (phase cycling variable), that is, what determines the end of the ventilatory assistance to the inspiratory effort of the patient [19, 20]

The optimization of mechanical ventilation derives from the coordination between the physiological variables of the patient and the technological ones of the ventilator with the aim of optimizing gaseous exchange and reducing the work of breathing. Therefore, patient-ventilator synchrony is a goal that can be achieved by interpreting the ventilatory needs and the mechanical characteristics of the respiratory system of each individual patient and setting the ventilator accordingly. PVA appears whenever a mismatch between the three physiologic variables characterizing spontaneous breathing (respiratory drive, ventilatory requirements, and timing of the breathing pattern) and the three technologic variables characterizing ventilator function (inspiratory trigger, delivery mechanism, and cycle-off criterion) occurs.

There are several types of patient-ventilator asynchrony.

- Respiratory drive-ventilator inspiratory trigger asynchrony
- Ventilatory requirements-delivery mechanism asynchrony
- Inspiratory timing-ventilator cycling asynchrony

13.3 Respiratory Drive-Inspiratory Trigger Asynchrony

During partial ventilatory assistance, the inspiratory synchronization system (inspiratory trigger) detects the patient's inspiratory effort and activates a mechanical response. Thus, inspiratory effort is tracked to match patient effort with pressure, flow, or volume delivery. The coordination between the effort of the patient and the act of the ventilator takes place through the reading of mostly pneumatic signals (flow and pressure) within the respiratory circuit, which determine the opening of the inspiratory valve on request from the patient [21]. The goal of effective inspiratory triggering is to minimize the duration and intensity of muscle effort before the initiation of a mechanically supported breath [22]. Triggering asynchronies include auto-triggering, ineffective triggering, double triggering, and reverse triggering.

Auto-triggering can be defined as a mandatory breath delivered in the absence of a patient's inspiratory effort [23]. The number of breaths monitored by the ventilator is higher than those initiated by the patient [24]. Auto-triggering can be generated by too sensitive inspiratory triggers; air leaks; an external signal, such as heart rate or water in the respiratory circuit; or low respiratory drive [25]. By analyzing volume, flow, and pressure waveforms on the mechanical ventilator display, auto-triggering can be detected as a cycle delivered by the ventilator without a prior airway pressure decrease (Fig. 13.1).

Ineffective triggering is defined as an inspiratory effort not followed by a ventilator breath. This asynchrony occurs when the patient's attempt to initiate a breath does not reach the ventilator's trigger threshold. In other words, the ventilator fails to detect the patient's inspiratory efforts [26]. The possible underlying mechanisms are recognized to be high levels of ventilator assistance, weak respiratory drive, a high PEEPi, and an excessively low ventilator trigger sensitivity [1, 6, 27, 28]. Ineffective triggering results in the patient's respiratory rate being higher than the ventilator's rate. Flow and pressure waveforms on the mechanical ventilator display show ineffective inspiratory efforts as a decrease in airway pressure associated with a simultaneous increase in air flow (Fig. 13.2). Most ineffective efforts are detected during mechanical expiration; however, they can also occur during inspiration, where they are characterized by an abrupt increase in inspiratory flow (pressure support ventilation, PSV) or a transient abrupt decrease in airway pressure (volume-controlled ventilation, VCV) that fails to trigger a full additional breath [29, 30].

Double-triggering is characterized by one single patient respiratory muscle effort supported by two mechanical cycles separated by a very short expiratory time. The interruption of the mechanical insufflation before the completion of the patient's effort generates a second triggered mechanical insufflation, after a brief exhalation phase [28, 31]. Double-triggering can be elicited by high patient ventilatory demand that causes two breaths to be triggered with a limited expiratory phase

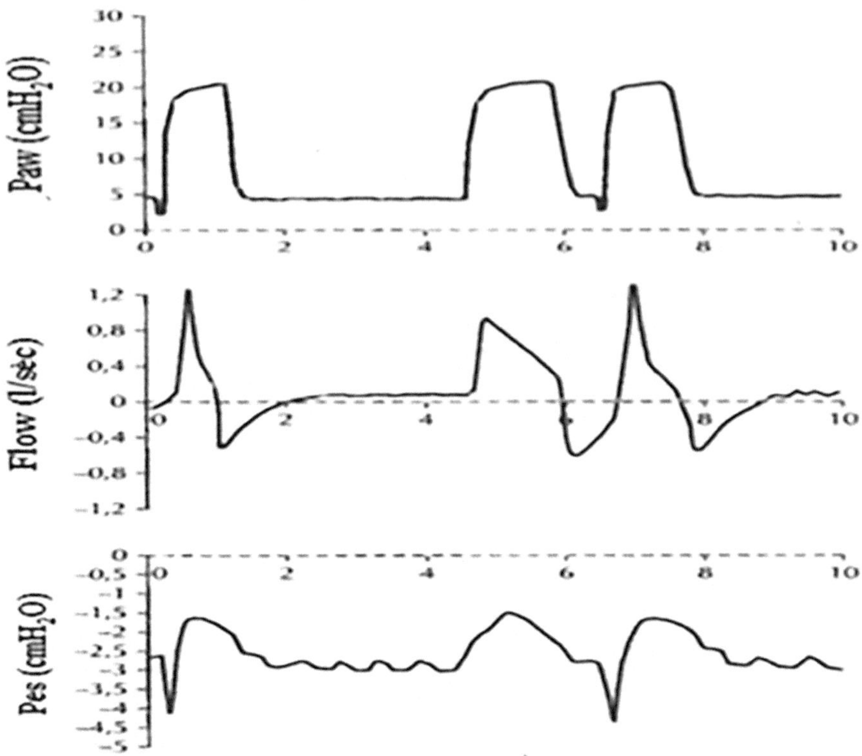

Fig. 13.1 Airway pressure, flow, and esophageal pressure traces during pressure support ventilation. The second breath can be observed to occur without inspiratory effort, i.e., with no deflection on the airway pressure or esophageal pressure trace. Note also the different flow-time profiles between triggered and auto-triggered breaths, a feature that characterizes the pressure support ventilation

caused by too short of a ventilator inspiratory time (Ti) compared with the patient's neural time. This problem can be addressed by increasing Ti in time-cycled mode, by adjusting the expiratory threshold time, or by optimizing the pressure rise time (i.e., the time taken to reach the targeted pressure set for the ventilator) [32].

Reverse triggering is a recently discovered form of PVA that occurs in heavily sedated patients. In this case, contrary to the usual triggering sequence (patient's effort switching on the ventilator-driven breath), the patient's respiratory center is activated in response to a passive insufflation of the lungs. This PVA originates in respiratory muscle contractions triggered by the ventilator [33, 34]. The underlying physiological mechanism of reverse triggering seems to be the activation of mechanoreceptors in the muscles and/or chest wall or complex spinal reflexes [35]. Esophageal pressure monitoring can help to detect this PVA: a drop in esophageal pressure can be related to diaphragmatic contractions triggered by ventilator insufflations [33]. Reverse triggering can result in stretching in the dependent lung.

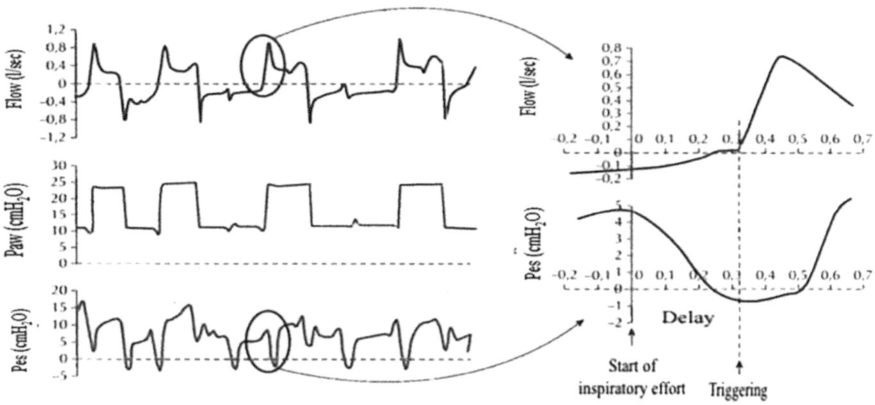

Fig. 13.2 Traces of airway pressure, flow, and esophageal pressure during pressure support ventilation. It can be observed that the onset of inspiratory effort corresponds to the point in which the expiratory flow suddenly decreases, whereas the inspiratory flow begins with a certain delay (trigger delay). Arrows indicate ineffective acts, identifiable as small increases in the expiratory flow trace, which correspond to slight deflections in the airway pressure trace

Proportional to negative intrathoracic pressure, stretching due to reverse triggering can be equivalent to that caused by applying 15 ml/kg tidal volume. Yoshida and coworkers recently demonstrated how reverse triggering can worsen pre-existing lung injury through a pendelluft effect from nondependent lung toward dependent lung due to poor transmission of the diaphragm contraction across the pleural surface [36]. Moreover, reverse triggering can result in increased strain and stretch due to breath stacking during double cycling caused by insufficient assistance [37].

13.4 Ventilatory Requirements-Delivery Mechanism Asynchrony

Gas delivery asynchrony occurs when ventilator-delivered flow, volume, and pressure are insufficient or excessive to meet the patient's ventilatory demand. The first case usually occurs when the flow is set by the operator and cannot be increased by patient spontaneous efforts, as occurs during VCV. However, insufficient inspiratory flow can also occur during pressure-controlled ventilation (PCV) and PSV when the set levels are insufficient to deliver the flow required by the patient. This type of asynchrony can be addressed by reducing patient's ventilatory demand (correction of fever, anxiety, pain, etc.) or increasing flow delivery by means of appropriate adjustments for each mode, observing patient comfort, accessory respiratory muscle use, and pressure waveform pattern. In patients on VCV, switching to PCV or PSV can be a good alternative. In fact, pressure-targeted breaths may more effectively match the patient's ventilatory requirements because flow is the dependent variable during constant pressure delivery. In addition, in PCV and PSV, an adjustment in airway pressurization rate directly affects flow delivery immediately after the respiratory cycle is triggered: rapid pressurization of the airways is coupled with high inspiratory flow only at the beginning of inspiration, thus reproducing the physiologic flow profile [38]. However, during a pressure-targeted breath, the setting for the time of pressure increase may influence the patient-ventilator interaction because its modification determines the dependent flow output [39, 40].

Excessive flow asynchrony occurs because of an exaggerated delivery of inspiratory flow. In some cases, excessive pressurization may occur, characterizing an overshoot of the flow in PCV or PSV. The best option consists of reducing flow delivery by reducing the set value in VCV or by reducing the applied pressure over PEEP or increasing the time of pressure increase in PCV and PSV [38].

13.5 Inspiratory Timing-Ventilator Cycling Asynchrony

Cycle asynchrony usually occurs when there is a mismatch between the patient's inspiratory time (i.e., neural time) and the ventilator's inspiratory time [27, 41].

Premature cycling occurs when the neural time is greater than the ventilator inflation time. The ventilator ends flow delivery, but the patient's inspiratory effort continues. If the patient's effort exceeds the trigger threshold, it can activate another breath, generating a double trigger. *Delayed cycling* occurs when the patient initiates the exhalation while the ventilator is still delivering flow. On waveform graphics, this is readily observable as a sharp pressure spike originated by recruitment of the expiratory muscles as an instinctive response to excessive muscle loading, which can be confirmed by palpating the abdominal muscles for activity [26].

A breath can be pressure-, time-, volume-, or flow-cycled. Although volume and pressure cycling are no longer used, a breath is defined as time-cycled when it is terminated after a given preset inspiratory time is reached (PCV or VCV). The breath is flow-cycled when the generated inspiratory flow decays from its peak by a fixed percentage (PSV) [40]. In ventilated patients with time-cycled breaths, it is necessary to monitor the patient's inspiratory flow and ratio of inspiratory time-to-total breath cycle to have correct ventilator cycling and optimal patient-ventilator synchrony. In ventilated patients with flow-cycled breaths, inspiratory time is determined exclusively by the time taken for the exponentially declining flow to reach the preset flow threshold value [42, 43]. The inspiratory flow threshold value, also called the expiratory trigger, then controls the transition from inspiration to expiration in these modalities under the postulate that the end of patient inspiration is followed by the inspiratory flow decay. To correct premature cycling, the threshold should be decreased, and, to correct delayed cycling, the threshold should be increased [38, 39, 44].

13.6 Detection of PVA

Although patient-ventilator asynchrony is very common, studying this phenomenon remains a challenge in daily clinical practice [6, 45]. Patient-ventilator asynchronies have been evaluated with several methods, such as the observation of waveforms on the ventilator screen, standardized and automatic dedicated software, or additional signals (i.e., ultrasonography, electrical impedance tomography) [46].

Pressure, volume, and flow waveforms are displayed in real time on the screen of ventilators. Visual inspection of these waveforms is the most common method adopted in routine clinical practice. This method, in fact, does not require the use of additional catheters, which can be considered difficult to position and a source of further discomfort for the patient and air leaks during noninvasive ventilation (NIV). There are limitations in the detection of asynchronies from ventilator waveform inspection. First, the ability of physicians, even experts, to detect asynchrony can be poor and does not allow for easy, reliable, and sensitive detection of asynchronies. Second, because asynchronies can happen at any time, it is not possible to continuously track for asynchronies. Third, some types of asynchronies such as reverse triggering are not easily detected by the inspection of pressure, flow, or volume waveforms only [45, 47].

Most of the clinical studies assessing asynchronies used offline breath by breath analysis. Online assessment only was possible during short periods (from several minutes to few hours). This sparked interest in dedicated software designed to continuously detect asynchronies in real time. To date, few studies have reported the feasibility and results of this technology [47]. To date, few studies reported the feasibility and results of such technology. Younes and colleagues developed an automated algorithm using tidal volume, pressure, flow, and esophageal pressure (Peso) signals on one hand and estimated the values of elastance and resistance on the other. This method provides a real-time trace relating respiratory muscle activity to airway pressure and flow. Therefore, it provides real-time visual feedback on instantaneous patient-ventilator interaction and thus enables reliable detection of excessive on-delay, off-delay, and ineffective efforts [48].

Blanch and coworkers validated a software (Better Care) designed to detect ineffective efforts during expiration. The software captures digital output from several ventilators and associates each captured waveform with the parameter it represents (flow, pressure, or tidal volume). The signals are then tagged, converted to the specific standard, formatted, and stored in the hospital's image archiving and communication system for analysis. This algorithm is able to detect ineffective effort with an area under the receiving operating characteristics curve of 0.96 when the gold standard is experts' judgment [29, 49].

Sinderby and colleagues proposed another automated algorithm based on the analysis of electrical activity of the diaphragm (EAdi) and ventilator pressure waveforms and quantification of mismatch between the two waveforms. A new index of patient-ventilator interaction (NeuroSync index), which was standardized and automated, was compared to manual analysis. The authors found that NeuroSync index produced high test-retest and inter-rater reliability [50]. The same technology was used in patients with chronic obstructive pulmonary disease (COPD) under NIV. In this last study, there was a significant correlation between the number of wasted efforts and the NeuroSync index [51].

More recently, the application of diaphragmatic ultrasonography has been proposed to recognize patient-ventilator asynchronies during invasive mechanical ventilation [52]. This technique has also been tested in healthy volunteers undergoing NIV with induced asynchronies [53]. This method is based on monitoring the excursion of the diaphragm dome or its thickening in the zone of apposition, to define the presence of the patient's respiratory effort. Ultrasound imaging of the diaphragm was then coupled in real time with ventilator waveforms to accurately recognize and identify asynchronies [53].

Finally, electrical impedance tomography (EIT) has been applied in acute respiratory distress syndrome (ARDS) porcine model to study the "pendelluft" phenomenon in case of asynchronies with the ventilator [54]. No studies, however, have so far evaluated the distribution of lung air or ventilation in patients undergoing invasive mechanical ventilation or NIV with severe patient-ventilator asynchronies.

13.7 Management of PVA

Table 13.1 summarizes the different approaches that can be used to correct each type of asynchrony. Although sedation and analgesia are often used to treat asynchronies, this approach has several adverse effects. Deep sedation is an independent risk factor for ineffective inspiratory efforts [6, 55, 56]. Furthermore, deep sedation is associated with longer mechanical ventilation duration and ICU length of stay [57].

Adjusting ventilator settings seems to be a better approach. In a previous study that analyzed subjects with asynchronies treated without any intervention, increased sedation-analgesia, or changes in ventilator settings, authors found asynchronies significantly decreased only after changes in ventilator setting [55].

13.7.1 PSV

Three factors may influence patient-ventilator interaction during PSV:

- Expiratory trigger
- Airway pressurization rate (pressure ramp)
- Level of ventilator assistance

The expiratory trigger sensitivity can be fixed (default at 25% of peak flow) or can vary from 1% to 90% or from 5 to 25 L/min in some old ventilator software [58]. Setting the expiratory trigger at a higher percentage of peak inspiratory flow improves patient-ventilator synchrony and reduces inspiratory muscle effort and dynamic hyperinflation in patients with COPD [59, 60]. On the other hand, setting

Table 13.1 Strategies for Management of PVA

Asynchrony	Action
Auto-triggering	Check trigger sensitivity Check for leaks and water in the ventilator circuit Decrease sedation
Ineffective triggering	Check trigger sensitivity Decrease sedation Decrease level of ventilator assistance Decrease inspiratory time Counterbalance auto-PEEP by using external PEEP Check for dyspnea Consider proportional modes
Double triggering	Increase ventilator inspiratory time (VCV or PCV) or decrease the cycling threshold percentage of peak flow (PSV)
Reverse triggering	Decrease sedation
Insufficient inspiratory flow	In VCV, increase inspiratory flow or switch to PCV or PSV In PCV or PSV, increase level of ventilator assistance and airway pressurization rate Decrease respiratory drive and patient's ventilatory demand (correction of fever, anxiety, pain, etc.)
Excessive inspiratory flow	In VCV, decrease inspiratory flow In PCV or PSV, decrease level of ventilator assistance and airway pressurization rate
Premature cycling	Increase ventilator inspiratory time (VCV or PCV), or decrease the cycling threshold percentage of peak flow (PSV)
Delayed cycling	Decrease ventilator inspiratory time (VCV or PCV), or increase the cycling threshold percentage of peak flow (PSV)

the expiratory trigger at a lower percentage of peak inspiratory flow improves patient-ventilator synchrony and decreases the work of breathing in patients with ARDS [61]. During NIV, air leaks may cause an abnormal prolongation of the mechanical inspiratory time at the expense of a patient's expiration requirements (inspiratory hang-up). Therefore, the correct setting of the expiratory trigger, the choice of an appropriate interface, and the use of ventilators with air leaks compensating software are essential to reduce the occurrence of PVA whenever ventilators are used to deliver NIV [62–70].

The setting of airway pressurization rate (pressure ramp) can affect the expiratory threshold by modifying the dependent inspiratory flow [71–74]. In fact, a rapid increase in pressure can lead to a particularly high peak inspiratory flow, which can then cause premature termination of inspiration when the fixed percentage criterion for expiratory cycle is reached [60, 74]. Prinianakis and colleagues evaluated the effects of varying the rate of pressure change during NIV PSV on the respiratory pattern of COPD patients, as well as inspiratory effort, arterial blood gases, ventilation tolerance, and the amount of air leak. No significant changes in respiratory pattern and arterial blood gases were observed between the different pressure slopes, but the pressure-time product of the diaphragm, an estimate of its metabolic rate, decreased significantly with increasing pressurization rate. Interestingly, air leaks increased, and patients' tolerance to ventilation was significantly lower with the rate of pressure change being faster [75].

During NIV, the level of ventilator assistance affects patient-ventilator interactions, primarily through effects on the generation of air leaks. Since, as mentioned above, air leaks can lead to changes in the inspiratory flow profile, their reduction by lowering to a PSV level of 1 or 2 cm H_2O has been shown to improve patient-ventilator interaction [31, 63, 76].

In recent years, researchers have proposed to vary the level of pressure support breath by breath to restore the physiological variability of respiratory activity, thereby improving patient-ventilator interaction [77].

Variable PSV is a recently introduced mode of assisted ventilation that has shown reduction in patient-ventilator asynchronies [78, 79]. Variable PSV has also shown to have comparable effects to neurally adjusted ventilatory assist (NAVA) on patient-ventilator synchrony [80].

13.7.2 PAV and PAV+

During proportional assisted ventilation (PAV), the ventilator generates pressure in proportion to the patient-generated flow and volume; the ventilator amplifies patient effort without imposing any ventilatory or pressure targets, and ventilator-generated pressure rises as long as inspiratory muscle effort is produced by the patient [81, 82]. During this mode of ventilation, the clinician adjusts the percentage of flow-assisted or volume-assisted ventilation after determining the patient's resistance and elastance, with the goal of reducing patient's work of breathing [83–85]. Despite the exciting potential of this technique, no large-scale studies have demonstrated an improvement in patient outcome with PAV compared with other modes of ventilation. Several studies performed during invasive ventilation showed that PAV improves patient-ventilator synchrony at the start of inspiration, but not necessarily at the end [86–91]. Furthermore, PAV was shown to be comfortable and tolerated in patients with moderate acute respiratory failure (ARF) during NIV, which may be in part attributable to improvement of patient-ventilator synchrony [92, 93]. However, in a more recent study comparing PAV with PSV in patients with exacerbated COPD treated with NIV, PAV did not improve patient-ventilator interaction [94]. Compared with PAV, PAV+ provides a continuous measurement of the patient's elastance and resistance according to the method described by Younes and coworkers. The physician is only required to set only a given percentage of the overall pressure requirement [83–85, 95–97].

During invasive ventilation, PAV+ appears to reduce the incidence of patient-ventilator asynchronies considerably compared with conventional PAV [98]. Furthermore, as compared to PSV, PAV+ decreases the setting time and responds automatically to changes in sedative doses [99, 100].

13.7.3 NAVA

With neural-adjusted ventilatory assist (NAVA), the electrical activity of the diaphragm (EAdi) is estimated by a dedicated esophageal catheter with electrical sensors and used for triggering, to deliver proportional inspiratory support, and for cycling; the inspiratory support delivered by the ventilator is adjusted by the NAVA level, or NAVA gain, a factor by which EAdi is multiplied to determine the pressure that will be applied to the airways. Therefore, patient effort, estimated by the EAdi waveform, determines triggering, pressurization, and cycling in NAVA, and the only parameter that must be set by the clinician is the NAVA level [32, 33, 101, 102]. Several studies have shown that NAVA can efficiently optimize patient-ventilator synchrony during NIV, decreasing ineffective efforts and premature and delayed cycling compared with PSV [103–106]. Furthermore, compared with PSV, NAVA improves patient-ventilator synchrony even in infants and children [107]. NAVA has a big advantage over the other proportional modes, as air leaks do not interfere with its proper functioning [108]. Finally, recent meta-analyses also confirm that NAVA improves patient-ventilator synchrony; however, its impact on clinical outcomes is still uncertain, and further studies are needed [109–111].

13.8 Conclusion

PVA occurs commonly during mechanical ventilatory support. Despite this, it continues to be an unrecognized, underestimated, and inappropriately treated phenomenon in the clinical setting.

Patient-ventilator synchrony is a goal that can be achieved by understanding of the principles of respiratory physiology and respiratory system mechanics of each individual patient and setting the ventilator accordingly. And it is precisely toward this goal that the rapid evolution of technologies aimed at detecting and solving problems concerning patient-ventilator interaction must be directed.

References

1. Leung P, Jubran A, Tobin MJ. Comparison of assisted ventilator modes on triggering, patient effort, and dyspnea. Am J Respir Crit Care Med. 1997;155:1940–8. https://doi.org/10.1164/ajrccm.155.6.9196100. PMID: 9196100.
2. Tobin MJ, Jubran A, Laghi F. Patient-ventilator interaction. Am J Respir Crit Care Med. 2001;163:1059–63. https://doi.org/10.1164/ajrccm.163.5.2005125. PMID: 11316635.
3. Ranieri VM. Optimization of patient-ventilator interactions: closed-loop technology to turn the century. Intensive Care Med. 1997;23:936–9. https://doi.org/10.1007/s001340050434. PMID: 9347363.
4. Dick CR, Sassoon CS. Patient-ventilator interactions. Clin Chest Med. 1996;17:423–38. https://doi.org/10.1016/s0272-5231(05)70325-7. PMID: 8875005.
5. Gilstrap D, MacIntyre N. Patient-ventilator interactions. Implications for clinical management. Am J Respir Crit Care Med. 2013;188:1058–68. https://doi.org/10.1164/rccm.201212-2214CI. PMID: 24070493.

6. de Wit M, Pedram S, Best AM, Epstein SK. Observational study of patient-ventilator asynchrony and relationship to sedation level. J Crit Care. 2009;24:74–80. https://doi.org/10.1016/j.jcrc.2008.08.011. Epub 2009 Jan 17. PMID: 19272542; PMCID: PMC2676917.
7. Beitler JR, Sands SA, Loring SH, Owens RL, Malhotra A, Spragg RG, Matthay MA, Thompson BT, Talmor D. Quantifying unintended exposure to high tidal volumes from breath stacking dyssynchrony in ARDS: the BREATHE criteria. Intensive Care Med. 2016;42:1427–36. https://doi.org/10.1007/s00134-016-4423-3.
8. Pohlman MC, McCallister KE, Schweickert WD, Pohlman AS, Nigos CP, Krishnan JA, Charbeneau JT, Gehlbach BK, Kress JP, Hall JB. Excessive tidal volume from breath stacking during lung-protective ventilation for acute lung injury. Crit Care Med. 2008;36:3019–23. https://doi.org/10.1097/CCM.0b013e31818b308b. PMID: 18824913.
9. Gea J, Zhu E, Gáldiz JB, Comtois N, Salazkin I, Fiz JA, Grassino A. Consecuencias de las contracciones excéntricas del diafragma sobre su función [Functional consequences of eccentric contractions of the diaphragm]. Spanish. Arch Bronconeumol. 2009;45:68–74. https://doi.org/10.1016/j.arbres.2008.04.003. PMID: 19232267.
10. Mead J. Control of respiratory frequency. J Appl Physiol. 1960;15:325–36.
11. Mead J, Whittenberger JL. Physical properties of human lungs measured during spontaneous respiration. J Appl Physiol. 1953;5:779–96.
12. Whitelaw WA, Derenne JP, Milic-Emili J. Occlusion pressure as a measure of respiratory center output in conscious man. Respir Physiol. 1975;23:181–99. https://doi.org/10.1016/0034-5687(75)90059-6. PMID: 1144940.
13. Hubmayr RD, Abel MD, Rehder K. Physiologic approach to mechanical ventilation. Crit Care Med. 1990;18:103–13. https://doi.org/10.1097/00003246-199001000-00022. PMID: 2403503.
14. Ranieri VM, Mascia L, Petruzzelli V, Bruno F, Brienza A, Giuliani R. Inspiratory effort and measurement of dynamic intrinsic PEEP in COPD patients: effects of ventilator triggering systems. Intensive Care Med. 1995;21:896–903. https://doi.org/10.1007/BF01712330. PMID: 8636521.
15. Alberti A, Gallo F, Fongaro A, Valenti S, Rossi A. P0.1 is a useful parameter in setting the level of pressure support ventilation. Intensive Care Med. 1995;21:547–53. https://doi.org/10.1007/BF01700158. PMID: 7593895.
16. Ward ME, Corbeil C, Gibbons W, Newman S, Macklem PT. Optimization of respiratory muscle relaxation during mechanical ventilation. Anesthesiology. 1988;69:29–35. https://doi.org/10.1097/00000542-198807000-00005. PMID: 3389564.
17. Puddy A, Younes M. Effect of inspiratory flow rate on respiratory output in normal subjects. Am Rev Respir Dis. 1992;146:787–9. https://doi.org/10.1164/ajrccm/146.3.787. PMID: 1519864.
18. Georgopoulos D, Mitrouska I, Bshouty Z, Anthonisen NR, Younes M. Effects of non-REM sleep on the response of respiratory output to varying inspiratory flow. Am J Respir Crit Care Med. 1996;153:1624–30. https://doi.org/10.1164/ajrccm.153.5.8630612. PMID: 8630612.
19. Laghi F, Karamchandani K, Tobin MJ. Influence of ventilator settings in determining respiratory frequency during mechanical ventilation. Am J Respir Crit Care Med. 1999;160:1766–70. https://doi.org/10.1164/ajrccm.160.5.9810086. PMID: 10556154.
20. Banner MJ, Blanch PB, Gabrielli A. Tracheal pressure control provides automatic and variable inspiratory pressure assist to decrease the imposed resistive work of breathing. Crit Care Med. 2002;30:1106–11. https://doi.org/10.1097/00003246-200205000-00024. PMID: 12006809.
21. Sassoon CS. Mechanical ventilator design and function: the trigger variable. Respir Care. 1992;37:1056–69. PMID: 10145700.
22. Hill LL, Pearl RG. Flow triggering, pressure triggering, and autotriggering during mechanical ventilation. Crit Care Med. 2000;28:579–81. https://doi.org/10.1097/00003246-200002000-00054. PMID: 10708209.
23. Fabry B, Guttmann J, Eberhard L, Bauer T, Haberthür C, Wolff G. An analysis of desynchronization between the spontaneously breathing patient and ventilator during inspiratory pres-

sure support. Chest. 1995;107:1387–94. https://doi.org/10.1378/chest.107.5.1387. PMID: 7750336.
24. Gonzalez-Bermejo J, Janssens JP, Rabec C, Perrin C, Lofaso F, Langevin B, Carlucci A, Lujan M, SomnoNIV group. Framework for patient-ventilator asynchrony during long-term non-invasive ventilation. Thorax. 2019;74:715–7. https://doi.org/10.1136/thoraxjnl-2018-213022. Epub 2019 Apr 26. PMID: 31028239.
25. Imanaka H, Nishimura M, Takeuchi M, Kimball WR, Yahagi N, Kumon K. Autotriggering caused by cardiogenic oscillation during flow-triggered mechanical ventilation. Crit Care Med. 2000;28:402–7. https://doi.org/10.1097/00003246-200002000-00019. PMID: 10708174.
26. Subirà C, de Haro C, Magrans R, Fernández R, Blanch L. Minimizing asynchronies in mechanical ventilation: current and future trends. Respir Care. 2018;63:464–78. https://doi.org/10.4187/respcare.05949. Epub 2018 Feb 27. Erratum in: Respir Care. 2019 Mar;64(3):e1. PMID: 29487094.
27. Parthasarathy S, Jubran A, Tobin MJ. Cycling of inspiratory and expiratory muscle groups with the ventilator in airflow limitation. Am J Respir Crit Care Med. 1998;158:1471–8. https://doi.org/10.1164/ajrccm.158.5.9802014. Erratum in: Am J Respir Crit Care Med 1999 Mar;159(3):1023. PMID: 9817695.
28. Thille AW, Rodriguez P, Cabello B, Lellouche F, Brochard L. Patient-ventilator asynchrony during assisted mechanical ventilation. Intensive Care Med. 2006;32:1515–22. https://doi.org/10.1007/s00134-006-0301-8. Epub 2006 Aug 1. PMID: 16896854.
29. Blanch L, Sales B, Montanya J, Lucangelo U, Garcia-Esquirol O, Villagra A, Chacon E, Estruga A, Borelli M, Burgueño MJ, Oliva JC, Fernandez R, Villar J, Kacmarek R, Murias G. Validation of the Better Care® system to detect ineffective efforts during expiration in mechanically ventilated patients: a pilot study. Intensive Care Med. 2012;38:772–80. https://doi.org/10.1007/s00134-012-2493-4.
30. Epstein SK. How often does patient-ventilator asynchrony occur and what are the consequences? Respir Care. 2011;56:25–38. https://doi.org/10.4187/respcare.01009. PMID: 21235836.
31. Vignaux L, Vargas F, Roeseler J, Tassaux D, Thille AW, Kossowsky MP, Brochard L, Jolliet P. Patient-ventilator asynchrony during non-invasive ventilation for acute respiratory failure: a multicenter study. Intensive Care Med. 2009;35:840–6. https://doi.org/10.1007/s00134-009-1416-5. Epub 2009 Jan 29. PMID: 19183949.
32. Mulqueeny Q, Ceriana P, Carlucci A, Fanfulla F, Delmastro M, Nava S. Automatic detection of ineffective triggering and double triggering during mechanical ventilation. Intensive Care Med. 2007;33:2014–8. https://doi.org/10.1007/s00134-007-0767-z. Epub 2007 Jul 5. PMID: 17611736.
33. Akoumianaki E, Lyazidi A, Rey N, Matamis D, Perez-Martinez N, Giraud R, Mancebo J, Brochard L, Richard JM. Mechanical ventilation-induced reverse-triggered breaths: a frequently unrecognized form of neuromechanical coupling. Chest. 2013;143:927–38. https://doi.org/10.1378/chest.12-1817. PMID: 23187649.
34. Murias G, de Haro C, Blanch L. Does this ventilated patient have asynchronies? Recognizing reverse triggering and entrainment at the bedside. Intensive Care Med. 2016;42:1058–61. https://doi.org/10.1007/s00134-015-4177-3. Epub 2015 Dec 16. PMID: 26676866.
35. Pham T, Telias I, Piraino T, Yoshida T, Brochard LJ. Asynchrony consequences and management. Crit Care Clin. 2018;34:325–41. https://doi.org/10.1016/j.ccc.2018.03.008. PMID: 29907268.
36. Yoshida T, Amato MBP, Kavanagh BP. Understanding spontaneous vs. ventilator breaths: impact and monitoring. Intensive Care Med. 2018;44:2235–8. https://doi.org/10.1007/s00134-018-5145-5. Epub 2018 Mar 24. PMID: 29574574.
37. Yoshida T, Nakamura MAM, Morais CCA, Amato MBP, Kavanagh BP. Reverse triggering causes an injurious inflation pattern during mechanical ventilation. Am J Respir Crit Care Med. 2018;198:1096–9. https://doi.org/10.1164/rccm.201804-0649LE. PMID: 29953244.

38. Holanda MA, Vasconcelos RDS, Ferreira JC, Pinheiro BV. Patient-ventilator asynchrony. J Bras Pneumol. 2018;44:321–33. https://doi.org/10.1590/S1806-37562017000000185. Epub 2018 Jul 6. Erratum in: J Bras Pneumol. 2018 Sep 03;: PMID: 30020347; PMCID: PMC6326703.
39. Kacmarek RM, Chipman D. Basic principles of ventilator machinery. In: Tobin MJ, editor. Principles and practice of mechanical ventilation. 2nd ed. New York: McGraw-Hill; 2006. p. 53–95.
40. Chatburn RL. Classification of mechanical ventilators. In: Tobin MJ, editor. Principles and practice of mechanical ventilation. 2nd ed. New York: McGraw-Hill; 2006. p. 37–52.
41. Tobin MJ, Yang KL, Jubran A, Lodato RF. Interrelationship of breath components in neighboring breaths of normal eupneic subjects. Am J Respir Crit Care Med. 1995;152:1967–76. https://doi.org/10.1164/ajrccm.152.6.8520764. PMID: 8520764.
42. Ranieri VM, Giuliani R, Mascia L, Grasso S, Petruzzelli V, Puntillo N, Perchiazzi G, Fiore T, Brienza A. Patient-ventilator interaction during acute hypercapnia: pressure-support vs. proportional-assist ventilation. J Appl Physiol (1985). 1996;81:426–36. https://doi.org/10.1152/jappl.1996.81.1.426. PMID: 8828695.
43. Brochard L. Pressure support ventilation. In: Tobin MJ, editor. Principles and practice of mechanical ventilation. New York: McGraw-Hill; 1994. p. 239–57.
44. Hess DR. Ventilator waveforms and the physiology of pressure support ventilation. Respir Care. 2005;50:166–86; discussion 183-6. PMID: 15691390.
45. Colombo D, Cammarota G, Alemani M, Carenzo L, Barra FL, Vaschetto R, Slutsky AS, Della Corte F, Navalesi P. Efficacy of ventilator waveforms observation in detecting patient-ventilator asynchrony. Crit Care Med. 2011;39:2452–7. https://doi.org/10.1097/CCM.0b013e318225753c. PMID: 21705886.
46. Longhini F, Bruni A, Garofalo E, Tutino S, Vetrugno L, Navalesi P, De Robertis E, Cammarota G. Monitoring the patient-ventilator asynchrony during non-invasive ventilation. Front Med (Lausanne). 2023;9:1119924. https://doi.org/10.3389/fmed.2022.1119924. PMID: 36743668; PMCID: PMC9893016.
47. Dres M, Rittayamai N, Brochard L. Monitoring patient-ventilator asynchrony. Curr Opin Crit Care. 2016;22:246–53. https://doi.org/10.1097/MCC.0000000000000307. PMID: 27070802.
48. Younes M, Brochard L, Grasso S, Kun J, Mancebo J, Ranieri M, Richard JC, Younes H. A method for monitoring and improving patient: ventilator interaction. Intensive Care Med. 2007;33:1337–46. https://doi.org/10.1007/s00134-007-0681-4. Epub 2007 May 31. PMID: 17541554.
49. Blanch L, Villagra A, Sales B, Montanya J, Lucangelo U, Luján M, García-Esquirol O, Chacón E, Estruga A, Oliva JC, Hernández-Abadia A, Albaiccta GM, Fernández-Mondejar E, Fernández R, Lopez-Aguilar J, Villar J, Murias G, Kacmarek RM. Asynchronies during mechanical ventilation are associated with mortality. Intensive Care Med. 2015;41:633–41. https://doi.org/10.1007/s00134-015-3692-6. Epub 2015 Feb 19. PMID: 25693449.
50. Sinderby C, Liu S, Colombo D, Camarotta G, Slutsky AS, Navalesi P, Beck J. An automated and standardized neural index to quantify patient-ventilator interaction. Crit Care. 2013;17:R239. https://doi.org/10.1186/cc13063. PMID: 24131701; PMCID: PMC4056567.
51. Doorduin J, Sinderby CA, Beck J, van der Hoeven JG, Heunks LM. Automated patient-ventilator interaction analysis during neurally adjusted non-invasive ventilation and pressure support ventilation in chronic obstructive pulmonary disease. Crit Care. 2014;18:550. https://doi.org/10.1186/s13054-014-0550-9. PMID: 25307894; PMCID: PMC4207887.
52. Soilemezi E, Vasileiou M, Spyridonidou C, Tsagourias M, Matamis D. Understanding patient-ventilator asynchrony using diaphragmatic ultrasonography. Am J Respir Crit Care Med. 2019;200:e27–8. https://doi.org/10.1164/rccm.201901-0054IM. PMID: 30908924.
53. Vivier E, Haudebourg AF, Le Corvoisier P, Mekontso Dessap A, Carteaux G. Diagnostic accuracy of diaphragm ultrasound in detecting and characterizing patient-ventilator asynchronies during noninvasive ventilation. Anesthesiology. 2020;132:1494–502. https://doi.org/10.1097/ALN.0000000000003239. PMID: 32205549.

54. Wittenstein J, Huhle R, Leiderman M, Möbius M, Braune A, Tauer S, Herzog P, Barana G, de Ferrari A, Corona A, Bluth T, Kiss T, Güldner A, Schultz MJ, Rocco PRM, Pelosi P, Gama de Abreu M, Scharffenberg M. Effect of patient-ventilator asynchrony on lung and diaphragmatic injury in experimental acute respiratory distress syndrome in a porcine model. Br J Anaesth. 2023;130:e169–78. https://doi.org/10.1016/j.bja.2021.10.037. Epub 2021 Nov 10. PMID: 34895719.
55. Chanques G, Kress JP, Pohlman A, Patel S, Poston J, Jaber S, Hall JB. Impact of ventilator adjustment and sedation-analgesia practices on severe asynchrony in patients ventilated in assist-control mode. Crit Care Med. 2013;41:2177–87. https://doi.org/10.1097/CCM.0b013e31828c2d7a. PMID: 23782972.
56. de Haro C, Magrans R, López-Aguilar J, Montanyà J, Lena E, Subirà C, Fernandez-Gonzalo S, Gomà G, Fernández R, Albaiceta GM, Skrobik Y, Lucangelo U, Murias G, Ochagavia A, Kacmarek RM, Rue M, Blanch L, Asynchronies in the Intensive Care Unit (ASYNICU) Group. Effects of sedatives and opioids on trigger and cycling asynchronies throughout mechanical ventilation: an observational study in a large dataset from critically ill patients. Crit Care. 2019;23:245. https://doi.org/10.1186/s13054-019-2531-5. PMID: 31277722; PMCID: PMC6612107.
57. Barr J, Fraser GL, Puntillo K, Ely EW, Gélinas C, Dasta JF, Davidson JE, Devlin JW, Kress JP, Joffe AM, Coursin DB, Herr DL, Tung A, Robinson BR, Fontaine DK, Ramsay MA, Riker RR, Sessler CN, Pun B, Skrobik Y, Jaeschke R, American College of Critical Care Medicine. Clinical practice guidelines for the management of pain, agitation, and delirium in adult patients in the intensive care unit. Crit Care Med. 2013;41:263–306. https://doi.org/10.1097/CCM.0b013e3182783b72. PMID: 23269131.
58. Tassaux D, Michotte JB, Gainnier M, Gratadour P, Fonseca S, Jolliet P. Expiratory trigger setting in pressure support ventilation: from mathematical model to bedside. Crit Care Med. 2004;32:1844–50. https://doi.org/10.1097/01.ccm.0000138561.11634.6f. PMID: 15343011.
59. Tassaux D, Gainnier M, Battisti A, Jolliet P. Impact of expiratory trigger setting on delayed cycling and inspiratory muscle workload. Am J Respir Crit Care Med. 2005;172:1283–9. https://doi.org/10.1164/rccm.200407-880OC. Epub 2005 Aug 18. PMID: 16109983.
60. Chiumello D, Polli F, Tallarini F, Chierichetti M, Motta G, Azzari S, Colombo R, Rech R, Pelosi P, Raimondi F, Gattinoni L. Effect of different cycling-off criteria and positive end-expiratory pressure during pressure support ventilation in patients with chronic obstructive pulmonary disease. Crit Care Med. 2007;35:2547–52. https://doi.org/10.1097/01.CCM.0000287594.80110.34. PMID: 17893630.
61. Tokioka H, Tanaka T, Ishizu T, Fukushima T, Iwaki T, Nakamura Y, Kosogabe Y. The effect of breath termination criterion on breathing patterns and the work of breathing during pressure support ventilation. Anesth Analg. 2001;92:161–5. https://doi.org/10.1097/00000539-200101000-00031. PMID: 11133620.
62. Stell IM, Paul G, Lee KC, Ponte J, Moxham J. Noninvasive ventilator triggering in chronic obstructive pulmonary disease. A test lung comparison. Am J Respir Crit Care Med. 2001;164:2092–7. https://doi.org/10.1164/ajrccm.164.11.2011147. PMID: 11739140.
63. Calderini E, Confalonieri M, Puccio PG, Francavilla N, Stella L, Gregoretti C. Patient-ventilator asynchrony during noninvasive ventilation: the role of expiratory trigger. Intensive Care Med. 1999;25:662–7. https://doi.org/10.1007/s001340050927. PMID: 10470568.
64. Hotchkiss JR, Adams AB, Dries DJ, Marini JJ, Crooke PS. Dynamic behavior during noninvasive ventilation: chaotic support? Am J Respir Crit Care Med. 2001;163:374–8. https://doi.org/10.1164/ajrccm.163.2.2004004. PMID: 11179109.
65. Nava S, Bruschi C, Rubini F, Palo A, Iotti G, Braschi A. Respiratory response and inspiratory effort during pressure support ventilation in COPD patients. Intensive Care Med. 1995;21:871–9. https://doi.org/10.1007/BF01712327. PMID: 8636518.
66. Yamada Y, Du HL. Analysis of the mechanisms of expiratory asynchrony in pressure support ventilation: a mathematical approach. J Appl Physiol (1985). 2000;88:2143–50. https://doi.org/10.1152/jappl.2000.88.6.2143. PMID: 10846029.

67. Mehta S, McCool FD, Hill NS. Leak compensation in positive pressure ventilators: a lung model study. Eur Respir J. 2001;17:259–67. https://doi.org/10.1183/09031936.01.17202590. PMID: 11334129.
68. Bruni A, Garofalo E, Pelaia C, Messina A, Cammarota G, Murabito P, Corrado S, Vetrugno L, Longhini F, Navalesi P. Patient-ventilator asynchrony in adult critically ill patients. Minerva Anestesiol. 2019;85:676–88. https://doi.org/10.23736/S0375-9393.19.13436-0. Epub 2019 Feb 13. PMID: 30762325.
69. Garofalo E, Bruni A, Pelaia C, Liparota L, Lombardo N, Longhini F, Navalesi P. Recognizing, quantifying and managing patient-ventilator asynchrony in invasive and noninvasive ventilation. Expert Rev Respir Med. 2018;12:557–67. https://doi.org/10.1080/17476348.2018.1480941. Epub 2018 May 31. PMID: 29792537.
70. Al Otair HA, BaHammam AS. Ventilator- and interface-related factors influencing patient-ventilator asynchrony during noninvasive ventilation. Ann Thorac Med. 2020;15:1–8. https://doi.org/10.4103/atm.ATM_24_19. Epub 2020 Jan 2. PMID: 32002040; PMCID: PMC6967144.
71. Richard JC, Carlucci A, Breton L, Langlais N, Jaber S, Maggiore S, Fougère S, Harf A, Brochard L. Bench testing of pressure support ventilation with three different generations of ventilators. Intensive Care Med. 2002;28:1049–57. https://doi.org/10.1007/s00134-002-1311-9. Epub 2002 May 30. PMID: 12185424.
72. Bonmarchand G, Chevron V, Ménard JF, Girault C, Moritz-Berthelot F, Pasquis P, Leroy J. Effects of pressure ramp slope values on the work of breathing during pressure support ventilation in restrictive patients. Crit Care Med. 1999;27:715–22. https://doi.org/10.1097/00003246-199904000-00023. PMID: 10321660.
73. Chatmongkolchart S, Williams P, Hess DR, Kacmarek RM. Evaluation of inspiratory rise time and inspiration termination criteria in new-generation mechanical ventilators: a lung model study. Respir Care. 2001;46:666–77. PMID: 11403698.
74. Chiumello D, Pelosi P, Croci M, Bigatello LM, Gattinoni L. The effects of pressurization rate on breathing pattern, work of breathing, gas exchange and patient comfort in pressure support ventilation. Eur Respir J. 2001;18:107–14. https://doi.org/10.1183/09031936.01.00083901. PMID: 11510780.
75. Prinianakis G, Delmastro M, Carlucci A, Ceriana P, Nava S. Effect of varying the pressurisation rate during noninvasive pressure support ventilation. Eur Respir J. 2004;23:314–20. https://doi.org/10.1183/09031936.03.00010203. PMID: 14979510.
76. Spahija J, de Marchie M, Albert M, Bellemare P, Delisle S, Beck J, Sinderby C. Patient-ventilator interaction during pressure support ventilation and neurally adjusted ventilatory assist. Crit Care Med. 2010;38:518–26. https://doi.org/10.1097/CCM.0b013e3181cb0d7b. PMID: 20083921.
77. Tobin MJ, Mador MJ, Guenther SM, Lodato RF, Sackner MA. Variability of resting respiratory drive and timing in healthy subjects. J Appl Physiol (1985). 1988;65:309–17. https://doi.org/10.1152/jappl.1988.65.1.309. PMID: 3403474.
78. Spieth PM, Güldner A, Huhle R, Beda A, Bluth T, Schreiter D, Ragaller M, Gottschlich B, Kiss T, Jaber S, Pelosi P, Koch T, Gama de Abreu M. Short-term effects of noisy pressure support ventilation in patients with acute hypoxemic respiratory failure. Crit Care. 2013;17:R261. https://doi.org/10.1186/cc13091. PMID: 24172538; PMCID: PMC4056040.
79. Ball L, Sutherasan Y, Fiorito M, Dall'Orto A, Maiello L, Vargas M, Robba C, Brunetti I, D'Antini D, Raimondo P, Huhle R, Schultz MJ, Rocco PRM, Gama de Abreu M, Pelosi P. Effects of different levels of variability and pressure support ventilation on lung function in patients with mild-moderate acute respiratory distress syndrome. Front Physiol. 2021;22:725738. https://doi.org/10.3389/fphys.2021.725738. PMID: 34744766; PMCID: PMC8569865.
80. Vargas M, Buonanno P, Sica A, Ball L, Iacovazzo C, Marra A, Pelosi P, Servillo G. Patient-ventilator synchrony in neurally-adjusted ventilatory assist and variable pressure support ventilation. Respir Care. 2022;67:503–9. https://doi.org/10.4187/respcare.08921. Epub 2022 Feb 28. PMID: 35228305.

81. Younes M, Puddy A, Roberts D, Light RB, Quesada A, Taylor K, Oppenheimer L, Cramp H. Proportional assist ventilation. Results of an initial clinical trial. Am Rev Respir Dis. 1992;145:121–9. https://doi.org/10.1164/ajrccm/145.1.121. PMID: 1731574.
82. Navalesi P, Hernandez P, Wongsa A, Laporta D, Goldberg P, Gottfried SB. Proportional assist ventilation in acute respiratory failure: effects on breathing pattern and inspiratory effort. Am J Respir Crit Care Med. 1996;154:1330–8. https://doi.org/10.1164/ajrccm.154.5.8912744. PMID: 8912744.
83. Younes M, Webster K, Kun J, Roberts D, Masiowski B. A method for measuring passive elastance during proportional assist ventilation. Am J Respir Crit Care Med. 2001;164:50–60. https://doi.org/10.1164/ajrccm.164.1.2010068. PMID: 11435238.
84. Younes M, Kun J, Masiowski B, Webster K, Roberts D. A method for noninvasive determination of inspiratory resistance during proportional assist ventilation. Am J Respir Crit Care Med. 2001;163:829–39. https://doi.org/10.1164/ajrccm.163.4.2005063. PMID: 11282753.
85. Farré R, Mancini M, Rotger M, Ferrer M, Roca J, Navajas D. Oscillatory resistance measured during noninvasive proportional assist ventilation. Am J Respir Crit Care Med. 2001;164:790–4. https://doi.org/10.1164/ajrccm.164.5.2102049. PMID: 11549534.
86. Giannouli E, Webster K, Roberts D, Younes M. Response of ventilator-dependent patients to different levels of pressure support and proportional assist. Am J Respir Crit Care Med. 1999;159:1716–25. https://doi.org/10.1164/ajrccm.159.6.9704025. PMID: 10351909.
87. Du HL, Ohtsuji M, Shigeta M, Chao DC, Sasaki K, Usuda Y, Yamada Y. Expiratory asynchrony in proportional assist ventilation. Am J Respir Crit Care Med. 2002;165:972–7. https://doi.org/10.1164/ajrccm.165.7.2103049. PMID: 11934724.
88. Ranieri VM, Grasso S, Mascia L, Martino S, Fiore T, Brienza A, Giuliani R. Effects of proportional assist ventilation on inspiratory muscle effort in patients with chronic obstructive pulmonary disease and acute respiratory failure. Anesthesiology. 1997;86:79–91. https://doi.org/10.1097/00000542-199701000-00012. PMID: 9009943.
89. Bigatello LM, Nishimura M, Imanaka H, Hess D, Kimball WR, Kacmarek RM. Unloadiing of the work of breathing by proportional assist ventilation in a lung model. Crit Care Med. 1997;25:267–72. https://doi.org/10.1097/00003246-199702000-00012. PMID: 9034262.
90. Appendini L, Purro A, Gudjonsdottir M, Baderna P, Patessio A, Zanaboni S, Donner CF, Rossi A. Physiologic response of ventilator-dependent patients with chronic obstructive pulmonary disease to proportional assist ventilation and continuous positive airway pressure. Am J Respir Crit Care Med. 1999;159:1510–7. https://doi.org/10.1164/ajrccm.159.5.9804130. PMID: 10228119.
91. Wrigge H, Golisch W, Zinserling J, Sydow M, Almeling G, Burchardi H. Proportional assist versus pressure support ventilation: effects on breathing pattern and respiratory work of patients with chronic obstructive pulmonary disease. Intensive Care Med. 1999;25:790–8. https://doi.org/10.1007/s001340050954. PMID: 10447535.
92. Gay PC, Hess DR, Hill NS. Noninvasive proportional assist ventilation for acute respiratory insufficiency. Comparison with pressure support ventilation. Am J Respir Crit Care Med. 2001;164:1606–11. https://doi.org/10.1164/ajrccm.164.9.2011119. PMID: 11719297.
93. Fernández-Vivas M, Caturla-Such J, González de la Rosa J, Acosta-Escribano J, Alvarez-Sánchez B, Cánovas-Robles J. Noninvasive pressure support versus proportional assist ventilation in acute respiratory failure. Intensive Care Med. 2003;29:1126–33. https://doi.org/10.1007/s00134-003-1768-1. Epub 2003 Jun 12. PMID: 12802487.
94. Zhang J, Luo Q, Chen R. Patient-ventilator interaction with noninvasive proportional assist ventilation in subjects with COPD. Respir Care. 2020;65:45–52. https://doi.org/10.4187/respcare.06430. Epub 2019 Sep 24. PMID: 31551283.
95. Rusterholtz T, Bollaert PE, Feissel M, Romano-Girard F, Harlay ML, Zaehringer M, Dusang B, Sauder P. Continuous positive airway pressure vs. proportional assist ventilation for noninvasive ventilation in acute cardiogenic pulmonary edema. Intensive Care Med. 2008;34:840–6. https://doi.org/10.1007/s00134-008-0998-7. Epub 2008 Jan 23. PMID: 18214425.

96. Grasso S, Puntillo F, Mascia L, Ancona G, Fiore T, Bruno F, Slutsky AS, Ranieri VM. Compensation for increase in respiratory workload during mechanical ventilation. Pressure-support versus proportional-assist ventilation. Am J Respir Crit Care Med. 2000;161:819–26. https://doi.org/10.1164/ajrccm.161.3.9902065. PMID: 10712328.
97. Wysocki M, Richard JC, Meshaka P. Noninvasive proportional assist ventilation compared with noninvasive pressure support ventilation in hypercapnic acute respiratory failure. Crit Care Med. 2002;30:323–9. https://doi.org/10.1097/00003246-200202000-00010. PMID: 11889302.
98. Xirouchaki N, Kondili E, Vaporidi K, Xirouchakis G, Klimathianaki M, Gavriilidis G, Alexandopoulou E, Plataki M, Alexopoulou C, Georgopoulos D. Proportional assist ventilation with load-adjustable gain factors in critically ill patients: comparison with pressure support. Intensive Care Med. 2008;34:2026–34. https://doi.org/10.1007/s00134-008-1209-2. Epub 2008 Jul 8. PMID: 18607562.
99. Xirouchaki N, Kondili E, Klimathianaki M, Georgopoulos D. Is proportional-assist ventilation with load-adjustable gain factors a user-friendly mode? Intensive Care Med. 2009;35:1599–603. https://doi.org/10.1007/s00134-009-1524-2. Epub 2009 Jun 16. PMID: 19529915.
100. Costa R, Spinazzola G, Cipriani F, Ferrone G, Festa O, Arcangeli A, Antonelli M, Proietti R, Conti G. A physiologic comparison of proportional assist ventilation with load-adjustable gain factors (PAV+) versus pressure support ventilation (PSV). Intensive Care Med. 2011;37:1494–500. https://doi.org/10.1007/s00134-011-2297-y. Epub 2011 Jul 1. PMID: 21720909.
101. Sinderby C, Beck J, Spahija J, de Marchie M, Lacroix J, Navalesi P, Slutsky AS. Inspiratory muscle unloading by neurally adjusted ventilatory assist during maximal inspiratory efforts in healthy subjects. Chest. 2007;131:711–7. https://doi.org/10.1378/chest.06-1909. PMID: 17356084.
102. Terzi N, Piquilloud L, Rozé H, Mercat A, Lofaso F, Delisle S, Jolliet P, Sottiaux T, Tassaux D, Roesler J, Demoule A, Jaber S, Mancebo J, Brochard L, Richard JC. Clinical review: update on neurally adjusted ventilatory assist–report of a round-table conference. Crit Care. 2012;16:225. https://doi.org/10.1186/cc11297. PMID: 22715815; PMCID: PMC3580602.
103. Cammarota G, Olivieri C, Costa R, Vaschetto R, Colombo D, Turucz E, Longhini F, Della Corte F, Conti G, Navalesi P. Noninvasive ventilation through a helmet in postextubation hypoxemic patients: physiologic comparison between neurally adjusted ventilatory assist and pressure support ventilation. Intensive Care Med. 2011;37:1943–50. https://doi.org/10.1007/s00134-011-2382-2. Epub 2011 Oct 18. PMID: 22005826.
104. Piquilloud L, Tassaux D, Bialais E, Lambermont B, Sottiaux T, Roeseler J, Laterre PF, Jolliet P, Revelly JP. Neurally adjusted ventilatory assist (NAVA) improves patient-ventilator interaction during non-invasive ventilation delivered by face mask. Intensive Care Med. 2012;38:1624–31. https://doi.org/10.1007/s00134-012-2626-9. Epub 2012 Aug 3. PMID: 22885649.
105. Schmidt M, Dres M, Raux M, Deslandes-Boutmy E, Kindler F, Mayaux J, Similowski T, Demoule A. Neurally adjusted ventilatory assist improves patient-ventilator interaction during postextubation prophylactic noninvasive ventilation. Crit Care Med. 2012;40:1738–44. https://doi.org/10.1097/CCM.0b013e3182451f77. PMID: 22610179.
106. Bertrand PM, Futier E, Coisel Y, Matecki S, Jaber S, Constantin JM. Neurally adjusted ventilatory assist vs pressure support ventilation for noninvasive ventilation during acute respiratory failure: a crossover physiologic study. Chest. 2013;143:30–6. https://doi.org/10.1378/chest.12-0424. PMID: 22661448.
107. Vignaux L, Grazioli S, Piquilloud L, Bochaton N, Karam O, Levy-Jamet Y, Jaecklin T, Tourneux P, Jolliet P, Rimensberger PC. Patient-ventilator asynchrony during noninvasive pressure support ventilation and neurally adjusted ventilatory assist in infants and children. Pediatr Crit Care Med. 2013;14:e357–64. https://doi.org/10.1097/PCC.0b013e3182917922. PMID: 23863816.

108. Sinderby C, Beck J. Neurally adjusted ventilatory assist in non-invasive ventilation. Minerva Anestesiol. 2013;79:915–25. Epub 2013 Apr 5. PMID: 23558763.
109. Sehgal IS, Dhooria S, Aggarwal AN, Behera D, Agarwal R. Asynchrony index in pressure support ventilation (PSV) versus neurally adjusted ventilator assist (NAVA) during non-invasive ventilation (NIV) for respiratory failure: systematic review and meta-analysis. Intensive Care Med. 2016;42:1813–5. https://doi.org/10.1007/s00134-016-4508-z. Epub 2016 Aug 25. PMID: 27562243.
110. Pettenuzzo T, Aoyama H, Englesakis M, Tomlinson G, Fan E. Effect of neurally adjusted ventilatory assist on patient-ventilator interaction in mechanically ventilated adults: a systematic review and meta-analysis. Crit Care Med. 2019;47(7):e602–9. https://doi.org/10.1097/CCM.0000000000003719. PMID: 30882481.
111. Chen C, Wen T, Liao W. Neurally adjusted ventilatory assist versus pressure support ventilation in patient-ventilator interaction and clinical outcomes: a meta-analysis of clinical trials. Ann Transl Med. 2019;7:382. https://doi.org/10.21037/atm.2019.07.60. PMID: 31555696; PMCID: PMC6736804.

Part V

Ventilatory Strategies and Procedural Measures

CPAP/BIPAP: Settings and Indications in Interventional Procedures

14

Maciej Ogonowski

14.1 Introduction

Continuous positive airway pressure (CPAP) and bilevel positive airway pressure (BIPAP) are two noninvasive ventilation techniques that have been commonly used to treat different respiratory conditions.

CPAP is a type of noninvasive treatment, where a flow generator provides a constant level of pressure to the airway, which is maintained throughout the respiratory cycle.

BIPAP is a type of positive-pressure ventilation, which provides two levels of positive pressure—inspiratory positive airway pressure (IPAP) and expiratory positive airway pressure (EPAP).

14.2 Indications for CPAP and BiPAP Therapy

CPAP therapy allows for maintaining the airway patency throughout the respiratory cycle. That is why the most common indications for CPAP therapy are moderate to severe obstructive sleep apnea (OSA) as well as mild OSA accompanied by symptoms such as sleepiness, fatigue, insomnia, or comorbid conditions like hypertension, coronary artery disease, stroke, congestive heart failure, or type 2 diabetes [1]. CPAP therapy is also a first-line treatment in central sleep apnea related to chronic heart failure [2]. While CPAP therapy can be used in obesity hypoventilation syndrome, acute respiratory failure, and neuromuscular disorders that affect pulmonary muscles, BiPAP is generally recommended for these conditions.

M. Ogonowski (✉)
Department of Pneumonology, Faculty of Medical Sciences in Katowice, Medical University of Silesia, Katowice, Poland
e-mail: mogonowski@gcm.pl

© The Author(s), under exclusive license to Springer Nature Switzerland AG 2025

K. Panda et al. (eds.), *Noninvasive Ventilatory Approaches in Interventional Procedures*, Noninvasive Ventilation. The Essentials,
https://doi.org/10.1007/978-3-032-05328-2_14

14.3 CPAP's Most Important Settings

14.3.1 Pressure

The pressure setting for CPAP devices is typically expressed in centimeters of water (cm H_2O). It is the pressure of delivered air that is necessary to maintain airway patency. Usually, it ranges between 4 and 20 cm H_2O [3], depending on the severity of patient's sleep apnea.

To determine the optimal pressure setting, a manual titration study or an auto-titration study might by conducted. In a manual titration study, CPAP is started at a low level, and then, the pressure is gradually increased until upper airway obstruction is eliminated. In an auto-titration study, an auto-titrating continuous positive airway pressure (APAP) device is used, which automatically detects respiratory events and delivers higher or lower levels of pressure. Patient uses APAP machine for a few days, and then, a physician reads the data from the device and the CPAP pressure is set to the pressure needed to eliminated 90% of obstructive events.

APAP machines may also be used for treatment—they adjust delivered pressure on a daily basis which increases patient's comfort and therefore increase patient's adherence to therapy.

It is important to note that the pressure setting should be regularly adjusted as the patient's condition evolves. That is why regular follow-up appointments are essential to monitor the patient's condition.

14.3.2 Ramp Time

This describes how long will it take for a CPAP machine to achieve the prescribed pressure settings. It should be adjusted to suit the patient's comfort, and it is normally set between 10 and 30 min. The ramp time might be disabled in certain situations, for example, if a patient wants to use the CPAP machine during daytime naps. This feature is also turned off if a physician needs to use the CPAP machine for immediate therapeutic uses, for example, in CPAP-assisted bronchoscopy.

14.3.3 Humidity

Humidity settings for CPAP machines may be tailored to prevent dryness and irritation of the patient's airway during therapy [4]. Actually, the most common reasons for low acceptance and adherence rates of CPAP therapy include its side effects such as nasal congestion or dryness of the nose or throat [5]. These factors can be largely prevented by humidifying the inspired air, which allows for a better adherence to the treatment and an improved quality of patient's life [6]. The optimal humidity level required depends on the patient's individual needs and preferences. Humidifiers are typically well tolerated. However, in certain situations, such as allergies to substances used in them or excessive mucus production in the airways, some patients may prefer not to use a humidifier.

14.4 BiPAP's Most Important Settings

14.4.1 IPAP, EPAP, Pressure Support

The range of pressure settings for inspiratory and expiratory pressures is usually between 4–30 and 2–20 cm H_2O, respectively. Pressure support (PS) is the difference between IPAP and EPAP—normally it is set between 4 and 20 cm H_2O.

14.4.2 Respiratory Rate

This is the number of breaths delivered per minute. Usually, it is set between 14 and 20 breaths/min, but the desired number of breaths varies based on the patient's underlying disease. Allowing a fewer number of breaths per minute makes the expiration phase longer, leading to more efficient removal of CO_2, which is beneficial for patients with COPD. In patients with neuromuscular diseases, this parameter is usually set to 16–20 breaths per minute. This higher rate helps prevent respiratory fatigue and ensures sufficient ventilation to support their respiratory needs. The respiratory rate is also sometimes initially set at a higher value in hyperventilated patients, as it allows for better compliance with therapy. Gradually, the physician decreases the respiratory rate to the desired level as the patient becomes accustomed to the therapy.

14.4.3 Fraction of Inspired Oxygen (FiO_2)

The FiO_2 that is delivered by BiPAP machine can be between 21% and 100%, and it is set based on patient condition in order to achieve desired oxygen saturation levels. Some BiPAP machines allow to have this parameter set fixed, while in others, FiO_2 achieved is a by-product of oxygen flow rate and the circuit that has been used.

14.4.4 Inspiratory-to-Expiratory Ratio (I:E Ratio)

The I:E ratio represents the proportions assigned to the inspiratory and expiratory phases. On BiPAP machines, it is not possible to set this parameter to a fixed value. Instead, the I:E ratio achieved is a by-product of respiratory rate and inspiration time. Typically, an I:E ratio of 1:2 to 1:3 is desired for chronic obstructive respiratory disease (COPD), while an I:E ratio of 1:1 is preferred for OHS and neuromuscular diseases [7]. This is why, in COPD cases, a shorter inspiratory time and lower respiratory rate are set, allowing for a longer expiration time. Conversely, in neuromuscular diseases, a longer inspiration time, and higher respiratory rates are chosen. The impact of inspiration time and respiratory rate on I:E ratio has been presented on Figs. 14.1 and 14.2.

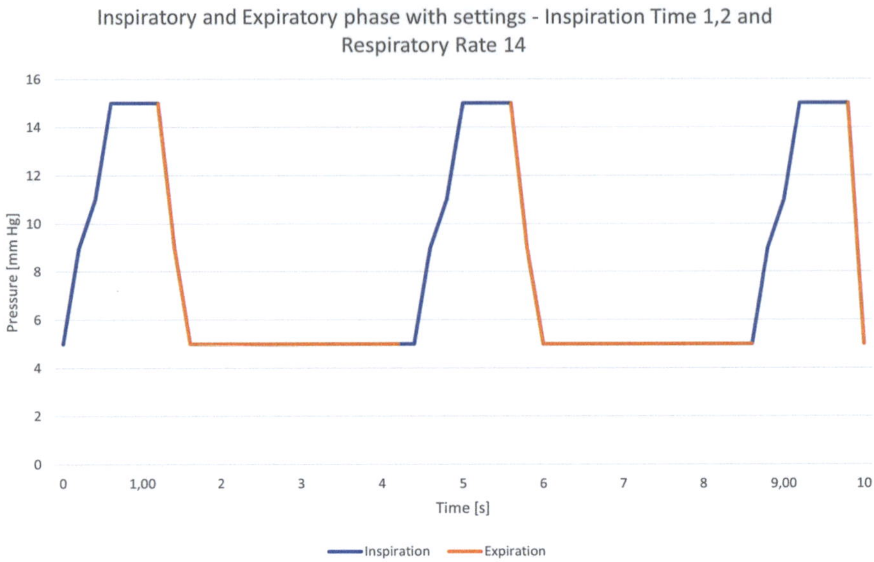

Fig. 14.1 Inspiratory and expiratory phase with settings—inspiration time 1, 2 and respiratory rate 14

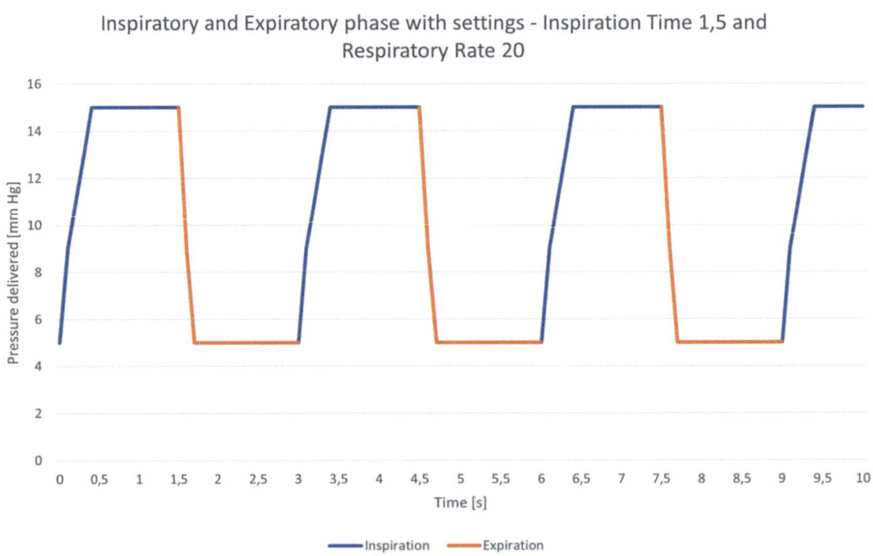

Fig. 14.2 Inspiratory and expiratory phase with settings—inspiration time 1, 5 and respiratory rate 20

14.5 CPAP and BiPAP in Interventional Procedures

- Although flexible bronchoscopy (FOB) is considered a safe procedure, it can give rise to complications such as hypoxemia, bronchospasm, and pulmonary edema. To minimize these risks, noninvasive ventilation techniques, such as CPAP or BiPAP, can be utilized. First attempts to do so date back to 1999 when Maitre et al. [8] used CPAP while performing bronchoscopy in order to reduce hypoxemia during procedure. Hypoxemic patients have been found to tolerate FOB better with CPAP than with oxygen supplementation alone. Furthermore, the incidence of subsequent respiratory complications, such as respiratory failure or the need for intubation, was much higher when patients did not receive CPAP. In the group that was supplemented with only oxygen, 4 out of 15 patients required mechanical ventilation, whereas none of the 15 patients who received CPAP required it. Notably, the use of CPAP does not extend the duration of the exam. It is usually suggested to use 5 cm H_2O pressure when using CPAP or the parameters that patient was accustomed to beforehand [9–11]. CPAP can also be used in variations of bronchoscopy such as endobronchial ultrasound-guided transbronchial needle aspiration (EBUS-TBNA). Tapan et al. [12] have demonstrated that in patients undergoing EBUS-TBNA, the group receiving nasal continuous positive airway pressure (nCPAP) in addition to oxygen demonstrated a significantly shorter mean desaturation time and a significantly higher lowest saturation compared to the control group receiving oxygen alone. BiPAP may also be used as a support for bronchoscopy—it is usually set with IPAP 8–20 cm H_2O and EPAP 8–14 cm H_2O (and adjusted accordingly to the patient's condition). FiO_2 is usually set in order to reach O_2 saturation above 90% [11, 13]. Pinto et al. [14] conducted a study that compared efficacy of FOB that was performed with CPAP vs BiPAP—results of this study suggest that there was no significant advantage of BiPAP over CPAP; however, it is worth noting that the population included in the study was relatively small (15 patients).
- Drug-induced sleep endoscopy (DISE) is a diagnostic modality utilized to assess the degree and patterns of upper airway obstruction in patients suffering from OSA [15]. DISE is performed by inducing sleep through the administration of propofol and midazolam, following which a flexible endoscope is introduced via the nostril. Subsequently, continuous positive airway pressure therapy with a face mask is initiated, with a starting pressure of 4–6 cm H_2O, and increased gradually until upper airway obstruction is reduced or a 16 cm H_2O CPAP pressure is achieved [16, 17]. This approach holds potential as an alternative to the conventional manual CPAP titration and may be employed as a diagnostic tool for exploring the reasons behind CPAP treatment failure.
- Percutaneous endoscopic gastrostomy (PEG) tube placement is a treatment offered to patients with amyotrophic lateral sclerosis (ALS) who suffer from dysphagia or accelerated weight loss. However, patients with ALS often have impaired pulmonary function and are at an increased risk of complications during the procedure. In light of this, studies have been conducted to explore the use of noninvasive ventilation (NIV) to facilitate PEG tube placement. In a study

carried out by Czell et al. [18], patients who underwent the procedure were initiated on BiPAP in spontaneous mode, with initial settings of IPAP at 15 cm H_2O and EPAP at 5 cm H_2O. These settings were then increased during the PEG placement procedure. The study found that the utilization of BiPAP was associated with a reduced rate of complications. These findings highlight the potential benefits of incorporating NIV in PEG tube placement for ALS patients with impaired pulmonary function.
- The use of CPAP has been studied for its effectiveness in treating postoperative hypoxemia and reducing postoperative pulmonary complications in patients undergoing major abdominal surgeries [19]. In a large, randomized, controlled trial, usage of CPAP, in the postoperative period of a large abdominal surgery, has been compared with standard oxygen therapy [20]. CPAP pressure in this study has been set at 7.5 cm H_2O. The results showed these patients had lower intubation rate and lower rate of pneumonia. A meta-analysis carried out by Ireland et al. [21] showed that usage of CPAP in a postoperative period in those undergoing major abdominal surgeries may reduce postoperative atelectasis, pneumonia, and reintubation rates. It is worth noting that the effects of CPAP usage on mortality is uncertain and that studies carried out so far lack the data on adverse effects of positive airway therapy in this setting.

14.6 CPAP or BiPAP

As advancements in medical knowledge and technology continue to emerge, it is foreseeable that new applications for noninvasive ventilation techniques during invasive procedures will be discovered. These developments may necessitate further exploration into the use of CPAP and BiPAP in innovative ways. Therefore, it is important to think whether physicians should use CPAP or BiPAP in the pursuit of these new solutions.

To determine whether CPAP or BiPAP is more suitable for a particular scenario, several factors need to be evaluated. These include the patient's underlying condition, the invasiveness of the procedure, the level of respiratory support required, and any potential contraindications or complications associated with each technique.

BiPAP is a method that enables control over both the inspiratory and expiratory phases. Furthermore, the transition from BiPAP in spontaneous mode to spontaneous/timed or timed mode is relatively swift. This allows physicians to promptly respond and adjust the therapy according to the patient's evolving needs. Such flexibility ensures that patients receive the appropriate level of assistance and care, promoting their overall respiratory well-being. Consequently, it is likely that in the future, BiPAP mode will be utilized more frequently to assist invasive or novel procedures. On the other hand, CPAP mode, particularly in the APAP variant, also offers advantages. It is relatively easy to set up, making it more feasible to introduce in locations lacking specialized physicians in noninvasive ventilation.

14.7 Conclusion

CPAP and BiPAP are two ventilation methods that have proven to be valuable in assisting invasive procedures. Currently, their utilization relies on expert opinions due to the absence of official guidelines in this field. To establish optimal practices, it is crucial to conduct further studies, preferably in a prospective and controlled environment, that would compare the efficacy of these methods among comparable groups of patients.

References

1. Epstein LJ, Kristo D, Strollo PJ Jr, Friedman N, Malhotra A, Patil SP, Ramar K, Rogers R, Schwab RJ, Weaver EM, Weinstein MD, Adult Obstructive Sleep Apnea Task Force of the American Academy of Sleep Medicine. Clinical guideline for the evaluation, management and long-term care of obstructive sleep apnea in adults. J Clin Sleep Med JCSM Off Publ Am Acad Sleep Med. 2009;5:263–76.
2. Aurora RN, Chowdhuri S, Ramar K, et al. The treatment of central sleep apnea syndromes in adults: practice parameters with an evidence-based literature review and meta-analyses. Sleep. 2012;35:17–40.
3. Kushida CA, Chediak A, Berry RB, Brown LK, Gozal D, Iber C, Parthasarathy S, Quan SF, Rowley JA, Positive Airway Pressure Titration Task Force; American Academy of Sleep Medicine. Clinical guidelines for the manual titration of positive airway pressure in patients with obstructive sleep apnea. J Clin Sleep Med JCSM Off Publ Am Acad Sleep Med. 2008;4:157–71.
4. Esquinas Rodriguez AM, Scala R, Soroksky A, BaHammam A, de Klerk A, Valipour A, Chiumello D, Martin C, Holland AE. Clinical review: humidifiers during non-invasive ventilation – key topics and practical implications. Crit Care. 2012;16:203.
5. Pépin JL, Leger P, Veale D, Langevin B, Robert D, Lévy P. Side effects of nasal continuous positive airway pressure in sleep apnea syndrome. Study of 193 patients in two French sleep centers. Chest. 1995;107:375–81.
6. Soudorn C, Muntham D, Reutrakul S, Chirakalwasan N. Effect of heated humidification on CPAP therapy adherence in subjects with obstructive sleep apnea with nasopharyngeal symptoms. Respir Care. 2016;61:1151–9.
7. Davidson AC, Banham S, Elliott M, et al. BTS/ICS guideline for the ventilatory management of acute hypercapnic respiratory failure in adults. Thorax. 2016;71:ii1–ii35.
8. Maitre B, Jaber S, Maggiore SM, Bergot E, Richard JC, Bakthiari H, Housset B, Boussignac G, Brochard L. Continuous positive airway pressure during fiberoptic bronchoscopy in hypoxemic patients. A randomized double-blind study using a new device. Am J Respir Crit Care Med. 2000;162:1063–7.
9. Antonelli M, Conti G, Rocco M, Arcangeli A, Cavaliere F, Proietti R, Meduri GU. Noninvasive positive-pressure ventilation vs. conventional oxygen supplementation in hypoxemic patients undergoing diagnostic bronchoscopy. Chest. 2002;121:1149–54.
10. Scala R, Naldi M, Maccari U. Early fiberoptic bronchoscopy during non-invasive ventilation in patients with decompensated chronic obstructive pulmonary disease due to community-acquired-pneumonia. Crit Care. 2010;14:R80.
11. Esquinas A, Zuil M, Scala R, Chiner E. Bronchoscopy during non-invasive mechanical ventilation: a review of techniques and procedures. Arch Bronconeumol. 2013;49:105–12.
12. Oral Tapan O, Genc S, Tertemiz KC, Ozgen Alpaydin A, Itil BO, Iyilikci Karaoglan L. The effect of oxygen application with nCPAP for the prevention of desaturation during EBUS-TBNA. Int J Clin Pract. 2021;75:e14045.

13. Sircar M, Jha OK, Chabbra GS, Bhattacharya S. Noninvasive ventilation-assisted bronchoscopy in high-risk hypoxemic patients. Indian J Crit Care Med. 2019;23:363–7.
14. Pinto T, Gonçalves M, Magalhães A, Winck JC. Efficacy of noninvasive positive pressure ventilation during fiberoptic bronchoscopy: bi-level vs CPAP valve. Eur Respir J. 2011;38:p2069.
15. Croft CB, Pringle M. Sleep nasendoscopy: a technique of assessment in snoring and obstructive sleep apnoea. Clin Otolaryngol Allied Sci. 1991;16:504–9.
16. Civelek S, Emre IE, Dizdar D, Cuhadaroglu C, Eksioglu BK, Eraslan AK, Turgut S. Comparison of conventional continuous positive airway pressure to continuous positive airway pressure titration performed with sleep endoscopy. Laryngoscope. 2012;122:691–5.
17. Dieleman E, Veugen CCAFM, Hardeman JA, Copper MP. Drug-induced sleep endoscopy while administering CPAP therapy in patients with CPAP failure. Sleep Breath Schlaf Atm. 2021;25:391–8.
18. Czell D, Bauer M, Binek J, Schoch OD, Weber M. Outcomes of percutaneous endoscopic gastrostomy tube insertion in respiratory impaired amyotrophic lateral sclerosis patients under noninvasive ventilation. Respir Care. 2013;58:838–44. https://doi.org/10.4187/respcare.02024.
19. Benditt JO. Novel uses of noninvasive ventilation. Respir Care. 2009;54:212–22.
20. Squadrone V, Coha M, Cerutti E, et al. Continuous positive airway pressure for treatment of postoperative hypoxemia. A randomized controlled trial. JAMA. 2005;293:589–95.
21. Ireland CJ, Chapman TM, Mathew SF, Herbison GP, Zacharias M. Continuous positive airway pressure (CPAP) during the postoperative period for prevention of postoperative morbidity and mortality following major abdominal surgery. Cochrane Database Syst Rev. 2014;2014:CD008930.

Nasal High-Flow Oxygen Therapy: Settings and Indications

15

Patrycja Rzepka Wrona

15.1 Introduction

Patients with hypoxemia receive oxygen supplementation, which often is provided with the use of low-flow nasal cannula (LFNC).

This method has its limitations, as it can only provide oxygen flow up to 6 L/min, which equates to maximum FiO_2 of 0.45. A greater flow results in irritation of mucosa and increase in nasal bleedings.

Flow rate through LFNC directly translates to FiO_2. To increase FiO_2, oxygen flow rate must be increased. Its another limitation is high level of gas leak as LFNC is an open system. This limits efficacy of supplemental oxygen therapy delivered with LFNC.

High-flow nasal cannula (HFNC) therapy is a system of oxygen supplementation which can deliver 21–100% heated and humidified oxygen at a flow rate of up to 60 L/min. Flow rate, FiO_2, and gas temperature can be titrated independently. HFNC allows for greater control over FiO_2 delivery than LFNC.

15.2 Objectives

- Identify the advantages of HFNC oxygen therapy.
- Identify indications for this method of oxygen therapy.
- Choose the most adequate settings for specific clinical situation.

P. R. Wrona (✉)
Department of Lung Diseases and Tuberculosis, Faculty of Medical Sciences in Zabrze, Medical University of Silesia in Katowice, Katowice, Poland

© The Author(s), under exclusive license to Springer Nature Switzerland AG 2025

K. Panda et al. (eds.), *Noninvasive Ventilatory Approaches in Interventional Procedures*, Noninvasive Ventilation. The Essentials,
https://doi.org/10.1007/978-3-032-05328-2_15

15.3 Indications for HFNC

15.3.1 Acute Hypoxemic Respiratory Failure

Pneumonia frequently leads to acute hypoxemic failure. HFNC, in this clinical setting, has several advantages based on pathophysiology of the disease:

- Flow of humidified and heated gas results in mobilization of low respiratory tract secretions, improving cough reflex and allowing for sputum suction, if needed.
- Oxygen demands are met because of precise FiO_2 titration and low leak.
- Delivery of positive end-expiratory pressure (PEEP) from flow rate up to 60 L/min improves end-expiratory lung volumes.

Patients with an acute exacerbation of chronic obstructive pulmonary disease (COPD-AE) resulting from low respiratory tract infections are a specific population, as noninvasive ventilation (NIV) was proved to reduce mortality and need for endotracheal intubation [1].

15.3.2 Community-Acquired Pneumonia (CAP)

HFNC lowers 90-day all-cause mortality, even after adjustment for disease severity, compared to NIV and standard oxygen supplemental therapy. Moreover, it reduces intubation rates in patients with severe respiratory failure ($PaO_2/FiO_2 \leq 200$) [2, 3].

15.3.3 Post-extubation

Patients who benefit from HFNC are these who have low risk of reintubation within 72 h from extubation [4], namely:

- Age < 65 years
- Acute Physiology and Chronic Health Evaluation II scale (APACHE II) < 12 when extubated
- Ventilated for < 7 days
- Are able to manage respiratory tract secretions
- Nonobese
- No airway patency issues
- Intubated for reason other than congestive heart failure
- 0–1 comorbidities

Patients treated with HFNC had significantly lower risk of reintubation compared to these treated with LFNC.

15.3.4 Preoxygenation Before Intubation

As opposed to oxygen therapy with use of a bag mask or NIV, HFNC does not need to be removed during intubation. It provides continued oxygen supplementation and, most probably, continued positive end-expiratory pressure during apneic period of intubation. HFNC is superior to LFNC as preoxygenation prior to intubation in critically ill patients [5].

15.3.5 Do-Not-Resuscitate (DNR) Patients with Respiratory Failure

DNR patients with hypoxemia and hypercapnia ($pCO_2 < 65$ mmHg) can be treated with HFNC with effective oxygenation [6]. The majority of these patients will not require escalation to NIV. HFNC is also well tolerated in this setting and can be used in end-of-life care outside the intensive care unit (palliative therapy).

15.3.6 Cardiogenic Pulmonary Edema

High-quality data regarding benefits of HFNC in this clinical setting is not abundant. However, HFNC may increase intrathoracic pressure due to PEEP and increase in end-expiratory lung volume. It is estimated that every 10 L/min of flow delivered to a patient who is breathing with mouth closed equals 1 cm H_2O of PEEP [7]. It seems reasonable to offer this treatment modality to patients unable to tolerate continuous positive airway pressure (CPAP) therapy or NIV.

15.4 HFNC Settings

Settings of HFNC may be titrated and controlled independently, to tailor the therapy according to the patient's needs and clinical settings.

15.4.1 Flow

Inspiratory demand of an adult in respiratory distress may range from 30 to 120 L/min [8], depending on the frequency of breathing and anatomical and functional dead space. Increase in flow causes washout of anatomical dead space. Therefore, a greater fraction of minute ventilation is used for gas exchange. HFNC does not increase instrumental dead space, as opposed to NIV. This is why HFNC does not require an increase in respiratory rate or tidal volume to maintain alveolar ventilation. This may explain the decrease in respiratory rate observed in patients with acute respiratory failure receiving high-flow oxygen therapy and lack of instrumental dead space may explain reduction of pCO_2.

During HFNC, CO_2 is not rebreathed, as may be the case during oxygen therapy with an oxygen mask at low flow.

As stated above, increase in flow results in an increase in PEEP. PEEP increase also depends on the size of nasal prongs and leaks resulting from lack of proper adjustment.

It is suggested to start with flow at 50 L/min, which can be either reduced or increased according to patient's tolerance.

15.4.2 Humidification and Temperature

Proper humidification and adjustment of temperature allow for the reduction in inspiratory resistance. Inhalation of cold air, both in healthy people and patients with asthma/bronchial hyperreactivity, activates osmoreceptors in nasal mucosa, which consequently induces bronchospasm through activation of muscarinic receptors [9].

Temperature should be titrated according to patient's comfort. Higher temperatures are required along with the increase in air flow.

15.4.3 FiO_2

Depending on the device type, FiO_2 can be an independently titrated parameter or a parameter which depends directly on the flow. Turbine devices supply oxygen with low-pressure system, and such devices just monitor FiO_2. An increase in flow results in reduction of FiO_2, and the other way around.

Nevertheless, FiO_2 should be titrated based on the SpO_2 target. It is recommended to maintain SpO_2 in the range of 88–92% in hypercapnic patients with COPD and hypoxemic respiratory drive, whereas in other clinical cases, SpO_2 is usually recommended to be maintained in the range of 94–96%, excluding specific clinical situations, e.g., acute respiratory failure during pregnancy.

15.5 Summary

HFNC is a valuable option of management of respiratory distress. It is well-tolerated by patients due to their ability to speak and eat during therapy. Correct use and careful bedside monitoring may reduce the risk of endotracheal intubation, invasive ventilation, and, importantly, morbidity and mortality.

References

1. Ralf E, Heine A, Obst A, et al. Acute COPD exacerbation treatment with noninvasive ventilation. Sci Rep. 2023;13:6586. https://doi.org/10.1038/s41598-023-33871-z.
2. Frat JP, Thille AW, Mercat A, et al. High-flow oxygen through nasal cannula in acute hypoxemic respiratory failure. N Engl J Med. 2015;372:2185–96.
3. Ni YN, Luo J, Yu H, et al. Can high-flow nasal cannula reduce the rate of endotracheal intubation in adult patients with acute respiratory failure compared with conventional oxygen therapy and noninvasive positive pressure ventilation? A systematic review and meta-analysis. Chest. 2017;151:764–75.
4. Hernández G, Vaquero C, González P, et al. Effect of postextubation high flow nasal cannula use conventional oxygen therapy on reintubation in low-risk patients a randomized clinical trial. JAMA. 2016;315:1354–61.
5. Ni YN, Luo J, Yu H, et al. The effect of high-flow nasal cannula in reducing the mortality and the rate of endotracheal intubation when used before mechanical ventilation compared with conventional oxygen therapy and noninvasive positive pressure ventilation. A systematic review and meta-analysis. Am J Emerg Med. 2018;36:226–33.
6. Peters SG, Holets SR, Gay PC. High-flow nasal cannula therapy in do-not-intubate patients with hypoxemic respiratory distress. Respir Care. 2013;58:597–600. http://rc.rcjournal.com/content/58/4/597.short.
7. Frat JP, Coudroy R, Marjanovic N, Thille AW. High-flow nasal oxygen therapy and noninvasive ventilation in the management of acute hypoxemic respiratory failure. Ann Transl Med. 2017;5:297.
8. Lodeserto FJ, Lettich TM, Rezaie SR. High-flow nasal cannula: mechanisms of action and adult and pediatric indications. Cureus. 2018;10:e3639. https://doi.org/10.7759/cureus.3639. PMID: 30740281; PMCID: PMC6358040.
9. On LS, Boonyongsunchai P, Webb S, Davies L, Calverley PM, Costello RW. Function of pulmonary neuronal M(2) muscarinic receptors in stable chronic obstructive pulmonary disease. Am J Respir Crit Care Med. 2001;163:1320–5.

16 Biphasic Cuirass Ventilation in Procedures

Megan M. Rashid

16.1 Introduction and Historical Perspective

Positive-pressure ventilation is ubiquitous in the hospital setting, utilized to improve oxygenation and ventilation, decrease work of breathing, improve ventilation/perfusion matching, and increase minute ventilation, particularly in the settings of acute hypoxic or hypercarbic respiratory failure or volume overload in acute systolic heart failure [1]. However, it comes with its own distinct disadvantages, as the increases in intrathoracic pressure lead to decreased venous return, increased pulmonary vascular resistance and subsequent increases in right ventricular afterload and therefore right ventricular work, and decreased left ventricular stroke volume with decreased cardiac output [2]. These hemodynamic perturbations are often poorly tolerated in the setting of cardiogenic shock or right ventricular failure, as the increased intrapulmonary pressures can worsen cardiac function [3], requiring the use of inotropes or vasopressors to help offset these effects [2]. Typically, positive-pressure ventilation can be administered noninvasively, via a face mask or nasal mask, but if clinical status does not improve relatively quickly, the patient may require endotracheal intubation and invasive mechanical ventilation. Further, some patients may not tolerate a facial mask (either due to agitation, claustrophobia, or facial deformity) [4]. Particularly in the periprocedural arena, these noninvasive administration devices can interfere with the proceduralists' positioning or access to the airway (e.g., in the bronchoscopy suite). Other options do exist, including negative-pressure ventilation devices, which are considered to be more physiologic than positive-pressure

M. M. Rashid (✉)
Department of Anesthesiology, Virginia Commonwealth University Health System, Richmond, VA, USA
e-mail: Megan.rashid@vcuhealth.org

© The Author(s), under exclusive license to Springer Nature Switzerland AG 2025

K. Panda et al. (eds.), *Noninvasive Ventilatory Approaches in Interventional Procedures*, Noninvasive Ventilation. The Essentials,
https://doi.org/10.1007/978-3-032-05328-2_16

ventilation, with robust implications in the anesthesia world, as the cuirass devices become more portable and convenient.

The medical community has been developing a usable version of a negative-pressure ventilator since the mid-1800s. The first US patent application for such a device was in 1864 [5], but the most popular version was the iron lung, with peak prevalence during the worldwide polio epidemic in the 1940s and 1950s. This technology was eventually all but phased out through the 1960s as the easier-to-deliver intermittent positive-pressure ventilation became more prominent, but many scholars agree that the decrease in physiologic derangements with negative-pressure ventilation likely has some role in medicine [6]. These bulky devices eventually evolved into the more convenient cuirass design, in which two domed plastic shells protect internal bladders, which are fitted onto the patient and connected to an external pump. The device works on a vacuum pump mechanism, in which consistent negative pressure within the cuirass causes the chest wall to expand, which decreases intrapulmonary pressure and results in air flow into the lungs [7]. Most devices in use today are biphasic and are capable of delivering both negative and positive pressure, which aids in both inhalation and exhalation and allows control over the inhalation/exhalation (I:E) ratio. Over the past two decades, we have made advances in patient monitoring, ventilator technology, and portability of increasingly flexible cuirasses, resulting in increased mentions in the literature of this mode of ventilation. The modern biphasic cuirass ventilator (BCV) is relatively easy to put on and take off a person, which is important when describing a rescue device. Gur et al. evaluated the ease of placement and initiation of ventilation of a BCV device on healthy volunteers mimicking the effects of nerve gas poisoning, half wearing protective gear and half without protective gear. They found that biphasic cuirass ventilation was easy to learn and execute even by nonmedical personnel, resulting in adequate first-pass placement on 11 out of 15 without protective gear and 8 out of 15 in protective gear, with an average of about 95 seconds for appropriate placement and initiation of adequate ventilation [8].

Modern BCVs are quite versatile, with multiple modes available for use, depending on specific pathophysiology. These ventilators can replicate most modes of positive-pressure ventilation, with the added benefit of actively assisting with expiration. They can provide controlled or synchronized biphasic mandatory ventilation, allowing for spontaneous breaths between mandatory breaths. They also can offer continuous negative pressure, which is akin to CPAP and can improve alveolar recruitment. High-frequency oscillation ventilation serves as an adjunct in hypoxic respiratory failure and can aid in pulmonary hygiene via secretions management and cough assistance. A special cardiac-cycle-synchronized mode is triggered based on EKG and has significant implications in advanced cardiac disease and timed magnetic resonance imaging of the heart [3].

16.2 Beneficial Effects of Biphasic Cuirass Ventilation

Multiple studies have examined the beneficial effects of biphasic cuirass ventilation, including McBride et al., wherein they evaluated the hemodynamic effects of intermittent mandatory ventilation and continuous negative-pressure ventilations in healthy volunteers utilizing pressure recording analytical methods (PRAM) via an arterial line [9]. They found a trend toward increased stroke volume (decreased heart rate with preserved cardiac output) and a significantly improved cardiac cycle efficiency (which describes the cardiocirculatory performance in terms of energy expenditure). Given the cardiovascular benefits of biphasic cuirass ventilation, it has also been utilized in multiple studies on the postoperative cardiac surgery population. In part two of their study of hemodynamic effects of BCV, McBride et al. utilized the same monitoring system as they intervened with BCV for 5 min in recently extubated cardiac surgery patients. They found a significant increase in stroke volume without alteration in heart rate, suggesting an increase in cardiac output [10].

The use of biphasic cuirass ventilation has been described broadly in patients with chronic pulmonary or neuromuscular disorders, including dystrophies, amyotrophic lateral sclerosis, cystic fibrosis, and central hypoventilation syndrome. The primary cause of death for this patient population is respiratory failure, usually after worsening dysphagia and inability to clear secretions, several respiratory infections, and subsequent restrictive lung disease, often requiring ongoing positive-pressure mechanical ventilation [7] and placement of tracheostomy. BCV could serve as a valuable resource toward the end of life, allowing for improvement in ventilation with concomitant improvement in quality of life (with native airway intact, able to eat, drink, and interact with people). Importantly, this also leaves them with autonomy later into their disease process, which enable them to discuss treatment options and participate in the decision-making for their own care plans, including uncomplicated discontinuation of therapy if their goals of care change [7].

In these progressive diseases, biphasic cuirass ventilation can help with weaning from temporary positive-pressure ventilation (e.g., after a course of pneumonia), delaying the need for a tracheostomy, and improving quality of life and mobility. Tada et al. discuss two cases of acute-on-chronic hypercapnic respiratory failure in patients with advanced directives inconsistent with intubation, who required injurious noninvasive positive-pressure ventilation that resulted in pneumothoraces and subsequent pneumomediastinum and subcutaneous emphysema. They were treated with a combination of noninvasive positive-pressure ventilation at lower settings assisted by concomitant biphasic cuirass ventilation to increase tidal volumes without worsening the pneumothoraces. Eventually, they were both weaned off of positive-pressure ventilation, without requiring intubation and invasive mechanical ventilation. These effects were thought to be due to improving global atelectasis and improving diaphragmatic strength over time [11].

Another population that could benefit from BCV are those with moderate to severe pulmonary hypertension secondary to chronic lung disease, as they have few options when it comes to improving symptomatology and quality of life. Most of these options are pharmaceutical, with various side effects that can limit their use, leaving an opportunity for other treatment modalities. Sato et al. studied the effects of a trial of serial intermittent biphasic cuirass ventilation sessions (1 h daily for 2 weeks) in a series of 17 patients in this population. They measured pulse oximetry before and after each daily session and performed a right heart catheterization at the beginning and end of the trial. Biphasic cuirass ventilation transiently improved oxygenation after each session and improved mean arterial pressures, pulmonary artery occlusion pressures, and pro-BNP levels at the end of the trial, all suggesting an improvement in circulatory function [12].

16.3 Risks of Biphasic Cuirass Ventilation

Though it has multiple benefits, the cuirass ventilator is not without risk. Particularly for patients who require its chronic use, the cuirass itself can cause skin breakdown, which could then act as a nidus for infection [7]. Further, sleep apnea syndrome and severe obesity do not lend themselves well to this intervention due to potential upper airway obstruction issues that the cuirass does not solve. In addition, obesity and severe kyphoscoliosis can interfere with the fit and, therefore, function of these devices, as they rely on an intact seal to function. Due to the abrupt changes in intra-thoracic and intra-abdominal pressures caused by the device, patients with rib fractures and recent abdominal surgery are not ideal candidates for BCV [4]. In the acute or periprocedural settings, it is vital to note that the airway is not secured, despite ventilation typically proceeding as planned. Therefore, the differential diagnosis of any hypoxia or hypercarbia needs to include obstruction, both by lower airway disease (e.g., bronchospasm) and upper airway issues (e.g., secretions). Monitoring of the patient can be difficult, particularly in oscillation mode, as end-tidal CO_2 is difficult to obtain, and the high-frequency oscillations interfere with pulse oximetry, EKG, and noninvasive blood pressure measurements [13].

16.4 Implications and Uses in the Hospital Setting

The potential uses for noninvasive biphasic cuirass ventilation in the acute care setting are numerous, particularly in environments with fewer resources. For example, Zitek et al. from the University of Nevada describe the use of BCV during an induction and intubation when the pulse oximetry was unreliable, with ventilation proceeding during instrumentation of airway, with transition to positive-pressure ventilation once the airway was secured [14]. Their experience could be extrapolated to any potentially difficult airway, to allow time for a surgeon to arrive at bedside prior to induction with medication or to allow the potential for awake fiberoptic intubation if needed. BCV could also be used in the setting of resuscitation, particularly in a mass casualty event. Gur et al. looked at biphasic cuirass ventilation compared to traditional bag-valve-mask ventilation in pigs in the acute phase of organophosphate poisoning. They exposed these pigs to organophosphates, then administered atropine to all of them but supported their ventilation in three different ways while waiting for recovery of muscle function. They found that mortality was significantly improved in the BCV group (0%) compared to the control group with no assistance with ventilation (67%) and the bag-mask ventilation group (71%) [15]. In this case, if one were met with a can't-intubate-can't-ventilate scenario, BCV could be used as a rescue intervention while attempting different modes of airway visualization and intubation or while waiting for the resolution of neuromuscular blockade and sedation.

This modality could theoretically revolutionize the anesthetic management of patients undergoing procedures involving manipulation of the airway, though the technique has not caught on globally. Upper airway procedures are famously difficult to manage from an anesthetic standpoint, with conflicting goals between the anesthesia team (control of the airway) and the surgical team (visualization and manual access to surgical site). Common methods utilized include intermittent ventilation via bag-mask ventilation or intermittent jet ventilation, both of which limit the time during which the surgeon can operate and can potentially lead to barotrauma or hypoventilation. However, cuirass ventilation allows for continuation of ventilation without interruption through the procedure [16]. Monks et al. describe a series of 41 patients undergoing microlaryngeal surgery during which they utilized a cuirass ventilator for its high-frequency oscillatory mode. They found no significant adverse effects, including no decrease in visualization as rated by the surgical team and no episodes of oxygen desaturations or increases in carbon dioxide tension [13].

Similar to the otolaryngology operating rooms, there are multiple opportunities for cuirass ventilation in places like the bronchoscopy suite, where the anesthesiologist's access to the airway is limited, with endotracheal intubation frequently interfering with anatomical access to the tissue the patient needs biopsied. These cases are often done with spontaneous ventilation, but patients often require a deep plane of anesthesia to blunt airway reflexes, which can lead to hypoventilation. Kanda et al. describe a series of 11 patients who received biphasic cuirass ventilation during rigid bronchoscopy in the setting of tracheal stenosis. For each patient, they measured the respiratory rate, tidal volume, and pulse oximetry saturation and found that BCV maintained oxygenation and ventilation during these procedures and was tolerated well in the setting of adequate anesthesia [17]. Further, in the more extreme cases of potential difficulty ventilating during any surgical procedure, the use of venovenous extracorporeal membrane oxygenation (ECMO) has been described to maintain oxygenation and ventilation. However, ECMO is invasive and resource-intensive, requiring heparinization (leading to increased risk of bleeding complications), an arterial line, and large bore central access (usually placed by a cardiac surgeon in the United States) and a specially trained perfusionist to run and monitor the pump. There also must be an intensive care unit with personnel credentialed in its use [16]. Hirade et al. describe a series of three patients in which they utilized biphasic cuirass ventilation as an alternative to ECMO during rigid bronchoscopy and tracheal stent placement without significant desaturations [18].

Though not well-described in the literature, the benefits of biphasic cuirass ventilation in a setting like the endoscopy suite are clear. Like the bronchoscopy suite, the proceduralist and the anesthesiologist are working in the same space, with conflicting goals—the endoscopist requires unhindered access to the esophagus for completion of the procedure, whereas the anesthesiologist would prefer more access to the airway for ventilatory support. Cuirass ventilation could provide the best of both worlds, with the added benefit of utilizing the high-frequency oscillation to help with clearance of secretions in the event of aspiration. These clearance mechanisms have been shown to be strong enough to be used during whole lung lavage under anesthesia in the setting of autoimmune pulmonary alveolar proteinosis (as an alternative to aggressive manual percussion) [19].

Another nonoperating room anesthetizing location that could benefit from cuirass ventilation is the radiation oncology suite. These interventions are not comfortable, and patients need to tolerate lying supine without moving for extended periods of time. Clinkscales et al. describe a case report in which a patient was scheduled for multiple sessions of radiation for right tonsillar squamous cell carcinoma. As his treatment progressed, he was no longer able to tolerate the supine position, and a tracheostomy was recommended for tolerance of future sessions. However, the patient wanted to try other methods first if able, so the radiation oncologists and pulmonologists worked together to recalculate the treatments for the use of a biphasic cuirass ventilator. The patient was able to complete his treatment without further issue, though the authors admit that the process was complex [20]. While this worked well in the setting of a head and neck cancer, the same method could be used for brachytherapy as well.

There are even implications for BCV to be used as a rescue in the setting of inadequate ventilation in an unplanned (or planned) general anesthetic. Sutliffe et al. describe a case report of a woman with a history of tracheal carcinoma who required radiation therapy and tracheostomy placement, with post-decannulation course complicated by severe tracheal stenosis. Her stenosis worsened during pregnancy, and she became significantly symptomatic in the third trimester. She presented to the hospital around 34 weeks with shortness of breath in the setting of an upper respiratory infection, with a computed tomography scan that showed multiple areas of tracheal stenosis, with the narrowest areas approaching 0.7 cm in diameter. The decision was made to urgently induce labor, for which neuraxial anesthesia was utilized. However, her delivery was complicated by postpartum hemorrhage requiring induction of general anesthesia for laparotomy and control of uterine bleeding. A 4.0 endotracheal tube failed to provide adequate ventilation until additional support was supplied by application of a cuirass ventilator set to high-frequency oscillation. At this point, the patient was able to be aggressively suctioned, as she had copious thick secretions affecting ventilation. Hemostasis was achieved by the surgical team, and she went through emergence and subsequent weaning from the BCV, ultimately being discharged home after about 2 weeks at her pre-pregnancy baseline [21].

In the postoperative arena, there are multiple instances of biphasic cuirass ventilation being used to facilitate weaning from a positive-pressure ventilator, often in the setting of injurious pressure support settings and subsequent barotrauma. Nishiyama et al. describe a case of a middle-aged woman with hereditary spinocerebellar degeneration in whom progressive muscle weakness resulted in a requirement for noninvasive positive-pressure requirement at home. This was complicated by the development of pneumonia requiring increasing pressure support, leading to the development of pneumothorax and acute hypercapnic respiratory failure requiring intubation with difficulty weaning from the ventilator and subsequent tracheostomy placement. Due to the pneumothorax and ongoing air leak, she had low tidal volumes despite aggressive increases in positive-pressure support, prompting the concomitant use of biphasic cuirass ventilation for both alveolar recruitment and chest physiotherapy. At the end of each daily hour-long treatment, her tidal volumes were significantly improved (189–328 mL), and after about a week, she was successfully weaned from both positive-pressure ventilation and supplemental oxygen [22].

16.5 Conclusion

As the convenience and portability of biphasic cuirass ventilation systems improve, there is an opportunity for their increased utilization. They are versatile, with implications that span the healthcare spectrum, including the medical home, prehospital, periprocedural areas, and intensive care settings.

References

1. Hore CT. Non-invasive positive pressure ventilation in patients with acute respiratory failure. Emerg Med Australas. 2002;14:281–95.
2. Corp A, Thomas C, Adlam M. The cardiovascular effects of positive pressure ventilation. BJA Educ. 2021;21:202–9.
3. Linton DM. Cuirass ventilation: a review and update. Crit Care Resusc. 2005;7:22–8.
4. Annunziata A, Calabrese C, Simioli F, Coppola A, Flora M, Marotta A, et al. Negative-pressure ventilation in neuromuscular diseases in the acute setting. J Clin Med. 2022;11:2589.
5. Jones A, et al. Improvement in vacuum apparatus for treating diseases. United States. 1864.
6. Woollam CH. The development of apparatus for intermittent negative pressure respiration. (2) 1919–1976, with special reference to the development and uses of cuirass respirators. Anaesthesia. 1976;31:666–85.
7. Onweni C, Rashid S, Goswami R, Treece J, Shipley LC, De Souza R, et al. Cuirass ventilation: an alternative home-based modality for chronic respiratory failure. Home Health Care Manag Pract. 2020;32:40–4.
8. Gur I, Eisenkraft A, Bar-Yishay E. The application of biphasic extrathoracic cuirass-assisted ventilation in normal subjects wearing chemical-biological-radiological-nuclear (CBRN) gas masks. Mil Med. 2017;182:e1801–e5.
9. McBride WT, Ranaldi G, Dougherty MJ, Siciliano T, Trethowan B, Elliott P, et al. The hemodynamic and respiratory effects of cuirass ventilation in healthy volunteers: part 1. J Cardiothorac Vasc Anesth. 2012;26:868–72.
10. McBride WT, Ranaldi G, Dougherty MJ, Siciliano T, Trethowan B, Elliott P, et al. The hemodynamic and respiratory effects of continuous negative and control-mode cuirass ventilation in recently extubated cardiac surgery patients: part 2. J Cardiothorac Vasc Anesth. 2012;26:873–7.

11. Tada M, Kadowaki T, Tsubouchi Y, Nishikawa E, Iwamoto S, Kobayashi K, et al. Concurrent use of biphasic cuirass ventilation and low-intensity noninvasive positive pressure ventilation. Clin Pulm Med. 2020;27:26–9.
12. Sato Y, Saeki N, Asakura T, Aoshiba K, Kotani T. Effects of extrathoracic mechanical ventilation on pulmonary hypertension secondary to lung disease. J Anesth. 2016;30:663–70.
13. Monks PS, Broomhead CJ, Dilkes MG, Mckelvie P. The use of the Hayek oscillator during microlaryngeal surgery. Anaesthesia. 1995;50:865–9.
14. Zitek T, Berkeley RP, Hodnick R, Davis K, Dadon N, Slattery DE. A novel technique to intubate patients without reliable pulse oximetry. Am J Emerg Med. 2018;36:2131.e1–2.
15. Gur I, Shapira S, Katalan S, Rosner A, Baranes S, Grauer E, et al. Biphasic cuirass ventilation is better than bag-valve mask ventilation for resuscitation following organophosphate poisoning. Toxicol Rep. 2015;2:40–5.
16. Mori H, Shono A, Hirade R, Nikai T, Saito Y. Biphasic cuirass ventilation during anesthesia for tracheobronchial stent insertion or removal by a rigid bronchoscope: a case report. A A Pract. 2018;10:198–200.
17. Kanda HMD. The clinical usefulness of biphasic cuirass ventilation in the prevention of hypoventilation during interventional bronchoscopy using a rigid bronchoscope. Chest. 2012;142:866A-B.
18. Hirade R, Shono A, Kanda H, Motooka A, Sakura S, Saito Y. Biphasic cuirass ventilation as an alternative to extracorporeal membrane oxygenation during tracheal stenting with rigid bronchoscope: 5AP4-1. Eur J Anaesthesiol. 2012;29:88.
19. Nakamura K, Omura S, Kajiura K, Ishigaki M. Removal of lung lavage fluid during whole-lung lavage using biphasic cuirass ventilation chest percussion in a patient with autoimmune pulmonary alveolar proteinosis. Lung India. 2019;36:540–2.
20. Clinkscales W, Spence M, Gleysteen J, Hayes N, Izaguirre E, Wakefield D, et al. Novel use of biphasic cuirass ventilation during definitive radiation therapy: a technical report. Pract Radiat Oncol. 2021;11:e276–e81.
21. Sutcliffe N, Remington SAM, Ramsay TM, Mason C. Severe tracheal stenosis and operative delivery. Anaesthesia. 1995;50:26–9.
22. Keiko Nishiyama YS, Sato T, Kodaka M, Nishimura Y, Komori M. Improvement of postoperative atelectasis in response to biphasic cuirass ventilation in a patient who was receiving non-invasive positive pressure ventilation at home. J Jpn Soc Intensive Care Med. 2012;19:247–8.

17 Pharmacology of Sedation for Noninvasive Ventilator Approaches

Habib Md Reazaul Karim

17.1 Introduction

Noninvasive ventilation (NIV) is gaining wider acceptance over time. It is being used for the management of acute respiratory failure (ARF) arising from exacerbation of chronic obstructive pulmonary disease (COPD), heart failure, cardiogenic pulmonary edema, acute hypoxemic respiratory failure, weaning from ventilation, and even for perioperative use with neuraxial anesthesia, as an adjunct for extubation and prevention of postoperative pulmonary complications [1–3]. The use of NIV for palliative care, do-not-intubate situations, home use for different causes, and even selective patients with altered consciousness has been described in the literature [4, 5]. Although noninvasive, the interface used and patient characteristics might lead to discomfort, intolerance, and even failure of NIV therapy. Studies have noted different intolerance rates ranging from 5% to 15% [6]. The intolerance rate also has been noted to differ for different interfaces. One study found the rate for nasal mask interface to be 34.3% and for facial masks to be 11.4% [7]. Such situations often require pharmacotherapy, and non-pharmacological measures might not be adequate. Sedatives have the properties to reduce anxiety and claustrophobia, and some of the sedatives also have analgesia. However, most of the pharmacological agents used have an impact on the cardiorespiratory system and consciousness level, which, on the other hand, might impact NIV therapy.

H. M. R. Karim (✉)
Anaesthesiology, Critical Care, and Pain Medicine, All India Institute of Medical Sciences, Guwahati, India

© The Author(s), under exclusive license to Springer Nature Switzerland AG 2025

K. Panda et al. (eds.), *Noninvasive Ventilatory Approaches in Interventional Procedures*, Noninvasive Ventilation. The Essentials,
https://doi.org/10.1007/978-3-032-05328-2_17

17.2 Rationale for Sedation in NIV

NIV has proven benefits over invasive ventilation in some specific disease conditions as it avoids tracheal intubation, maintains the ability to communicate, and reduces respiratory complications, sedation requirements, and hospitalization costs [8, 9]. Nevertheless, NIV requires acceptance of interface and patient cooperation. Feeling distressed due to the flow or dyspnea results in intolerance [10]. One semi-structured interview of the patients who received NIV therapy for ARF revealed that the therapy has an impact on cognitive and affective attitudes, and the patients described the therapy even as "I had the feeling that I was trapped" [11]. Intolerance leads to NIV failure, increased intubation rate, and higher mortality [10]. Sedation can reduce anxiety, promote sleep, and even modulate physiological responses to stress, facilitating NIV [12]. Therefore, cautious, titrated, and judicious use of sedation might reduce or treat the chances of NIV intolerance consequent to pain, discomfort, claustrophobia, or agitation in at-risk patients, improve success, and reduce the intubation and initiation of invasive ventilation [12].

17.3 Indication for Sedation in NIV

A recent Delphi consensus indicates that sedation should be considered in adult patients with hypoxemic or hypercapnic ARF that need to be managed for anxiety, agitation, delirium, dyspnea, and intolerance or pain [13]. A systematic review and international expert consensus also indicate that sedation pharmacotherapy should be considered only after failed non-pharmacological measures and should be used for patients with NIV intolerance due to anxiety, agitation, delirium, and pain [14].

17.4 Timing for Sedation in NIV Therapy

The current literature is inadequate to strongly suggest appropriate timing for starting sedation during NIV therapy. The Delphi consensus states that sedation can either be initiated at the start of NIV therapy to improve patient comfort and prevent intolerance or as a rescue therapy at the onset of intolerance [13]. However, the use of sedation for NIV therapy has conflicting results, especially for the impact on mortality, tracheal intubation rate, and even intolerance [14, 15]. A study found that analgosedation started within 8 h of initiation of NIV did not result in reduced intolerance or improved sedation [16]. Hence, initiation of sedation therapy as a rescue measure, especially after the application of non-pharmacological measures, appears to be the appropriate approach.

17.5 Which Drug Is Ideal?

An ideal drug should be safe, efficacious, selective in action with minimal side effects and drug interactions, easy to administer, and affordable. Applying the same principle, the ideal sedative for NIV therapy should provide effective analgosedation and still preserve ventilatory drive; promote sleep; maintain hemodynamics, airway patency, and reflexes; cause anxiolysis; and be devoid of delirium [14, 17]. It should also be widely available and easy to titrate and has a short duration of action, especially short context-sensitive half-time and organ-independent metabolism [14]. Unfortunately, the ideal drug is still theoretical, and there is still a lack of such sedative drugs for NIV therapy in current clinical practice [13, 14].

17.6 Pharmacology of Commonly Used Sedatives

A good number of drugs of different classes and mechanisms of action have been used for sedation. A few commonly used drugs are briefly mentioned below.

17.6.1 Propofol

Propofol (2,6-diisopropylphenol) is an intravenous potent hypnotic drug commonly used for induction of general anesthesia, procedural sedation, and critical care sedation. It is a γ-aminobutyric acid (GABA) receptor agonist which is an inhibitory neurotransmitter. The drug is soothing without causing any excitation phenomena and has favorable context-sensitive half-time for long-term infusion. The terminal half-life is also short and has anti-emetic, anti-nauseating action [18]. However, it is associated with bradycardia, hypotension, metabolic disturbances, and even propofol-related infusion syndrome (PRIS) when used for longer duration [18, 19]. PRIS is relatively a devastating condition, especially in children. The cumulative dose and duration play an important role. Fever, lipidemia, and hepatomegaly are commonly noted in children, but in adults, rhabdomyolysis and hyperkalemia are more frequent [19]. A mean infusion rate > 5 mg/kg/h in adults for more than 48 h is considered unsafe and a risk for PRIS [19]. The usual sedation dose for propofol is 100–150 μg/kg/min bolus, usually over 3–5 min, followed by 25–75 μg/kg/min maintenance infusion. The bolus dose should preferably be avoided in the elderly.

17.6.2 Midazolam

It is a short-acting sedative-hypnotic agent of the benzodiazepine group that increases the activity of GABA after binding with the GABA-A site, thereby suppressing neuronal excitability. It rapidly crosses the blood-brain barrier and has a wide therapeutic range. The metabolism depends highly on hepatic cytochrome P450 3A (CYP3A) enzyme activity; therefore, the pharmacokinetic and drug interaction is significantly evident in patients with CYP3A inhibitors or polymorphism [20]. The drug has an elimination half-life of 90–150 min and has an active metabolite, i.e., alpha-1 hydroxy midazolam. Although relatively cardio-stable, the drug has a significant effect on respiration and causes hiccups, nausea, and even delirium. Long-duration use is also associated with partially reversible memory loss. Acute angle-closure glaucoma is considered a contraindication for use, and the dose needs to be titrated closely in renal failure, hepatic failure, elderly, hypotensive patients, etc. [21]. The usual adult dose for intravenous sedation infusion is 0.3–1 μg/kg/min. A 1–2.5 mg bolus can be administered in healthy adults before initiating infusion and titration.

17.6.3 Fentanyl

Fentanyl is a potent synthetic opioid analgesic that also has a sedative effect. It exerts its action primarily through agonist activity at the μ-opioid receptor. Opioids also cause inhibition of periaqueductal gray GABAergic neurons and brainstem cholinergic circuits, thereby decreasing arousal and promoting sleep [22]. The drug is metabolized by the hepatic enzyme CYP3A, and the terminal elimination half-life is nearly 220–850 min. Increasing context-sensitive half-time is an issue with prolonged infusion [23]. The primary metabolite is norfentanyl, which is neither toxic nor active. Like midazolam, a drug interaction is evident with those inhibiting CYP3A, and the response is variable in patients with CYP3A polymorphism. Nausea, vomiting, itching, respiratory depression, and bradycardia are notable adverse events. The usual bolus dose is 0.5 μg/kg, followed by a maintenance dose of 1–7 μg/kg/h [24, 25]. Opioid-naïve patients usually require lower doses. Sepsis patients with acute kidney injury may predispose to overdosing and impacting ventilation, especially if on adaptive support ventilation [26].

17.6.4 Morphine

Morphine is a naturally occurring alkaloid that also acts through the μ-opioid receptor present in the brainstem and thalamus to produce analgesia and sedation. The elimination half-life is 2–3 h. A good amount of the drug is secreted unchanged in the urine, and it is metabolized in the liver to morphine-3 and morphine-6 glucuronide, which are pharmacologically active and have a longer duration of action. Some amount of metabolism is also noted in the kidney [27]. Therefore, both liver and hepatic dysfunction can impact the morphine pharmacokinetics. Intravenous administration releases a significant amount of histamine causing hypotension. Other significant side effects that might impact NIV therapy are respiratory depression, nausea, and vomiting. A bolus dose of 2.5–5 mg is advocated for sedation during NIV [28]. The usual dose for infusion in critical care for sedation is 10–100 μg/kg/h [29].

17.6.5 Remifentanil

Remifentanil is another synthetic highly potent μ-opioid receptor agonist with a fast onset and a short elimination half-life, i.e., 3–10 min. The metabolism is independent of renal or hepatic systems and is metabolized by plasma cholinesterases. Even the context-sensitive half-time is independent of infusion duration and is three to four in volunteers and patients, respectively [30]. Shortness of breath, blurred vision, light-headedness, chest pain, confusion, etc., are common side effects that might impact the NIV therapy. Although the drug has many favorable features as a sedative, the cost is a deterrent for routine use, especially in developing nations. A low dose of 0.05 μg/kg/min is usually enough to maintain analgosedation [31]. Another study determined the mean dose required for sedation during NIV as 0.1 ± 0.03 μg/kg/min [32]. A 1 μg/kg bolus can be administered over 30–60 min before.

17.6.6 Dexmedetomidine

Dexmedetomidine is a selective α2-adrenoreceptor agonist with an α2:α1 ratio of 1620:1. It has sedative, anxiolytic, and analgesic effects potentially beneficial during NIV intolerance. The sedation is produced through activation of α_2-receptors in the locus coeruleus, inducing a state mimicking natural sleep [33]. Although bolus administration leads to transient hypertension, it is a sympatholytic agent that results in significant bradycardia and hypotension. Patients on beta-blockers might have exaggerated hypotension and bradycardia. The drug, however, has minimal or no depression of respiratory function. The mean elimination half-life in healthy subjects is 2.5 h and can be as prolonged as 7.4 h in severe hepatic dysfunction [33]. The usual dose for sedation is 0.5–1 μg/kg bolus over 20 min, followed by 0.2–0.7 μg/kg/min infusion.

17.6.7 Ketamine

Ketamine exerts its analgesic, amnesic, and psychosensory action essentially through antagonism of the N-methyl D-aspartate receptor. It also potentializes GABA-A complex and acts on opioid receptors. However, the effect of such interaction resulting in analgesia is uncertain [34]. The drug is primarily metabolized in the liver to norketamine, which is also an active compound; the kidneys, intestines, and even lungs are also involved in the metabolism of the drugs. Kidney dysfunction has minimal impact on the ketamine pharmacokinetics, but drugs inducing cytochromes P450 system might lead to rapid metabolism. Elimination half-life is 2–3 h and depends on the liver's blood flow [34]. The usual starting dose is 0.5 mg/kg/h titrated to effect and usually requires 1–3 mg/kg/h. A dosage above 2.25 mg/kg/h usually results in adverse events like tachyarrhythmia and agitation [35]. Increases in secretion are also another concern during NIV therapy. Interestingly, ketamine preserves the pharyngeal and airway reflexes.

17.6.8 Remimazolam

Remimazolam is an ultrashort-acting benzodiazepine. Like other benzodiazepines, it acts through the GABA-A receptor to induce cell membrane hyperpolarization, thereby inhibiting neural activity. It has rapid onset, short duration of action, and predictable recovery. It also has organ-independent metabolism and undergoes rapid hydrolysis by nonspecific tissue esterase to inactivate metabolites [36]. The terminal elimination half-life in the compartmental model is shown as 60–80 min, recovery time is 10 min, and the context-sensitive half-time was 6.8 ± 2.4 min after 4 h infusion [37]. Hypotension, delayed emergence, re-sedation, anaphylaxis, blurred vision, headache, chest discomfort, and nausea are notable side effects that might impact the NIV therapy [38].

17.7 Effect of Sedatives on Human Organ Systems

A different group of sedative drugs has a different effect on the respiration. Opioids decrease the respiratory rate in both ventilated and non-ventilated patients. The reduction rate was higher in ventilated patients (95% CI 12–24% versus 15–37%) [39]. Propofol and benzodiazepines reduced the tidal volumes; propofol reduced it more (95% CI 17–40% versus 20–52%,) in spontaneously breathing patients. There was no change in tidal volume in assisted patients [39]. Compared to the placebo, dexmedetomidine did not significantly reduce the respiratory rate and saturation in surgical patients receiving ventilation; the partial pressure of oxygen to a fraction of inspired oxygen ratio was, however, better in dexmedetomidine [40]. Ketamine also has little or no effect on the tidal volume or respiratory rate; however, it has been shown to improve the inspiratory flow [39, 41]. Dexmedetomidine and propofol have also been noted to impair the hypoxic control of breathing in healthy volunteers and rarely even cause central apnea [42].

17.8 Which Agent Is Better?

Current literature is insufficient to indicate the best sedative agent for NIV therapy. A prospective randomized study comparing dexmedetomidine, remifentanil, and propofol sedation in patients intolerant to NIV therapy found that NIV failure, mortality, and length of stay were reduced with dexmedetomidine [43]. International expert opinion, the Delphi consensus, also favors dexmedetomidine as the emerging better choice [13, 14]. A recent meta-analysis also shows that compared to any other sedative and placebo, dexmedetomidine reduces the risk of delirium and the need for mechanical ventilation in acutely ill adults requiring NIV [44, 45]. However, dexmedetomidine also showed a higher risk of bradycardia and hypotension [44]. Contrarily, a retrospective study investigating data from 4,33,357 sedation shows higher odds of intubation and mortality with either dexmedetomidine alone or in combination with other agents as compared to opioids and benzodiazepines [15].

The retrospective study also noted that significant numbers of patients required more than one drug in different combinations [15]. A similar result was noted during the COVID-19 pandemic [46]. On the other hand, a recent multicenter randomized study enrolling post-cardiac surgical patients with NIV intolerance found that remifentanil might be better than dexmedetomidine [47]. Nevertheless, whatever drug is used, a protocolized and titrated use should be practiced [13, 14].

17.9 Sedation Scale, Optimal Sedation, and Sedative Drug Interactions

Many sedation scales are in clinical use; Richmond Agitation-Sedation Scale (RASS) is a structured, objective assessment that scales the agitation level and possible sedation. The scale uses terms and scores them with different scores from "+4 combative" to "−5 unarousable." The score is widely used and has been used to be reliable in medical, surgical, neuroscience, and coronary critical care patients. The score also showed excellent inter-rater reliability among physicians, nurses, and pharmacists [48]. Optimal sedation is a matter of debate. While multicenter observation studies with risk-adjusted regression analysis show that deeper sedation within the first 48 h in critically ill patients is associated with increased length of mechanical ventilation and hospital stay, the recent meta-analysis and trial sequential analysis of 4352 patients' data from 15 randomized trials found no difference between light and deeper sedation [49, 50]. The meta-analysis found similar serious adverse effects, delirium, and all-cause mortality [50]. Nevertheless, current guidelines and expert opinion advocate light sedation corresponding to RASS "0 to −2" and even "+1 to −2" by some researchers and guidelines [14, 51, 52]. While the meta-analysis did not show differences in serious side effects, the physician should keep the drug interactions in mind, especially when using multiple sedatives. For example, benzodiazepines and opioids may interact and produce exaggerated respiratory depression. Pharmacokinetics and dynamics of sedatives may also be affected by substances like alcohol. Further, antihistamines and other antidepressants influencing serotonin levels may also interact. Furthermore, drug metabolism at the hepatic enzyme levels may also affect the drug metabolisms of the drugs metabolized by hepatic oxidative pathways [53, 54].

17.10 Conclusion

Pharmacological sedation during NIV therapy is a double-edged sword. Rescue sedation for NIV intolerance appears to be the most appropriate use of sedation pharmacotherapy. The pharmacokinetics of individual drugs are critical, and the same appears to be favorable for dexmedetomidine and remifentanil sedation during NIV. Evidence for remimazolam sedation needs to be further studied. Nonetheless, all sedation must be protocolized and titrated to the desired effect.

References

1. Rochwerg B, Brochard L, Elliott MW, et al. Official ERS/ATS clinical practice guidelines: noninvasive ventilation for acute respiratory failure. Eur Respir J. 2017;50:1602426. https://doi.org/10.1183/13993003.02426-2016.
2. Corcione N, Karim H, Mina B, et al. Non-invasive ventilation during surgery under neuraxial anaesthesia: a pathophysiological perspective on application and benefits and a systematic literature review. Anaesthesiol Intensive Ther. 2019;51:289–98. https://doi.org/10.5114/ait.2019.88572.
3. Karim HMR, Agha M, Esquinas AM. Adjunct to extubation-noninvasive mechanical ventilation. In: Esquinas AM, Min B, Spadaro S, et al., editors. Pharmacology in noninvasive ventilation. Noninvasive ventilation. The essentials. Cham: Springer; 2023. p. 443–53. https://doi.org/10.1007/978-3-031-44626-9_43.
4. Diaz de Teran T, Barbagelata E, Cilloniz C, et al. Non-invasive ventilation in palliative care: a systematic review. Minerva Med. 2019;110:555–63. https://doi.org/10.23736/S0026-4806.19.06273-6.
5. Gonçalves G, Saeed H, Abdelrahim ME, et al. Non-invasive ventilation in patients with an altered level of consciousness. A clinical review and practical insights. Adv Respir Med. 2020;88:233–44. https://doi.org/10.5603/ARM.2020.0110.
6. Dres M, Demoule A. Noninvasive ventilation: do not tolerate intolerance. Respir Care. 2016;61:393–4. https://doi.org/10.4187/respcare.04693.
7. Kwok H, McCormack J, Cece R, Houtchens J, Hill NS. Controlled trial of oronasal versus nasal mask ventilation in the treatment of acute respiratory failure. Crit Care Med. 2003;31:468–73. https://doi.org/10.1097/01.CCM.0000045563.64187.20.
8. Luo F, Annane D, Orlikowski D, et al. Invasive versus non-invasive ventilation for acute respiratory failure in neuromuscular disease and chest wall disorders. Cochrane Database Syst Rev. 2017;12:CD008380. https://doi.org/10.1002/14651858.CD008380.pub2.
9. Lindenauer PK, Stefan MS, Shieh MS, Pekow PS, Rothberg MB, Hill NS. Outcomes associated with invasive and noninvasive ventilation among patients hospitalized with exacerbations of chronic obstructive pulmonary disease. JAMA Intern Med. 2014;174:1982–93. https://doi.org/10.1001/jamainternmed.2014.5430.
10. Liu J, Duan J, Bai L, Zhou L. Noninvasive ventilation intolerance: characteristics, predictors, and outcomes. Respir Care. 2016;61:277–84. https://doi.org/10.4187/respcare.04220.
11. Iosifyan M, Schmidt M, Hurbault A, et al. “I had the feeling that I was trapped”: a bedside qualitative study of cognitive and affective attitudes toward noninvasive ventilation in patients with acute respiratory failure. Ann Intensive Care. 2019;9:134. https://doi.org/10.1186/s13613-019-0608-6.
12. Cammarota G, Simonte R, De Robertis E. Comfort during non-invasive ventilation. Front Med (Lausanne). 2022;9:874250. https://doi.org/10.3389/fmed.2022.874250. Erratum in: Front Med (Lausanne) 2023 Apr 4;10:1193466. doi: 10.3389/fmed.2023.1193466.
13. Spinazzola G, Spadaro S, Ferrone G, et al. Management of analgosedation during noninvasive respiratory support: an expert Delphi consensus document developed by the Italian Society of Anesthesia, Analgesia, Resuscitation and Intensive Care (SIAARTI). J Anesth Analg Crit Care. 2024;4:68. https://doi.org/10.1186/s44158-024-00203-0.
14. Karim HMR, Šarc I, Calandra C, Spadaro S, Mina B, Ciobanu LD, et al. Role of sedation and analgesia during noninvasive ventilation: systematic review of recent evidence and recommendations. Indian J Crit Care Med. 2022;26:938–48.
15. Dunbar PJ, Peterson R, McGrath M, et al. Analgesia and sedation use during noninvasive ventilation for acute respiratory failure. Crit Care Med. 2024;52:1043–53. https://doi.org/10.1097/CCM.0000000000006253.
16. Devlin JW, Al-Qadheeb NS, Chi A, et al. Efficacy and safety of early dexmedetomidine during noninvasive ventilation for patients with acute respiratory failure: a randomised, double-

blind, placebo-controlled pilot study. Chest. 2014;145:1204–12. https://doi.org/10.1378/chest.13-1448.
17. Longrois D, Conti G, Mantz J, Faltlhauser A, Aantaa R, Tonner P. Sedation in noninvasive ventilation: do we know what to do (and why)? Multidiscip Respir Med. 2014;9:56. https://doi.org/10.1186/2049-6958-9-56.
18. Sahinovic MM, Struys MMRF, Absalom AR. Clinical pharmacokinetics and pharmacodynamics of propofol. Clin Pharmacokinet. 2018;57:1539–58. https://doi.org/10.1007/s40262-018-0672-3.
19. Hemphill S, McMenamin L, Bellamy MC, Hopkins PM. Propofol infusion syndrome: a structured literature review and analysis of published case reports. Br J Anaesth. 2019;122:448–59. https://doi.org/10.1016/j.bja.2018.12.025.
20. Peter JU, Dieudonné P, Zolk O. Pharmacokinetics, pharmacodynamics, and side effects of midazolam: a review and case example. Pharmaceuticals (Basel). 2024;17:473. https://doi.org/10.3390/ph17040473. PMID: 38675433; PMCID: PMC11054797.
21. Lingamchetty TN, Hosseini SA, Saadabadi A. Midazolam. [Updated 2023 Jun 5]. In: StatPearls [Internet]. Treasure Island: StatPearls Publishing, Available from: https://www.ncbi.nlm.nih.gov/books/NBK537321/.; 2024.
22. Montandon G, Horner RL. Electrocortical changes associating sedation and respiratory depression by the opioid analgesic fentanyl. Sci Rep. 2019;9:14122. https://doi.org/10.1038/s41598-019-50613-2.
23. Bird HE, Huhn AS, Dunn KE. Fentanyl absorption, distribution, metabolism, and excretion: narrative review and clinical significance related to illicitly manufactured fentanyl. J Addict Med. 2023;17:503–8. https://doi.org/10.1097/ADM.0000000000001185.
24. Muellejans B, Matthey T, Scholpp J, Schill M. Sedation in the intensive care unit with remifentanil/propofol versus midazolam/fentanyl: a randomised, open-label, pharmacoeconomic trial. Crit Care. 2006;10:R91. https://doi.org/10.1186/cc4939.
25. Gish EC, Harrison D, Gormley AK, Johnson PN. Dosing evaluation of continuous intravenous fentanyl infusions in overweight children: a pilot study. J Pediatr Pharmacol Ther. 2011;16:39–46.
26. Kukanti C, Karim HMR, Panda CK, Jain A. Fentanyl infusion in a multi-organ failure patient on adaptive support ventilation: a conundrum. Anaesth Pain Intensive Care. 2024;28:608–10. https://doi.org/10.35975/apic.v28i3.2044.
27. Christrup LL. Morphine metabolites. Acta Anaesthesiol Scand. 1997;41:116–22. https://doi.org/10.1111/j.1399-6576.1997.tb04625.x.
28. Davidson C, Banham S, Elliott M, et al. British Thoracic Society/Intensive Care Society Guideline for the ventilatory management of acute hypercapnic respiratory failure in adults. BMJ Open Respir Res. 2016;3:e000133. https://doi.org/10.1136/bmjresp-2016-000133.
29. Barr J, Fraser GL, Puntillo K, et al. Clinical practice guidelines for the management of pain, agitation, and delirium in adult patients in the intensive care unit. Crit Care Med. 2013;41:263–306. https://doi.org/10.1097/CCM.0b013e3182783b72.
30. Egan TD. Remifentanil pharmacokinetics and pharmacodynamics. Clin Pharmacokinet. 1995;29:80–94. https://doi.org/10.2165/00003088-199529020-00003.
31. Cavaliere F, Antonelli M, Arcangeli A, et al. A low-dose remifentanil infusion is well tolerated for sedation in mechanically ventilated, critically-ill patients. Can J Anaesth. 2002;49:1088–94. https://doi.org/10.1007/BF03017909. PMID: 12477685.
32. Constantin JM, Schneider E, Cayot-Constantin S, et al. Remifentanil-based sedation to treat noninvasive ventilation failure: a preliminary study. Intensive Care Med. 2007;33:82–7. https://doi.org/10.1007/s00134-006-0447-4.
33. Weerink MAS, Struys MMRF, Hannivoort LN, Barends CRM, Absalom AR, Colin P. Clinical pharmacokinetics and pharmacodynamics of dexmedetomidine. Clin Pharmacokinet. 2017;56:893–913. https://doi.org/10.1007/s40262-017-0507-7.
34. Mion G, Villevieille T. Ketamine pharmacology: an update (pharmacodynamics and molecular aspects, recent findings). CNS Neurosci Ther. 2013;19:370–80. https://doi.org/10.1111/cns.12099.

35. Umunna BP, Tekwani K, Barounis D, Kettaneh N, Kulstad E. Ketamine for continuous sedation of mechanically ventilated patients. J Emerg Trauma Shock. 2015;8:11–5. https://doi.org/10.4103/0974-2700.145414.
36. Kim KM. Remimazolam: pharmacological characteristics and clinical applications in anesthesiology. Anesth Pain Med (Seoul). 2022;17:1–11. https://doi.org/10.17085/apm.21115.
37. Schüttler J, Eisenried A, Lerch M, Fechner J, Jeleazcov C, Ihmsen H. Pharmacokinetics and pharmacodynamics of remimazolam (CNS 7056) after continuous infusion in healthy male volunteers: part I. Pharmacokinetics and clinical pharmacodynamics. Anesthesiology. 2020;132:636–51.
38. Kempenaers S, Hansen TG, Van de Velde M. Remimazolam and serious adverse events: a scoping review. Eur J Anaesthesiol. 2023;40:841–53. https://doi.org/10.1097/EJA.0000000000001902.
39. Quickfall D, Sklar MC, Tomlinson G, Orchanian-Cheff A, Goligher EC. The influence of drugs used for sedation during mechanical ventilation on respiratory pattern during unassisted breathing and assisted mechanical ventilation: a physiological systematic review and meta-analysis. EClinicalMedicine. 2024;68:102417. https://doi.org/10.1016/j.eclinm.2023.102417.
40. Venn RM, Hell J, Grounds RM. Respiratory effects of dexmedetomidine in the surgical patient requiring intensive care. Crit Care. 2000;4:302–8. https://doi.org/10.1186/cc712.
41. Suleiman A, Santer P, Munoz-Acuna R, et al. Effects of ketamine infusion on breathing and encephalography in spontaneously breathing ICU patients. J Intensive Care Med. 2023;38:299–306. https://doi.org/10.1177/08850666221119716.
42. Lodenius Å, Ebberyd A, Hårdemark Cedborg A, et al. Sedation with dexmedetomidine or propofol impairs hypoxic control of breathing in healthy male volunteers: a nonblinded, randomized crossover study. Anesthesiology. 2016;125:700–15. https://doi.org/10.1097/ALN.0000000000001236.
43. Altınkaya Çavuş M, Gökbulut Bektaş S, Turan S. Comparison of clinical safety and efficacy of dexmedetomidine, remifentanil, and propofol in patients who cannot tolerate non-invasive mechanical ventilation: a prospective, randomized, cohort study. Front Med (Lausanne). 2022;9:995799. https://doi.org/10.3389/fmed.2022.995799.
44. Lewis K, Piticaru J, Chaudhuri D, et al. Safety and efficacy of dexmedetomidine in acutely ill adults requiring noninvasive ventilation: a systematic review and meta-analysis of randomized trials. Chest. 2021;159:2274–88. https://doi.org/10.1016/j.chest.2020.12.052.
45. Yang B, Gao L, Tong Z. Sedation and analgesia strategies for non-invasive mechanical ventilation: a systematic review and meta-analysis. Heart Lung. 2024;63:42–50. https://doi.org/10.1016/j.hrtlng.2023.09.005.
46. Nayak P, Karim HMR. Requirement and response pattern for sedatives in COVID-19 patients requiring non–invasive ventilation: a pilot observation. Anaesth Pain Intensive Care. 2022;26:260–2. https://doi.org/10.35975/apic.v26i2.1809.
47. Hao GW, Wu JQ, Yu SJ, et al. Remifentanil vs. dexmedetomidine for cardiac surgery patients with noninvasive ventilation intolerance: a multicenter randomized controlled trial. J Intensive Care. 2024;12:35. https://doi.org/10.1186/s40560-024-00750-2.
48. Sessler CN, Gosnell MS, Grap MJ, Brophy GM, O'Neal PV, Keane KA, Tesoro EP, Elswick RK. The Richmond agitation-sedation scale: validity and reliability in adult intensive care unit patients. Am J Respir Crit Care Med. 2002;166:1338–44. https://doi.org/10.1164/rccm.2107138. PMID: 12421743.
49. Shehabi Y, Chan L, Kadiman S, Alias A, Ismail WN, Tan MA, et al. Sedation depth and long-term mortality in mechanically ventilated critically ill adults: a prospective longitudinal multicentre cohort study. Intensive Care Med. 2013;39:910–8. https://doi.org/10.1007/s00134-013-2830-2. Epub 2013 Jan 24. PMID: 23344834; PMCID: PMC3625407.
50. Ceric A, Holgersson J, May TL, Skrifvars MB, Hästbacka J, Saxena M, et al. Effect of level of sedation on outcomes in critically ill adult patients: a systematic review of clinical trials with meta-analysis and trial sequential analysis. EClinicalMedicine. 2024;71:102569. https://doi.org/10.1016/j.eclinm.2024.102569. PMID: 38572080; PMCID: PMC10990717.
51. Devlin JW, Skrobik Y, Gélinas C, Needham DM, Slooter AJC, Pandharipande PP, et al. Clinical practice guidelines for the prevention and management of pain, agitation/sedation, delirium,

immobility, and sleep disruption in adult patients in the ICU. Crit Care Med. 2018;46:e825–73. https://doi.org/10.1097/CCM.0000000000003299. PMID: 30113379.
52. Seo Y, Lee HJ, Ha EJ, Ha TS. 2021 KSCCM clinical practice guidelines for pain, agitation, delirium, immobility, and sleep disturbance in the intensive care unit. Acute Crit Care. 2022;37:1–25. https://doi.org/10.4266/acc.2022.00094. Epub 2022 Feb 28. PMID: 35279975; PMCID: PMC8918705.
53. Cushman P Jr. Sedative drug interactions of clinical importance. Recent Dev Alcohol. 1986;4:61–83. https://doi.org/10.1007/978-1-4899-1695-2_3.
54. Wang JS, DeVane CL. Pharmacokinetics and drug interactions of the sedative hypnotics. Psychopharmacol Bull. 2003;37:10–29.

Part VI

NIV Procedures: Patients Selection

18 High-Risk Patients Undergoing Sedation: Risk Factors and High Impact Comorbidities

Ewa Trejnowska

Procedural sedation (PS) includes techniques, medications, and maneuvers to help patients tolerate unpleasant or painful procedures and avoid unwanted procedure-associated memories [1, 2]. Since PS also aims to decrease pain perception and is generally obtained through administering analgesics combined with a sedative, PS can be considered procedural sedation analgesia (PSA) [2]. According to the American College of Emergency Physicians (ACEP), PS is a "technique of administering sedatives or dissociative agents with or without analgesics to induce a state that allows the patient to tolerate unpleasant procedures while maintaining cardiorespiratory function" [3].

Due to patients' varying sensitivities to medications and pre-existing comorbidities, they may slip to a deeper sedation level than anticipated. The American Society of Anesthesiologists (ASA) defined four levels of sedation, [4, 5] where level four corresponds to general anesthesia. Practically, the most commonly accepted terms for sedation depth are as follows:

- Minimal, or *anxiolysis*, in which the patient remains awake but relaxed and able to interact.
- Moderate, also termed *conscious sedation*, is when the patient has depressed consciousness but responds to verbal requests or reacts to touch. Breathing remains intact, and no support is needed.
- Deep, wherein the patient cannot be easily aroused but responds to repeated or painful stimuli. Breathing may be impaired and may need to be supported.
- Dissociative is a trance-like state wherein the patient remains awake but unaware of the pain and retains no memory of the event. They can follow commands, and their airway reflexes remain intact [2].

E. Trejnowska (✉)
Department of Cardiac Anaesthesia and Intensive Care, Silesian Centre for Heart Diseases in Zabrze, Faculty of Medical Sciences in Zabrze, Medical University of Silesia, Katowice, Poland

© The Author(s), under exclusive license to Springer Nature Switzerland AG 2025

K. Panda et al. (eds.), *Noninvasive Ventilatory Approaches in Interventional Procedures*, Noninvasive Ventilation. The Essentials,
https://doi.org/10.1007/978-3-032-05328-2_18

Although differences between the first two levels of sedation are not always evident, there is a higher risk of life-threatening adverse events mandating immediate and appropriate management whenever a patient reaches a deeper sedation level (levels 3 or 4).

18.1 Patients with Cardiovascular Diseases: General Principles

Taking a history, physical examination, and a preoperative risk assessment is recommended for patients undergoing planned noncardiac surgery (NCS), preferably at the NCS proposal. The initial evaluation should emphasize cardiovascular risk factors, diagnosed cardiovascular disease (CVD), and comorbidities. In addition, standard laboratory tests should be requested for those undergoing surgery with intermediate or high risk, with further risk assessment made based on the information gathered.

Depending on the risk associated with the patient and the surgery, electrocardiogram (ECG) recording, physical fitness assessment, or determination of biomarkers, including cardiac troponins and/or B-type natriuretic peptide (BNP)/N-terminal fragment of BNP propeptide (NT-proBNP), is recommended. If time permits, CVD treatment and cardiovascular risk factors should be optimized before NCS using relevant guidelines. Consideration should also be given to endovascular or videoendoscopic procedures for high cardiovascular risk patients undergoing vascular or pulmonary surgery, as they have a lower risk of perioperative complications.

The general principle is to cancel or postpone outpatient procedures requiring sedation for patients with serious and unstable medical conditions, a cardiovascular episode (myocardial infarction or coronary angioplasty) in the previous 3 months, and significant limitations in everyday activities or those unable to climb standard steps to the second floor without cardiovascular complaints. An exception can be made if the procedure is minor or noninvasive or if performed for emergency reasons and the potential benefits outweigh the procedural and sedation risks.

18.2 Risk Assessment

The patient's history of chronic diseases and their stability, medication history, and allergies increase the risk during sedation procedures. As such, it is essential to assess the risk of complications. The ASA Physical Status (class) scale is the most commonly used clinical assessment system [6].

- ASA class 1: Normal healthy patient with no organic, physiologic, or psychiatric disturbance, excluding the very young and very old; healthy with acceptable exercise tolerance
- ASA class 2: Patients presenting with mild systemic disease and no functional limitations; well-controlled disease involving one body system, including con-

trolled hypertension, diabetes without systemic effects, chronic obstructive pulmonary disease (COPD), mild obesity, or pregnancy, and if cigarette smoking is absent
- ASA class 3: Patients with severe systemic disease and some level of functional limitation; controlled disease involving more than one body system or one major system with no immediate danger of death, including controlled congestive heart failure (CHF), stable angina, prior heart attack, poorly controlled hypertension, morbid obesity, or chronic renal failure, or a bronchospastic disease with intermittent symptoms
- ASA class 4: Patients with severe systemic disease that represents a constant threat to life; at least one severe disease not well controlled or at end stage with a possible risk of death, including unstable angina, symptomatic COPD, symptomatic CHF, or hepatorenal failure
- ASA class 5: Moribund patients not expected to survive for over 24 h without the operation; imminent risk of death from multiorgan failure, sepsis syndrome with hemodynamic instability, hypothermia, or poorly controlled coagulopathy

Adding the letter "E" to a physical condition indicates an emergency procedure, where delaying treatment would lead to a significantly increased risk to life or body parts [2].

Since the most serious complication is respiratory failure due to airway obstruction or hypoventilation, a thorough knowledge of airway anatomy, its variations, and any history of airway anomalies is necessary. The most commonly used scale for assessing airway anatomy is the Mallampati scale [7, 8].

A thorough evaluation of potential ventilation difficulties is mandatory and should include any anatomical features that may affect airway management, including dysmorphic or asymmetric facial features, significant malnutrition or cachexia with sunken cheeks and missing teeth, and facial trauma. Limited neck extension and mouth opening of less than 4–5 cm, which limits access, needs to be assessed. Finally, obesity can be an obstacle to ventilation, even in the absence of previously considered factors [2]. The patient's vital signs should also be considered when making a decision. For example, a patient who cannot tolerate cessation of breathing or a drop in blood pressure may be better handled using a dissociative agent rather than moderate to deep sedation.

The management of sedation aims to:

1. Assess disease severity
2. Confirm the patient is in optimal condition before the procedure (there is a difference in qualification between emergency and elective surgery)
3. Select premedication on a patient-by-patient basis and dose drugs carefully
4. Carry out sedation and perioperative management using methods and medications that minimally impact comorbidities [9]

Hypertension

Stable hypertension with values at rest not exceeding 180 mmHg systolic pressure and 110 mmHg diastolic pressure is usually acceptable for outpatient procedures under sedation. Isolated systolic pressure ranging from 180 to 200 mmHg may be acceptable in the elderly if the diastolic pressure does not exceed 110 mmHg.

Management Patients with chronic hypertension undergoing elective NCS should avoid large fluctuations in blood pressure, especially hypotension, during the perioperative period [5]. Those with recently detected hypertension that is very high, or has non-strongly high values, require evaluation and therapy optimization before elective surgery under sedation with noninvasive ventilation (NIV) [10].

Circulatory Failure

Patients with unstable and progressive circulatory failure and dyspnea at rest or on slight exertion should generally not be qualified for minimally invasive procedures under sedation. Typically, dyspnea caused by circulatory failure increases in the supine position and decreases while standing. The most common causes of circulatory failure should be considered in the diagnosis, including ischemic heart disease, a history of myocardial infarction, cardiomyopathy, valvular defects, and cardiac arrhythmias. The New York Heart Association (NYHA) functional classification collates survival and quality of life and divides patients into four classes: class I, ordinary physical activity does not cause symptoms; class II, ordinary physical activity causes symptoms; class III, symptoms occur with less than ordinary activity; and class IV, inability to carry out any physical activity without discomfort and symptoms present at rest.

Management Postpone surgery until the patient's general condition is optimized, especially for NYHA classes III and IV.

History of Myocardial Infarction

The use of antiplatelet drugs in NCS patients should refer to the 2022 European Society of Cardiology (ESC) guidelines on cardiovascular assessment and management of patients undergoing NCS [5]. Patients taking antiplatelet drugs after elective percutaneous coronary intervention (PCI) should have elective NCS delayed for 6 months, and those suffering from acute coronary syndrome (ACS) require a 12-month delay. In addition, patients with clear ECG features of prior myocardial infarction (deep Q-waves in pre-cardiac leads or II+ III+ AvR) without a history of symptoms indicating a myocardial infarction should be referred to a cardiologist for a preoperative evaluation of cardiovascular capacity.

Angina Pectoris

Patients with ischemic heart disease can usually undergo outpatient procedures under sedation if they have been stable for at least 3 months and do not have regular angina attacks during light exertion (i.e., light housework and short walks on level ground), or at rest, or during the night, and therapy is optimal. If symptomatic, a cardiological evaluation is necessary; therapy should be adjusted, and the procedure rescheduled or implemented with perioperative invasive blood pressure measurement.

Management Maintaining sufficient arterial blood oxygenation, coronary perfusion pressure, and hemoglobin concentration, as well as minimizing myocardial oxygen consumption, is always the primary course of action in cases of myocardial ischemia [9].

Patients Treated with Anticoagulants for Cardiovascular Reasons
According to the recommendations on the use of antiplatelet drugs in the 2022 ESC guidelines on cardiovascular assessment and management of patients undergoing NCS [5], the risk of ischemia is low for patients taking acetylsalicylic acid (aspirin) for primary prevention, and aspirin can be discontinued before planned NCS. For warfarin and other oral anticoagulant treatments, the decision-making process should be individualized for each patient. Most surgical procedures, including sedation with NIV, can be safely performed with an international normalized ratio (INR) value of 2 or below. However, care should be taken to maximize the duration of reduced anticoagulant therapy in conditions such as atrial fibrillation, the presence of a mechanical heart valve, impaired cardiac function with an ejection fraction of less than 30%, or positive history of embolic diseases or episodes [5].

Management It is recommended to stop warfarin and other oral anticoagulants 3–4 days before the planned surgery, with daily monitoring of INR and use of low-molecular-weight heparin (LMWH) when the INR falls below 2.5. In the postoperative period, warfarin should resume while continuing LMWH until the INR reaches an acceptable value [10].

Valvular Defects
In valvular regurgitation cases (aortic or mitral), surgery eligibility, sedation, NIV, and complication risk should be assessed according to patient capacity, accounting for the general rules for people with circulatory insufficiency.

In cases of valvular stenosis, the risk of complications increases, even if clinical symptoms remain moderate. The patient should be referred for cardiac evaluation for any invasive procedure or those requiring sedation or anesthesia if they have aortic or mitral valve stenosis and impaired performance in daily activities [10].

Management For valvular regurgitation, it is advisable to maintain a relatively fast heart rate (HR), which, by shortening the time of the diastolic phase, reduces the volume of blood returning to the ventricle. Similarly, reducing the afterload (peripheral arterial pressure) reduces the aortic-ventricular gradient and can minimize the backflow of blood [9]. Valvular stenosis management aims to maintain sinus rhythm, a relatively slow HR, adequate intraventricular blood volume (*preload*), and systemic vascular resistance (SVR; *afterload*) [9].

Arrhythmias, Conduction Block, and Pacemaker Patients
The causes of rhythm disturbances should be assessed and, if possible, corrected. Additionally, ectopic ventricular beats and asymptomatic non-fixed tachyarrhythmias are not contraindications for sedated or ambulatory procedures. Patients with complete and symptomatic paroxysmal atrioventricular (AV) block should consult a cardiologist for indications of pacemaker implantation before any procedure. Patients undergoing pacemaker or implantable cardioverter defibrillator (ICD) implantation may be sedated and operated on as an outpatient.

Management Planning should consider the appropriate type of electrocoagulation for these patients and ensure that a pacemaker programming or a control device (magnet) is available [10].

18.3 High-Risk Patients Undergoing Sedation: The Impact of Sleep Apnea Syndrome

Sleep apnea syndrome (SAS) often remains unrecognized, probably occurs in around 4% of adult males and 2% of adult females, and is usually associated with obesity and hypertrophy of the palatine or pharyngeal tonsils in children. Although these patients do not present symptoms in daily life, the risk of respiratory arrest remains elevated, especially on the first night after surgery performed under sedation or general anesthesia or after taking opioids to treat postoperative pain. A meta-analysis reported difficulties with intubation in 12 studies and mask ventilation difficulties in six, with two studies reporting issues with intubation and mask ventilation and two reporting a failed supraglottic airway. Several studies reported more than one difficult airway outcome [11]. Although deaths from this cause are rare, a large US review reported eight such events [12].

Symptoms of SAS almost always include snoring, apnea (>10 s), frequent position changes in sleep, fatigue despite apparently normal sleep, morning headaches, and hypertension [13].

Management Difficulties with mask ventilation should be considered during sedation and NIV procedures in SAS patients. Several sizes of masks should be prepared, and facilities should be available to allow tight fitting of the mask during NIV. Early after procedure, SAS patients require CPAP or NIV treatment. During the hospital stay after surgery, the patient requires continuous monitoring during the night. A cardiac monitor with a pulse oximeter, respiratory rate measurement function, and an apnea alarm is optimal. In patients without gastrointestinal contraindications such as vomiting, CPAP/NIV device used on a daily basis by patient should be reintroduced early after extubating. In OSA or OSA/OHS and or OSA/COPD patients, regional anesthesia should be preferred with monitored PAP treatment during surgical procedure.

18.4 Conclusions

- Assess disease severity.
- Confirm the patient is in optimal condition before the procedure (there is a difference in qualification between emergency and elective surgery).
- Individualize sedation and perioperative management using methods and medications that minimally impact comorbidities.
- Consider the use of CPAP in non-intubated patients undergoing surgery as it reduces the risk of perioperative complications.

References

1. Cascella M, Fusco R, Caliendo D, et al. Anesthetic dreaming, anesthesia awareness and patient satisfaction after deep sedation with propofol target controlled infusion: a prospective cohort study of patients undergoing day case breast surgery. Oncotarget. 2017;8:79248–56.
2. Benzoni T, Cascella M. Procedural sedation. In: StatPearls [Internet]. Treasure Island: StatPearls Publishing; 2023. PMID: 31869149 Bookshelf ID: NBK551685.
3. Green SM, Roback MG, Krauss BS, et al. Unscheduled procedural sedation: a multidisciplinary consensus practice guideline. Ann Emerg Med. 2019;73:e51–65.
4. Hinkelbein J, Lamperti M, Akeson J, et al. European Society of Anaesthesiology and European Board of Anaesthesiology guidelines for procedural sedation and analgesia in adults. Eur J Anaesthesiol. 2017;35:6–24. https://doi.org/10.1097/eja.0000000000000683.
5. Halvorsen S, Mehilli J, Cassese S, Hall TS, Abdelhamid M, Barbato E, De Hert S, de Laval I, Geisler T, Hinterbuchner L, Ibanez B, Lenarczyk R, Mansmann UR, McGreavy P, Mueller C, Muneretto C, Niessner A, Potpara TS, Ristić A, Sade LE, Schirmer H, Schüpke S, Sillesen H, Skulstad H, Torracca L, Tutarel O, Van Der Meer P, Wojakowski W, Zacharowski K, ESC Scientific Document Group. 2022 ESC guidelines on cardiovascular assessment and management of patients undergoing non-cardiac surgery: developed by the task force for cardiovascular assessment and management of patients undergoing non-cardiac surgery of the European Society of Cardiology (ESC) Endorsed by the European Society of Anaesthesiology and Intensive Care (ESAIC). Eur Heart J. 2022;43:3826–924. https://doi.org/10.1093/eurheartj/ehac270.
6. American Society of Anesthesiologists. ASA physical classification system. [Cited December 6, 2013]. Available at http://www.asahq.org/Home/For-Members/Clinical-Information/ASA-Physical-Status-Classification-System/.
7. Long B, Koyfman A, Gottlieb M. Factors predicting difficult endotracheal intubation. Acad Emerg Med. 2019;26(11):1294–6.
8. Dyrbuś M, Oraczewska A, Szmigiel S, et al. Mallampati score is an independent predictor of active oxygen therapy in patients with COVID-19. J Clin Med. 2022;11:2958. https://doi.org/10.3390/jcm11112958. PMID: 35683347.
9. Khol BA, Rosenbaum SH, Fleisher LA. Anesthesiology clinics: anesthesia for patients too sick for anesthesia. Anesthesiol Clin. 2010;28:65–100.

10. Raeder J. Clinical ambulatory anesthesia. Cambridge: Syndicate of the press of the University of Cambridge; 2010. p. 42–4.
11. Memtsoudis SG, Cozowicz C, Nagappa M, et al. Society of anesthesia and sleep medicine guideline on intraoperative management of adult patients with obstructive sleep apnea. Anesth Analg. 2018;127:967–87. https://doi.org/10.1213/ANE.0000000000003434.
12. Lofsky A. Cases of sleep apnea syndrome. Anesth Pt Safety Found Newsl. 2002;17:24–5.
13. Chung SA, Yuan H, Chung F. A systemic review of obstructive sleep apnea and its implications for anesthesiologists. Anesth Analg. 2008;107:1543–63.

19 Risk Factors and Comorbidities. Chronic Pulmonary, Cardiac, and Neurologic Diseases

Przemysław Puz and Aleksandra Derra

19.1 Chronic Pulmonary Diseases

Noninvasive ventilation (NIV) is now considered the standard of care for managing exacerbations of chronic obstructive pulmonary disease (ECOPD) accompanied by hypercapnic respiratory failure. It is recommended when the arterial partial pressure of CO_2 is ≥6.5 and pH ≤7.35, despite optimal medical therapy. NIV effectively relieves the workload on respiratory muscles and improves alveolar ventilation, resulting in reduced respiratory effort and improved gas exchange. In cases of ECOPD with moderate respiratory acidosis, NIV has been shown to lower intubation rates, improve survival, and reduce the length of hospital stay when compared to medical care alone with a number needed to treat of 5 to prevent 1 intubation and 12 to prevent 1 death. It also has a role in more severe exacerbations where mechanical ventilation was traditionally the first-line therapy. Direct comparisons have demonstrated non-inferiority of NIV to mechanical ventilation in this context, along with a potentially lower rate of complications. However, it is important to note that failure rates are higher, emphasizing the critical role of an experienced clinician's judgment. If NIV is considered in these situations, it should be implemented in a setting where prompt intubation is readily available, if deemed necessary, or as an

P. Puz (✉)
Department of Neurology, School of Health Sciences, Medical University of Silesia in Katowice, Katowice, Poland

Department of Neurology, Upper-Silesian Medical Center of the Silesian Medical University in Katowice, Katowice, Poland
e-mail: ppuz@sum.edu.pl

A. Derra
Department of Neurology, Upper-Silesian Medical Center of the Silesian Medical University in Katowice, Katowice, Poland

© The Author(s), under exclusive license to Springer Nature Switzerland AG 2025

K. Panda et al. (eds.), *Noninvasive Ventilatory Approaches in Interventional Procedures*, Noninvasive Ventilation. The Essentials,
https://doi.org/10.1007/978-3-032-05328-2_19

agreed-upon ceiling of treatment. Currently, the use of NIV is not recommended in exacerbations with hypercapnia but no acidosis. A study analyzing a subgroup of patients with pH >7.35 suggested a reduced need for intubation without affecting mortality, while others have shown no significant benefit [1–4].

When considering the application of NIV, it is important to address the specific subgroup of patients with obstructive sleep apnea and COPD overlap syndrome. Although these patients could potentially benefit significantly from the intervention, they have often been systematically excluded from randomized controlled trials examining NIV in the context of chronic hypercapnic respiratory failure and COPD.

An additional consideration arises regarding the selection of the positive airway pressure modality strategy for this subgroup. In cases where obstructive sleep apnea is the predominant pathology in the overlap syndrome, it may be advisable to modify the approach and utilize continuous positive airway pressure instead of NIV, similar to the recommended approach for obesity hypoventilation syndrome with severe sleep apnea. Patients with the overlap syndrome exhibit lower 5-year survival rates compared to those with obstructive sleep apnea, even when receiving continuous positive airway pressure treatment [3–5]. However, a prospective cohort study demonstrated that continuous positive airway pressure treatment improved survival and reduced hospital admissions in patients with the overlap syndrome. The potential benefits of incorporating a high-intensity noninvasive ventilation strategy, combined with adequate end-expiratory pressure to maintain airway patency, remain unknown in this patient population. Determining the primary factor responsible for hypercapnic respiratory failure can be challenging when faced with patients presenting with obesity hypoventilation syndrome and COPD overlap. Nevertheless, the pragmatic goals of positive airway pressure treatment for obesity hypoventilation syndrome align with those for chronic hypercapnic respiratory failure and COPD, aiming to correct sleep hypoxemia, obstructive events, and hypercapnia. In the absence of robust clinical trials specific to this population, scientists generally lean toward employing high-intensity noninvasive ventilation when clinical evaluation suggests that COPD is the underlying cause of chronic hypercapnic respiratory failure and positive airway pressure treatment when obesity hypoventilation syndrome or obstructive sleep apnea predominates [5].

One of the primary challenges associated with the utilization of NIV in chronic pulmonary diseases is the notable failure rate, defined as persistent or worsening acidosis despite efforts to optimize delivery. It is crucial to promptly identify those who require intubation after unsuccessful NIV, as they face an elevated risk of mortality. Several physiological variables have proven highly predictive of failure if they do not show improvement within 1–2 h. Late failure cases also occur and are indicative of a particularly unfavorable prognosis. Previously identified factors that predict the need for intubation, such as severe hypoxemia, shock, or altered consciousness, are themselves intubation criteria and are inadequate predictors for making early intubation decisions. Earlier studies have indicated that patients meeting criteria for acute respiratory distress syndrome (ARDS) and experiencing severe hypoxemia are at an increased risk of requiring intubation compared to others [6, 7].

19.2 Neurologic Diseases

NIV has proven to be beneficial in patients with progressive neuromuscular diseases (NMDs) or significant abnormalities of the thoracic cage, offering improved survival rates and enhanced quality of life. NMDs are a heterogeneous group of disorders characterized by impairment at the level of motor neurons, peripheral nerve, neuromuscular junction, or skeletal muscle. These conditions can be acquired or inherited, presenting with varying ages of onset, clinical features, courses, and prognoses. If muscle weakness affects the diaphragm and accessory respiratory muscles, it can lead to RF at different stages of the patient's life, often exacerbated by severe scoliosis. A list of neuromuscular disorders associated with RF at birth or within the first year of life includes spinal muscular atrophy type 1 (SMA1), spinal muscular atrophy with respiratory distress (SMARD), congenital myotonic dystrophy (CDM), infantile-onset Pompe disease (IOPD), some mitochondrial diseases, certain congenital myopathies, some congenital muscular dystrophies, some congenital myasthenic syndromes, and neonatal myasthenia gravis (transient). Additionally, Duchenne muscular dystrophy (DMD), amyotrophic lateral sclerosis (ALS), some muscular dystrophies, and some myofibrillar myopathies represent a group of neuromuscular diseases in which RF is an unavoidable outcome. The NMDs associated with the development of RF frequently include spinal muscular atrophy type 2 (SMA2), myotonic dystrophy type 1 (DM1), late-onset Pompe disease (LOPD), Guillain-Barré syndrome (GBS), myasthenia gravis (MG), facioscapulohumeral muscular dystrophy (FSHD), some congenital muscular dystrophies, some limb-girdle muscular dystrophies, some congenital myopathies, and congenital myasthenic syndromes [8, 9].

The advantages of NIV in this patient population encompass enhancements in daytime blood gas levels, including hypercapnia reduction, decreased oxygen cost of breathing, heightened ventilatory response to elevated carbon dioxide levels, and improved lung compliance. Neuromuscular disorders can be categorized also as either slowly progressive or rapidly progressive. Slowly progressive conditions encompass nonprogressive diseases (e.g., poliomyelitis) or conditions with gradual progression (e.g., certain myopathies and muscular dystrophy). In these cases, physiological changes such as weight gain, chest infections, additional chronic cardiorespiratory pathologies, or sleep-disordered breathing can result in ventilatory decompensation, requiring early ventilatory support even without underlying disease progression. The mean survival period following development of diurnal hypercapnia in DMD is 9.7 months if ventilatory support is not provided. It is recommended to initiate NIV in symptomatic DMD patients with a daytime $PaCO_2$ of >6.0 kPa. There is no evidence that NIV is effective when started as prophylactic therapy before the development of diurnal hypercapnia. Restrictive RF is the primary cause of mortality in patients with amyotrophic lateral sclerosis (ALS), and in certain cases, it may even mark the disease's onset. It is an acquired disorder that tends to progress more rapidly. Consequently, psychological and physical adjustments are more challenging. Patients with ALS typically do not experience respiratory symptoms until their vital capacity is reduced to 50–60% of the predicted value.

The respiratory system is profoundly affected by spinal muscular atrophy (SMA), with the extent of muscle function loss determining the severity of the impact. Patients with SMA type 1 (non-sitters) and type 2 (sitters) require vigilant monitoring and proactive management of their respiratory status. Among the progressive disorders are Duchenne muscular dystrophy and motor neuron disorders, where NIV has demonstrated significant benefits [8, 9].

To prevent severe complications, it is crucial to identify individuals at high risk of RF and provide timely interventions such as inspiratory aids (e.g., NIV) and expiratory assistance. Therefore, a proactive clinical approach is recommended to detect pulmonary issues before respiratory compromise occurs. Early diagnosis of respiratory dysfunction may prevent the need for urgent/late initiation of NIV, which is associated with reduced compliance and survival.

Among these patients, forced vital capacity (FVC) serves as a valuable and easily measured parameter for monitoring respiratory muscle strength. Individuals with FVC values below 50–60% of the predicted value should receive training in protocols that enable effective home-based treatments, supervised by well-trained family members or healthcare professionals, particularly during respiratory exacerbations. Overnight oximetry or transcutaneous capnometry can be a useful tool for assessing nocturnal hypoventilation, as desaturation indicates potential respiratory issues during sleep.

NIV is recommended for patients with ALS who have daytime $PaCO_2$ levels exceeding 6 kPa. NIV may also be beneficial for patients with normal $PaCO_2$ levels but with severe dyspnea or orthopnea resulting from respiratory muscle weakness. However, NIV is unlikely to provide benefits for asymptomatic patients or those with significant bulbar weakness.

The use of polysomnography to determine the necessity for NIV and optimize settings remains a topic of debate, although it has been recommended in one consensus statement. According to recommendations from a consensus committee, initiation of NIV is recommended in patients with neuromuscular disease who exhibit symptoms such as fatigue, dyspnea, or morning headache, along with meeting one of the following physiological criteria: a $PaCO_2$ level of 45 mm Hg or higher and nocturnal oximetry showing oxygen saturation of 88% or less for at least 5 consecutive minutes. NIV can also be utilized to provide respiratory support during gastrostomy tube placement in patients with neuromuscular disease. Successful transition from intubation to NIV is possible for certain patients with neuromuscular disease, and some individuals who have undergone tracheostomy can be rarely but effectively decannulated and transitioned to NIV. In such cases, transitioning to NIV with a capped tracheostomy tube and subsequent decannulation can be considered as a viable option [10, 11].

Patients suffering from progressive neuromuscular disease also necessitate assistance with coughing to effectively eliminate pulmonary secretions and prevent recurring respiratory tract infections. Failure to do so can result in acute respiratory failure or transient hypoxemia-induced cardiac arrhythmias. In order to prevent malnutrition, gastrostomy is often contemplated for ventilator-dependent patients who encounter challenges with oral eating despite utilizing a mouthpiece interface. Tracheostomy is no longer considered necessary solely due to ventilator dependency. Unless there is a life-threatening acute condition, tracheostomy is typically reserved for cases where the patient expresses a preference, cannot effectively utilize NIV, or experiences unsuccessful outcomes with noninvasive cough assistance techniques, particularly in situations involving bulbar dysfunction, to prevent aspiration of secretions [8, 12].

In cases where NIV proves ineffective or is deemed unsuitable, temporary intubation should be considered. Contraindications to NIV include uncooperative patient, reduced level of consciousness, delirium with restlessness or agitation, severe dysphagia, excessive secretions not managed by mechanical cough assistance, severe hypoxemia (PaO_2 <60 mmHg with FiO_2 >0.6), undrained pneumothorax, respiratory arrest, cardiac arrest, cardiovascular instability (hypotension, dysrhythmias, acute myocardial infarction), non-respiratory organ failure (hemodynamic instability, severe encephalopathy, severe gastrointestinal bleeding), tracheoesophageal fistula, inability to protect airway or high risk of aspiration, and facial or head trauma or surgery. Mechanical ventilation and endotracheal intubation are associated with increased risk of infectious complications, thus making NIV the preferred method of ventilatory treatment. Nevertheless, there are also situations in which the patient's condition should be closely monitored because of high risk of NIV failure. Those situations sometimes require a decision to transition from NIV to invasive ventilation, such as respiratory arrest, respiratory rate >35 breaths/min, severe dyspnea with the use of accessory muscles paradoxical respiration, severe hypoxemia PaO_2 <40 mm Hg or PaO_2/FiO_2 <200, severe acidosis (pH <7.25), hypercapnia ($PaCO_2$ >60 mmHg), hypersomnolence, impaired mental status, and cardiovascular complications (hypotension, shock, heart failure) [8, 13].

Other uses of NIV in neurology are in myasthenia gravis exacerbation and Guillain-Barré syndrome with respiratory compromise. Approximately 20% of patients with myasthenia gravis (MG) experience myasthenic crisis, which can lead to ARF due to a combination of upper airway obstruction and acute hypoventilation resulting from profound weakness in bulbar and inspiratory muscles. Invasive ventilation via endotracheal intubation (ETI) has strong supporting evidence and is recommended in most published series, with reported mortality rates ranging between 4% and 6%. However, extubation failure may occur in up to 25% of patients, and the presence of atelectasis has been strongly associated with such failures. NIV may not be suitable for patients with ARF unless upper airway function is well preserved. Nevertheless, in cases of myasthenic crisis, NIV is considered desirable to reduce the risk of prolonged invasive mechanical ventilation (IMV) complications, including ventilator-associated pneumonia and other systemic complications. By applying NIV with a relatively low inspiratory pressure range of 10–16 cm H_2O, the need for ETI can be prevented in these patients. Severe hypercapnia ($PaCO_2$ >50 mmHg) and elevated serum bicarbonate levels upon admission have been identified as potential predictors of NIV failure. To facilitate the early identification of Guillain-Barré syndrome (GBS) patients at risk of developing acute respiratory failure (ARF) requiring ventilatory support, the "20/30/40 rule" has been suggested. According to this rule, intubation is recommended if the forced vital capacity (FVC) is less than 20 mL/kg, the maximum inspiratory pressure (MIP) is less than 30 cm H_2O, and the maximal expiratory pressure (MEP) is less than 40 cm H_2O. However, the use of NIV in patients with GBS is not considered safe due to the following reasons: (a) patients typically remain extremely weak and require full ventilator assistance for an extended period, and (b) the manifestations of dysautonomia worsen as respiratory failure becomes more severe. Consequently, 25–50% of GBS patients may necessitate ETI and IMV [8, 14–16].

NIV is a useful alternative therapy to mechanical ventilation in many different neurological conditions causing acute/chronic respiratory failure. It may also have roles in preventing the development of respiratory failure in recently extubated ICU patients and in the postoperative period and also as a palliative treatment for patients with progressive neurological conditions.

19.3 Cardiac Diseases

Pulmonary edema is a common cause of acute RF, second only to pneumonia. Most patients with acute heart failure (AHF) syndromes exhibit some degree of pulmonary edema, either interstitial or alveolar. As a result, approximately 90% of AHF patients experience dyspnea, but less than half of them present with RF as evidenced by blood gas analysis, such as hypoxemia, hypercapnia, acidosis, or a combination of these factors. Among the different AHF syndromes, significant RF is primarily observed in acute cardiogenic pulmonary edema (ACPE), cardiogenic shock (CS), and cases associated with other lung abnormalities [17].

ACPE is characterized by a rapid increase in pulmonary capillary hydrostatic pressure and trans-vascular fluid filtration, surpassing the lymphatic interstitial drainage capacity. This leads to the accumulation of interstitial and alveolar fluid, impairing gas exchange and causing a shunt effect, ultimately resulting in respiratory failure. Without prompt therapeutic intervention, ACPE can rapidly progress to cardiorespiratory collapse within hours or even minutes. The diagnosis of ACPE requires several clinical criteria, including acute respiratory distress, orthopnea, physical examination findings, and respiratory failure. Initial bedside assessment based on these criteria allows for urgent initiation of therapies. However, the diagnosis should be further confirmed using additional criteria specific to AHF, such as clear signs of pulmonary congestion on imaging (chest radiography or CT scan), presence of multiple B-lines on lung ultrasound, elevated pulmonary capillary pressure on catheterization, increased total lung water on pulse contour and thermodilution analysis, evidence of elevated filling pressures on echocardiography, and significant elevation of natriuretic peptides. Key clinical findings in ACPE include respiratory distress and respiratory failure. It is important to note that other AHF scenarios characterized by interstitial or mild alveolar edema without significant respiratory distress or respiratory failure would not be classified as ACPE. The genesis of ACPE involves various factors, including the rate and speed of alveolar fluid filtration, microvascular membrane permeability, alterations in sodium chloride and water reabsorption, inflammation, and individual genetic susceptibility. Patients with ACPE often present with hypertension upon admission; these cases more commonly exhibit preserved left ventricular ejection fraction (EF), hypercapnia, and a lower heart rate, which are associated with a better prognosis compared to those with lower blood pressure. Some patients may experience a rapid onset of symptoms, referred to as "flash ACPE," without prior clinical signs of fluid accumulation. In the case of CS, when it is secondary to left ventricular failure, acute respiratory failure is almost always present along with pulmonary edema and tissue hypoperfusion. In addition to pulmonary edema, reduced lung perfusion leads to an increase in pulmonary dead space, causing a ventilation-perfusion mismatch. The systemic circulatory failure in CS leads to metabolic acidosis (lactic acidemia), which increases the respiratory workload and reduces central venous oxygen content (SvO_2) due to an augmented arteriovenous difference. These abnormalities further exacerbate respiratory failure in CS. Other scenarios in AHF include the presence of comorbidities such as COPD, asthma, pneumonia, large pleural effusion, atelectasis, or pulmonary embolism, which can precipitate or worsen RF. Isolated right ventricular failure typically manifests as AF in cases of acute pulmonary thromboembolism or decompensated chronic pulmonary hypertension [17–19].

In cases of AHF syndromes, NIV is recommended for patients with ACPE. It may also be considered for other AHF patients with respiratory failure associated with lung disease and in some cases of CS after stabilizing blood pressure. CPAP is a simpler technique and is recommended as first-line therapy, particularly in prehospital settings or less well-equipped areas. Noninvasive pressure support ventilation is equally effective in ACPE and may be preferred, by experienced teams, in patients with significant hypercapnia. High-flow nasal cannula can be an alternative, especially for AHF patients requiring prolonged NIV, and it is a well-tolerated technique with broader potential indications [17, 20].

Positive-pressure ventilation, such as that provided by NIV, has several effects on oxygenation, the work of breathing, and cardiovascular function. The positive inspiratory pressure (PIP) in NIV leads to an increase in oxygenation and a decrease in the work of breathing. In terms of oxygenation, NIV improves alveolar ventilation, resulting in better gas exchange and a decrease in carbon dioxide levels. This contributes to improved oxygenation and a reduction in the effort required for breathing. However, positive-pressure ventilation affects heart-lung interactions and can have both hemodynamic and respiratory effects. It has a tendency to reduce cardiac output and blood pressure. In patients with AHF and elevated preload and afterload, positive-pressure ventilation can actually increase cardiac output by reducing both pre- and afterload. It can also reduce intrapulmonary shunting, improving overall respiratory function. On the other hand, in cases of isolated right ventricular (RV) dysfunction, positive-pressure ventilation may be detrimental. The increase in RV afterload caused by positive pressure can worsen RV failure or precipitate its onset. Therefore, the effects of positive-pressure ventilation on hemodynamics and respiratory function depend on the underlying condition and the patient's individual characteristics. Close monitoring and careful assessment are necessary to ensure that positive-pressure ventilation is beneficial and does not exacerbate any existing cardiac or respiratory issues [17, 21, 22].

Before initiating NIV, contraindications should be considered, including cardiac or respiratory arrest, anatomical abnormalities that prevent proper fitting of the interface, inability to maintain a patent airway (uncontrolled agitation, coma, or obtunded mental status), refractory hypotension, relative mild agitation or poor cooperation, mild hypotension, upper gastrointestinal hemorrhage or vomiting, inability to expectorate copious secretions, recent upper gastrointestinal or airway surgery, multiorgan failure, and isolated right ventricular failure. Risk factors for NIV failure, such as lung infection, altered mental status, hypotension, high severity scores, copious secretions, extremely high respiratory rate, and severe hypoxemia despite high FiO_2, should be also considered. NIV is typically discontinued when satisfactory recovery has been achieved (usually 2–5 h in ACPE) or if signs of NIV failure are observed, such as no reduction in respiratory rate or carbon dioxide levels, no improvement in pH or oxygenation (SpO_2 or PaO_2/FiO_2), signs of fatigue, or neurological or underlying disease impairment [17, 23].

AMI is a common cause of ACPE. However, there is no established relationship between NIV use and the risk of AMI. Some early studies suggested a potential association, but subsequent trials, case-control studies, and meta-analyses have not reproduced those results. The use of NIV in patients with AMI has been shown to be safe in various studies, including those involving patients with type II AMI or non-ST-segment elevation myocardial infarction (non-STEMI). However, it should be noted that patients with ST-segment elevation myocardial infarction (STEMI) have not been extensively included in trials assessing the use of NIV. Additionally, recent data have shown no benefit of oxygen therapy in patients with suspected AMI without hypoxemia. Further research is needed to determine the role of NIV in patients with STEMI [17].

19.4 Summary

NIV has emerged as a cornerstone in the management of chronic and acute respiratory failure across various conditions, including COPD, neuromuscular diseases, OHS, and acute heart failure syndromes. Its ability to optimize respiratory muscle workload, enhance alveolar ventilation, and reduce hypercapnia has made it an effective alternative to invasive ventilation in appropriately selected patients.

In the context of those illness exacerbations, NIV significantly reduces the need for intubation, improves survival, and shortens hospital stays. However, its efficacy is closely tied to appropriate patient selection and timely intervention. While promising results have been observed in patients with COPD and OHS overlap syndrome, further research is needed to refine the optimal ventilation strategies for this subgroup.

Overall, the role of NIV continues to expand, offering a noninvasive approach to improving patient outcomes in chronic and acute respiratory failure. Future studies should focus on optimizing NIV protocols, determining individualized treatment strategies, and evaluating its long-term impact on patient survival and quality of life.

References

1. Wollsching-Strobel M, Bauer IA, Baur JJ, Majorski DS, Magnet FS, Storre JH, Windisch W, Schwarz SB. The impact of non-invasive ventilation on sleep quality in COPD patients. J Clin Med. 2022;11(18):5483. https://doi.org/10.3390/jcm11185483.
2. Masip J, Peacock WF, Price S, Cullen L, Martin-Sanchez FJ, Seferovic P, Maisel AS, Miro O, Filippatos G, Vrints C, Christ M, Cowie M, Platz E, McMurray J, DiSomma S, Zeymer U, Bueno H, Gale CP, Lettino M, Tavares M, Ruschitzka F, Mebazaa A, Harjola VP, Mueller C. Acute Heart Failure Study Group of the Acute Cardiovascular Care Association and the Committee on Acute Heart Failure of the Heart Failure Association of the European Society of Cardiology. Indications and practical approach to non-invasive ventilation in acute heart failure. Eur Heart J. 2018;39(1):17–25. https://doi.org/10.1093/eurheartj/ehx580.
3. Conti G, Antonelli M, Navalesi P, Rocco M, Bufi M, Spadetta G, et al. Noninvasive vs. conventional mechanical ventilation in patients with chronic obstructive pulmonary disease after failure of medical treatment in the ward: a randomized trial. Intensive Care Med. 2002;28:1701–7.
4. Jurjevic M, Matic I, Sakic-Zdravcevic K, Sakic S, Danic D, Bukovic D. Mechanical ventilation in chronic obstructive pulmonary disease patients, noninvasive vs. invasive method (randomized prospective study). Coll Antropol. 2009;33:791–7.
5. Hatipoğlu U, Aboussouan LS. Chronic hypercapnic respiratory failure and non-invasive ventilation in people with chronic obstructive pulmonary disease. BMJ Med. 2022;1(1):e000146.
6. MacLeod M, Papi A, Contoli M, et al. Chronic obstructive pulmonary disease exacerbation fundamentals: diagnosis, treatment, prevention and disease impact. Respirology. 2021;26:532–51.
7. Ambrosino N, Vagheggini G. Non-invasive ventilation in exacerbations of COPD. Int J Chron Obstruct Pulmon Dis. 2007;2(4):471–6.
8. Racca F, Vianello A, Mongini T, et al. Practical approach to respiratory emergencies in neurological diseases. Neurol Sci. 2020;41:497–508.
9. Ashalatha R. Role of non invasive ventilation in neurology clinical practice. Acta Sci Neurol. 2021;4(3):13–7.
10. Musson LS, Baxter SK, Norman P, O'Brien D, Elliott M, Bianchi S, Kaltsakas G, McDermott CJ, Stavroulakis T, Hobson EV. Delivery of noninvasive ventilation to people living with motor neuron disease in the UK. ERJ Open Res. 2023;9(2):00388–2022.
11. Hess DR. Noninvasive ventilation for neuromuscular disease. Clin Chest Med. 2018;39(2):437–47.
12. Prigent H, Fauroux B, Attarian S, Annane D, Lofaso F. Tracheostomy in ventilator-dependent patients with slowly progressive neuromuscular disease. Lancet Respir Med. 2023;11(5):410–1.
13. Boentert M, et al. Respiratory involvement in neuromuscular disorders. Curr Opin Neurol. 2017;30(5):529–37.
14. Seneviratne J, Mandrekar J, Wijdicks EF, Rabinstein AA. Predictors of extubation failure in myasthenic crisis. Arch Neurol. 2008;65:929–33.
15. Wu JY, Kuo PH, Fan PC, Wu HD, Shih FY, Yang PC. The role of non-invasive ventilation and factors predicting extubation outcome in myasthenic crisis. Neurocrit Care. 2009;10:35–42.
16. Mehta S. Neuromuscular disease causing acute respiratory failure. Respir Care. 2006;51:1016–21.
17. Masip J, Peacock WF, Price S, Cullen L, Martin-Sanchez FJ, Seferovic P, Maisel AS, Miro O, Filippatos G, Vrints C, Christ M, Cowie M, Platz E, McMurray J, DiSomma S, Zeymer U, Bueno H, Gale CP, Lettino M, Tavares M, Ruschitzka F, Mebazaa A, Harjola VP, Mueller C. Acute Heart Failure Study Group of the Acute Cardiovascular Care Association and the Committee on Acute Heart Failure of the Heart Failure Association of the European Society

of Cardiology. Indications and practical approach to non-invasive ventilation in acute heart failure. Eur Heart J. 2018;39(1):17–25.

18. Mark JJ, Choi DJ, Yoon CH, Oh IY, Lee JH, Ahn S, Yoo BS, Kang SM, Kim JJ, Baek SH, Cho MC, Jeon ES, Chae SC, Ryu KH, Oh BH. KorHF Registry. The prognostic value of arterial blood gas analysis in high-risk acute heart failure patients: an analysis of the Korean Heart Failure (KorHF) registry. Eur J Heart Fail. 2015;17:601–11.
19. Dickstein K, Cohen-Solal A, Filippatos G, McMurray JJV, Ponikowski P, Poole Wilson PA, Stromberg A, van Veldhuisen DJ, Atar D, Hoes AW, Keren A, Mebazaa A, Nieminen M, Priori SG, Swedberg K, Vahanian A, Camm J, DeCaterina R, Dean V, Dickstein K, Filippatos G, Funck-Brentano C, Hellemans I, Kristensen SD, McGregor K, Sechtem U, Silber S, Tendera M, Widimsky P, Zamorano JL, Tendera M, Auricchio A, Bax J, Bohm M, Corra U, della Bella P, Elliott PM, Follath F, Gheorghiade M, Hasin Y, Hernborg A, Jaarsma T, Komajda M, Kornowski R, Piepoli M, Prendergast B, Tavazzi L, Vachiery J-L, FWA V, Zamorano JL, Zannad F. ESC Committee for Practice Guidelines (CPG). ESC guidelines for the diagnosis and treatment of acute and chronic heart failure 2008: the task force for the diagnosis and treatment of acute and chronic heart failure 2008 of the European Society of Cardiology. Eur Heart J. 2008;29:2388–442.
20. Pinsky MR, Summer WR, Wise RA, Permutt S, Bromberger-Barnea B. Augmentation of cardiac function by elevation of intrathoracic pressure. J Appl Physiol. 1983;54:950–5.
21. Robin MJ. Advances in mechanical ventilation. N Engl J Med. 2001;344:1986–96.
22. Januzzi JL, Filippatos G, Nieminen M, Mihai GM. Troponin elevation in patients with heart failure: on behalf of the third universal definition of myocardial infarction global task force: heart failure section. Eur Heart J. 2012;33:2265–71.
23. Bello G, De Santis P, Antonelli M. Non-invasive ventilation in cardiogenic pulmonary edema. Ann Transl Med. 2018;6(18):355.

High-Risk Patients Undergoing Sedation for Endoscopy Procedures

20

Piotr Janowiak

20.1 Introduction

Sedation during endoscopic procedures is endorsed by a broad representation of medical societies, be it pulmonological [1], gastroenterological [2, 3], or anesthesiological [4, 5]. Although it is feasible to perform endoscopy without sedation [1, 3, 6], there are multiple arguments for its use. Sedative drugs improve patient's tolerance of the examination and thus allow for its greater length—if necessary. Improved tolerance allows greater patient cooperation, which may lead to better outcome of the endoscopy [3, 7] and greater willingness to repeat the procedure [6]. Although inducing deeper than anticipated state of sedation may be detrimental to the patient, the opposite, i.e., not using sedative drugs at all, can lead to adverse effects provoked by uncontrolled physiological reaction to the insertion of the endoscope [2]. Despite its potential for complications, procedural sedation is nonetheless safe. Adverse events, such as intubation, resuscitation, or others requiring intensive care unit (ICU) admission, occur only in 0–3% of the cases—including patients ranked ≥III on American Society of Anesthesiologists (ASA) physical status classification [8–13].

P. Janowiak (✉)
Department of Pulmonology, Faculty of Medicine, Medical University of Gdańsk, Gdańsk, Poland
e-mail: piotr.janowiak@gumed.edu.pl

© The Author(s), under exclusive license to Springer Nature Switzerland AG 2025

K. Panda et al. (eds.), *Noninvasive Ventilatory Approaches in Interventional Procedures*, Noninvasive Ventilation. The Essentials,
https://doi.org/10.1007/978-3-032-05328-2_20

20.2 Monitoring During Sedation

It is a general consensus that periprocedural sedation should, in most cases, be maintained at a moderate level, with preserved airway patency and spontaneous ventilation [4] which corresponds to score of 2–3 in modified Ramsay Sedation Scale (MRSS) [14]; level 2 in American Society of Anesthesiologists Sedation Scale (ASASS); or level 3 in Modified Observer's Alertness/Sedation scale (MOAA-S) [6]. This level of anesthesia can be safely maintained by a properly trained proceduralist, capable of performing basic airway maneuvers and proficient in pharmacological treatment of sedation side effects [3, 7]. However, it is advised that a separate person, responsible solely for monitoring the patient, should be present in the endoscopy room at the time of the procedure [5]. Because sedation is a continuum and patient's sedation depth is prone to change during the procedure, personnel should be prepared to address unexpected changes in sedation level. Furthermore, location where endoscopic sedation is carried out should provide immediate availability of an anesthesiologist—if a need for such an assistance arises [4]. If deeper levels of sedation are needed, e.g., for long and complex endoscopies, a commonly accepted consensus requires that the procedure should, by definition, be overseen by an anesthesiologist [3, 5]. Anesthesiologist supervision in other indications remains controversial. The European Society of Anesthesiology (ESA) guidelines state that every patient with chronic renal or hepatic failure, with severe cardiovascular disease, obstructive sleep apnea (OSA)—both documented and strongly suspected—BMI >40, ASA physical status III–IV, or older than 70 years, should have procedural sedation managed by an anesthesiologist [4]. In contrast to the abovementioned, the ASA recommends that only in severely sick or medically unstable patients, anesthesiologist consultation should be obtained. Regardless of the guidelines, one should remember that ASA physical status higher than II [8, 10, 12], male sex [10], and increased BMI [10] are independent risk factors for sedation complications.

Safe sedation requires continuous monitoring. Vital parameters such as noninvasive blood pressure (NIBP), heart rate (HR), and peripheral pulse oximetry (SpO_2) should be determined before the procedure [5] and monitored continuously throughout the procedure with NIBP measured at least in 5 min intervals [4, 5]. Joint recommendations of Indian Chest Society, National College of Chest Physicians and Indian Association for Bronchology also recommend continuous monitoring of respiratory rate (RR) [6]. Continuous electrocardiographic (ECG) monitoring is strongly advised in patients with clinically significant cardiovascular disease [1, 5]; however, ESA guidelines recommend it in all patients who are subjected to endoscopic sedation [4]. Furthermore, patient monitoring must not be limited to vital parameters—continuous observation for qualitative clinical signs and frequent assessment of depth of sedation are also mandatory [4, 5] especially that vital sign measures do not necessarily correlate with sedation depth [13]. Recommended sedation scales include MRSS, ASASS, and MOAA-S [4].

Both European and American societies of anesthesiology endorse continuous capnography for additional evaluation of ventilation in all patients subjected to procedural sedation [4, 5]. Studies show that measuring end-tidal carbon dioxide during both pulmonary and gastroenterological endoscopies might allow for earlier detection of apnea than pulse oximetry, on average 31.0–38.6 s before SpO2 drop [15, 16]. This, in turn, may lead to early, preventive intervention. Some studies indeed show that using side-stream capnography can lead to a reduction of hypoxemia episodes [11, 16, 17], but this is not a consistent finding [18, 19]. On the other hand, a retrospective study on a large number of inpatient and outpatient gastrointestinal endoscopies showed that capnography use was associated with a 47% odds reduction in death for inpatient population and a 61% odds reduction in pharmacological rescue events for outpatient population [20]. Nonetheless, it has been raised that capnography use in gastroenterological suites should be limited to procedures requiring either deep or long sedation or to higher-risk patients, classified at least as ASA III [21]. Despite ongoing debate, pulmonary societies have not issued any recommendations regarding its use during bronchoscopy [1]. Nonetheless, one should take into consideration that patients with pre-existing lung diseases are prone to the accumulation of pCO2, that pCO2 accumulation is common during bronchoscopy, and that the sole presence of endoscope in the airways impacts ventilation [22–24].

Patient monitoring should not be limited solely to the time of the procedure. According to the European and American societies of anesthesiology, post-endoscopy monitoring should take at least 30 min and include, at a minimum, NIBP, ECG, and pulse oximetry along with continuous visual observation [4, 5]. However, in a study by Dreher et al., patients with respiratory failure who underwent sedated bronchoscopy needed at least 2 h for pCO2 levels to drop to baseline level [23]. Furthermore, it is known that senile patients and patients with pre-existing lung diseases or other severe chronic diseases such as chronic renal failure (CRF) or chronic liver failure (CLF) might require more time to recover from sedation [1, 4, 13]. Post-procedural monitoring time should then be tailored to individual patient's needs.

20.3 Drugs For Sedation During Endoscopy

Attaining a moderate level of sedation typically requires a combination of two types of drugs: a hypnotic and an analgesic [4, 5]. Both gastrointestinal endoscopy and bronchoscopy guidelines typically endorse a combination of benzodiazepine and an opioid [1, 3]. Short-acting drugs with rapid onset are preferred; among benzodiazepines, midazolam or, newly approved, remimazolam [25]; among opioids, fentanyl and remifentanil [26]. Sedation induced by the abovementioned drugs can be reversed with flumazenil, which should be readily available in endoscopy suite along with an opioid antagonist—naloxone. Bronchoscopy studies show that the combination of opioid and benzodiazepine, compared to benzodiazepine alone, improves patient's comfort and reduces cough intensity and pain connected with the insertion of the endoscope. Furthermore, it allows for the reduction of total dosage of sedative agents delivered with the opioid [1]. These advantages are attainable without increase in side effects. Dreher et al., in their prospective bronchoscopy study on 30 patients, did not detect significant differences regarding transcutaneous pCO2 values, minimum SpO2, and recovery time between midazolam and combination of midazolam and alfentanil. In another combined sedation study, a randomized, double-blind, placebo-controlled trial by Stolz et al. on 120 patients, combination of midazolam and hydrocodone, compared to midazolam alone, reduced cough scores without negative impact on SpO2 [27]. Furthermore, midazolam and fentanyl can be used in combination in patients with severe cardiovascular disease or chronic renal failure (CRF). However, this combination is discouraged by ESA in CRF patients on the grounds of increased risk of adverse events—with mono-sedation as a preferred option [4].

Midazolam is not without disadvantages. As pointed out by Gan et al., its half-life is prolonged in the elderly, obesity, and hepatic impairment. The elderly are also more susceptible to its central nervous system depressant effects. Free fraction of midazolam is increased in patients with reduced serum albumin concentration—not an uncommon finding in the elderly or in patients with renal or hepatic impairment. Furthermore, its lipophilicity facilitates accumulation in adipose tissue, along with its metabolites, especially in CRF patients [28].

Other common drug combination, for better patient tolerance, includes propofol and opioids [1, 4]. Propofol has certain advantages over midazolam—its duration of action is shorter (4–8 min vs 10–20 min after intravenous bolus) and more predictable [4, 28]. Furthermore, liver or renal failure does not significantly alter propofol pharmacokinetics. However, similar to midazolam, propofol has lower clearance in the elderly patients. Despite its advantages, propofol is restricted for use by anesthesiologists in many countries [7]. It is a respiratory and circulatory depressant, with a narrow therapeutic range which does not have a reversal agent. It comes to no surprise that its usage by professionals without formal training in general anesthesia is controversial. Evidence for its use in endoscopy suite is conflicting. On one hand, European Society of Gastrointestinal Endoscopy (ESGE) supports the administration of propofol-based sedation without anesthesiologist supervision in selected patients planned to undergo short endoscopic procedure, i.e., in patients classified as ASA I–II, with airways assessed as 1–2 in Mallampati score, who do not present increased risk of airway obstruction and do not receive narcotic analgesics chronically. In this selected population, sedation with propofol, compared to other hypnotics, should provide better tolerance of the procedure with decreased time to sedation and quicker recovery without increase in adverse effects [2]. However, in a prospective, observational study on 307 endobronchial ultrasound (EBUS) patients, Viedma et al. showed that propofol-based sedation produced more complications such as hypotension, desaturation or bradypnea than midazolam-based sedation, despite better cough, pain, and dyspnea control [29]. Furthermore, in the recent meta-analysis by Ou et al., combination of alfentanil and propofol was connected with the increase in the rate of hypoxemia incidents during bronchoscopies [30].

Benzodiazepines, opioids, and propofol can cause collapse of the upper airways [31], which, along with respiratory depressant effect, might be detrimental to the obese patients or to OSA patients [4]. This is especially true for benzodiazepines in which the use in these groups is discouraged [32]. In this particular populations, dexmedetomidine, an α2-agonist with sedative, anxiolytic, and mild analgesic effects, might be an alternative in selected cases. Like other sedatives, dexmedetomidine impacts ventilation but only to a mild degree, allowing for maintaining spontaneous ventilation [33]. Furthermore, its impact on upper airways is minimal [31]. However, it might produce a strong influence on the cardiovascular system, leading to an emergence of bradycardia and hypotension [33]. It is also worth underlining that its use outside ICU is off-label in many countries [26]. Nonetheless, dexmedetomidine-based sedation potential was explored in endoscopic procedures with mixed results [34–38]. Some studies reported that, compared to other hypnotics, sedation with dexmedetomidine was tied to significant hemodynamic instability, prolonged recovery, and inadequate sedation, be it during esophageal, colorectal, or pulmonary endoscopy [34, 35, 38]. Furthermore, its delayed onset of action, after 6–10 min, questions the validity of its use in shorter endoscopic procedures [26].

20.4 Summary

Taking the abovementioned into consideration, certain recommendations can be formulated for high-risk patients. Any patient of ASA physical status III or higher should be treated as such. A designated member of the medical team, responsible solely for monitoring the depth of anesthesia, should assist with periprocedural sedation. In selected cases, especially in medically unstable patients, sedation ought to be supervised by an anesthesiologist. Sedation monitoring should not only include basic vital parameters (NIBP, HR, SpO2, RR) but also continuous ECG, qualitative clinical signs, and, where available, capnography. After the endoscopy, patient should be transferred to a designated space where supervised monitoring can be continued until sedation effects wear off. Sedation drugs should be tailored according to patient comorbidities and to the abilities of the responsible medical team. Chosen drugs should be delivered by continuous infusion or in small, incremental doses titrated to the desired level of anesthesia. Sufficient time should be allowed between subsequent doses or infusion rates, especially in patients with prolonged arm-brain circulation time [33].

References

1. Strohleit D, Galetin T, Kosse N, et al. Guidelines on analgosedation, monitoring, and recovery time for flexible bronchoscopy: a systematic review. BMC Pulm Med. 2021;21:1–13.
2. Dumonceau JM, Riphaus A, Schreiber F, et al. Non-anesthesiologist administration of propofol for gastrointestinal endoscopy: European Society of Gastrointestinal Endoscopy, European Society of Gastroenterology and Endoscopy Nurses and associates guideline–updated June 2015. Endoscopy. 2015;47:1175–89.
3. Early DS, Lightdale JR, Vargo JJ, et al. Guidelines for sedation and anesthesia in GI endoscopy. Gastrointest Endosc. 2018;87:327–37.

4. Hinkelbein J, Lamperti M, Akeson J, et al. European Society of Anaesthesiology and European Board of Anaesthesiology guidelines for procedural sedation and analgesia in adults. Eur J Anaesthesiol. 2018;35:6–24.
5. Apfelbaum JL, Gross JB, Connis RT, et al. Practice guidelines for moderate procedural sedation and analgesia 2018: a report by the American Society of Anesthesiologists Task Force on Moderate Procedural Sedation and Analgesia, the American Association of Oral and Maxillofacial Surgeons, American College of Radiology, American Dental Association, American Society of Dentist Anesthesiologists, and Society of Interventional Radiology. Anesthesiology. 2018;128:437–79.
6. Mohan A, Madan K, Hadda V, et al. Guidelines for diagnostic flexible bronchoscopy in adults: Joint Indian Chest Society/National College of chest physicians (I)/Indian association for bronchology recommendations. Lung India. 2019;36:S37–89.
7. Kern M, Kerner T, Tank S. Sedation for advanced procedures in the bronchoscopy suite: proceduralist or anesthesiologist? Curr Opin Anesthesiol. 2017;30:490–5.
8. Behrens A, Kreuzmayr A, Manner H, et al. Acute sedation-associated complications in GI endoscopy (ProSed 2 study): results from the prospective multicentre electronic registry of sedation-associated complications. Gut. 2019;68:445–52.
9. Dang D, Robinson PC, Winnicki S, et al. The safety of flexible fibre-optic bronchoscopy and proceduralist-administered sedation: a tertiary referral centre experience. Intern Med J. 2012;42:300–5.
10. Coté GA, Hovis RM, Ansstas MA, et al. Incidence of sedation-related complications with propofol use during advanced endoscopic procedures. Clin Gastroenterol Hepatol. 2010;8:137–42.
11. Beitz A, Riphaus A, Meining A, et al. Capnographic monitoring reduces the incidence of arterial oxygen desaturation and hypoxemia during propofol sedation for colonoscopy: a randomized, controlled study (ColoCap Study). Off J Am Coll Gastroenterol | ACG. 2012;107:1205–12.
12. Berzin TM, Sanaka S, Barnett SR, et al. A prospective assessment of sedation-related adverse events and patient and endoscopist satisfaction in ERCP with anesthesiologist-administered sedation. Gastrointest Endosc. 2011;73:710–7.
13. Pastis NJ, Hill NT, Yarmus LB, et al. Correlation of vital signs and depth of sedation by modified observer's assessment of alertness and sedation (MOAA/S) scale in bronchoscopy. J Bronchology Interv Pulmonol. 2022;29:54–61.
14. Du Rand IA, Blaikley J, Booton R, Chaudhuri N, Gupta V, Khalid S, Mandal S, Martin J, Mills J, Navani N, Rahman NM. British Thoracic Society guideline for diagnostic flexible bronchoscopy in adults: accredited by NICE. Thorax. 2013;68:i1–i44.
15. Cacho G, Pérez-Calle JL, Barbado A, et al. Capnography is superior to pulse oximetry for the detection of respiratory depression during colonoscopy. Rev Esp Enferm Dig. 2010;102:86–9.
16. Ishiwata T, Tsushima K, Terada J, et al. Efficacy of end-tidal capnography monitoring during flexible bronchoscopy in nonintubated patients under sedation: a randomized controlled study. Respiration. 2018;96:355–62.
17. Qadeer MA, Vargo JJ, Dumot JA, et al. Capnographic monitoring of respiratory activity improves safety of sedation for endoscopic cholangiopancreatography and ultrasonography. Gastroenterology. 2009;136:1568–76.
18. Mehta PP, Kochhar G, Albeldawi M, et al. Capnographic monitoring in routine EGD and colonoscopy with moderate sedation: a prospective, randomized, controlled trial. Am J Gastroenterol. 2016;111:395–404.
19. Barnett S, Hung A, Tsao R, et al. Capnographic monitoring of moderate sedation during low-risk screening colonoscopy does not improve safety or patient satisfaction: a prospective cohort study. Off J Am Coll Gastroenterol | ACG. 2016;111:388–94.
20. Jopling MW, Qiu J. Capnography sensor use is associated with reduction of adverse outcomes during gastrointestinal endoscopic procedures with sedation administration. BMC Anesthesiol. 2017;17:157.

21. Wadhwa V, Gupta K, Vargo JJ. Monitoring standards in sedation and analgesia: the odyssey of capnography in sedation for gastroenterology procedures. Curr Opin Anaesthesiol. 2019;32:453–6.
22. Ishiwata T, Tsushima K, Fujie M, et al. End-tidal capnographic monitoring to detect apnea episodes during flexible bronchoscopy under sedation. BMC Pulm Med. 2017;17:1–5.
23. Dreher M, Ekkernkamp E, Storre JH, et al. Sedation during flexible bronchoscopy in patients with pre-existing respiratory failure: midazolam versus midazolam plus alfentanil. Respiration. 2010;79:307–14.
24. Grendelmeier P, Tamm M, Jahn K, et al. Flexible bronchoscopy with moderate sedation in COPD: a case–control study. Int J Chron Obstruct Pulmon Dis. 2017;12:177.
25. Finlay JE, Leslie K. Sedation/analgesia techniques for nonoperating room anesthesia: new drugs and devices. Curr Opin Anesthesiol. 2021;34:678–82.
26. Goudra BG, Singh PM, Borle A, et al. Anesthesia for advanced bronchoscopic procedures: state-of-the-art review. Lung. 2015;193:453–65.
27. Stolz D, Chhajed PN, Leuppi JD, et al. Cough suppression during flexible bronchoscopy using combined sedation with midazolam and hydrocodone: a randomised, double blind, placebo controlled trial. Thorax. 2004;59:773–6.
28. Gan TJ. Pharmacokinetic and pharmacodynamic characteristics of medications used for moderate sedation. Clin Pharmacokinet. 2006;45:855–69.
29. Cases Viedma E, Andreo García F, Flandes Aldeyturriaga J, et al. Tolerance and safety of 5 models of sedation during endobronchial ultrasound. Arch Bronconeumol. 2016;52:5–11.
30. Ou Y, Feng M, Hu B, et al. The impact of alfentanil supplementation on the sedation of bronchoscopy: a meta-analysis of randomized controlled trials. Medicine. 2022;101:e27401.
31. Ehsan Z, Mahmoud M, Shott SR, et al. The effects of anesthesia and opioids on the upper airway: a systematic review. Laryngoscope. 2016;126:270–84.
32. Memtsoudis SG, Cozowicz C, Nagappa M, et al. Special article: society of anesthesia and sleep medicine guideline on intraoperative management of adult patients with obstructive sleep apnea. Anesth Analg. 2018;127:967.
33. José RJ, Shaefi S, Navani N. Sedation for flexible bronchoscopy: current and emerging evidence. Eur Respir Rev. 2013;22:106 LP – 116.
34. Jalowiecki P, Rudner R, Gonciarz M, et al. Sole use of dexmedetomidine has limited utility for conscious sedation during outpatient colonoscopy. Anesthesiology. 2005;103:269–73.
35. Eberl S, Preckel B, Bergman JJ, et al. Satisfaction and safety using dexmedetomidine or propofol sedation during endoscopic oesophageal procedures. Eur J Anaesthesiol. 2016;33:631–7.
36. Goyal R, Hasnain S, Mittal S, et al. A randomized, controlled trial to compare the efficacy and safety profile of a dexmedetomidine-ketamine combination with a propofol-fentanyl combination for ERCP. Gastrointest Endosc. 2016;83:928–33.
37. Lu Z, Li W, Chen H, et al. Efficacy of a dexmedetomidine–remifentanil combination compared with a midazolam–remifentanil combination for conscious sedation during therapeutic endoscopic retrograde cholangio-pancreatography: a prospective, randomized, single-blinded preliminary trial. Dig Dis Sci. 2018;63:1633–40.
38. Pertzov B, Krasulya B, Azem K, et al. Dexmedetomidine versus propofol sedation in flexible bronchoscopy: a randomized controlled trial. BMC Pulm Med. 2022;22:1–6.

21 NIV Procedures: Complications and Safety

Aleksandra Oraczewska

Noninvasive ventilation (NIV) is the most modern method of respiratory support. Its use brings incredible results in the treatment of type I and type II respiratory failure (RF) and has also become a common treatment for acute and chronic RF. Although NIV is considered a safe method of respiratory support, the use of this method is associated with some complications. Compared to conventional invasive mechanical ventilation, noninvasive mechanical ventilation has the advantage of reducing patient discomfort, treatment complications, and mortality. However, NIV is associated with frequent unpleasant or even life-threatening complications, so patients should be carefully screened beforehand to reduce the potential risk. All serious side effects of NIV are potentially life-threatening and can occur in all patients, but are strongly related to the patient's condition, cooperation, and concomitant diseases. Less serious complications may be related to the specific NIV interfaces and the patient's tolerance [1]. Failure of NIV depends on several factors, e.g., delayed NIV, inadequate ventilatory pressure, inexperience of the clinical team, and, most importantly, the clinical condition of the patient. The basis of well-applied NIV therapy is a skilled team that not only prepares the NIV equipment appropriately, but also explains to the patient, in a simple and clear way, the method application and rationale for the therapy [2, 3].

A. Oraczewska (✉)
Department of Lung Diseases and Tuberculosis, Faculty of Medical Sciences in Zabrze, Medical University of Silesia in Katowice, Katowice, Poland

© The Author(s), under exclusive license to Springer Nature Switzerland AG 2025

K. Panda et al. (eds.), *Noninvasive Ventilatory Approaches in Interventional Procedures*, Noninvasive Ventilation. The Essentials,
https://doi.org/10.1007/978-3-032-05328-2_21

21.1 Major NIV Complications

1. *Barotrauma*

Barotrauma is a complication of mechanical ventilation and increases morbidity and mortality. The normal mechanism of human respiration is associated with negative pressure in the chest. In comparison, mechanical ventilation based on positive pressure, which is not physiological, can lead to barotrauma [1]. The definition of barotrauma is physical tissue damage caused by a pressure difference between an unventilated space inside the body and the surrounding gas or fluid. With NIV, the risk of barotrauma is significantly lower than with invasive ventilation. There are some patient groups with a higher risk of barotrauma, such as chronic obstructive pulmonary disease (COPD), asthma, interstitial lung disease (ILD), and acute respiratory distress syndrome (ARDS). To prevent barotrauma, the ARDSnet protocol recommends keeping the plateau pressure below 30 cm H_2O—defined by a type of disease and ideal body weight (IBW)—in patients receiving mechanical ventilation for ARDS treatment [4]. If higher PEEP is required, it should be increased slowly while closely monitoring peak inspiratory pressure and plateau pressure [5]. We also need to choose the right type and size of interface for NIV support.

2. *Pneumonia and Aspiration Pneumonia*

Individual studies and meta-analyses have found that NIV reduces the risk of pneumonia associated with IMV by a factor of three to five, especially in patients with concomitant diseases [1]. Aspiration pneumonia has been described in about 5% of NIV patients [6]. Ventilator-acquired pneumonia (VAP) is associated with a longer duration of mechanical ventilation. The estimated mortality rate for VAP is around 10%. In patients admitted to the hospital, the physiologic flora of the nasopharynx is rapidly replaced by Gram-negative bacteria and Staphylococcus aureus strains. The results of the study have shown that a biofilm rapidly forms on the endotracheal tube around the sealing cuff, providing a reservoir of pathogens for the developing infection of the bronchial tree [7]. The results of numerous studies confirm the hypothesis that colonization of the airways and digestive tract by pathogens is the main element in the pathogenesis of VAP. In this model, the microorganisms migrate from the pharynx to the bronchi and lungs and through the digestive system into the blood. Suggested strategies to reduce VAP include elevation of the patient's head (up to 45%), continuous suctioning of the airway, use of antiseptics such as chlorhexidine to decontaminate the oral cavity, use of probiotics, and enteral feeding. To protect against aspiration pneumonia, it is advisable to place the patient in a sitting position, optimize ventilatory support, wait at least half an hour after a meal, and use gastric drainage if necessary.

3. Hemodynamic Instability

Ventilation can have negative hemodynamic effects. It may be caused by increasing pressure in the thorax, which reduces preload and filling of the right and left ventricles [8]. Continuous positive airway pressure decreases cardiac output and stroke volume and increases systemic vascular resistance without altering heart rate and arterial pressure. To avoid hemodynamic instability, we must select the patient carefully, for example, avoid patients with uncontrolled cardiac arrhythmias and bleeding. We also need to ensure adequate hydration and optimize ventilatory support.

21.2 Minor NIV Complications

1. Aerophagia, Gastric Distension, and Vomiting

Aerophagia occurs in almost all patients in whom NIV is used, especially with masks covering the nose and mouth. Gastric distension is estimated to be between 5% and 30%. During breathing with NIV support, the tidal volume is distributed between the airway and the digestive tract, with the extent of distribution depending on airway resistance and gastric sphincter pressure. Over-inflation of the stomach is an undesirable phenomenon and is associated with complications. A distended stomach puts pressure on the lungs, which reduces their compliance and impairs ventilation. Insufflation of gastric contents facilitates vomiting and inhalation of gastric contents and can lead to serious complications (i.e., aspiration into the lungs, compartment syndromes, and hypertension, which can eventually lead to death). Airway pressures greater than 20–25 cm H_2O should be avoided. In addition, NIV should be inserted approximately half an hour after a meal, observation, and gastric examination in an almost seated position using a nasogastric tube.

2. Discomfort and Noise

Discomfort is still responsible for 12–33% of NIV failures [9]. To improve patient comfort, we need to explain the whole procedure clearly. The noise of NIV equipment is normal; the noise is much better tolerated in the mask than in the helmets. In some cases, doctors may consider light sedation, especially at the beginning of therapy, to improve compliance. Mask selection, sizing, and donning take time. Gently place the mask over the face and hold it without tight straps at first. Initial settings can also be mild, starting with CPAP and the lowest PS [1].

3. Dryness of the Throat, Nose, and Nosebleeds

During NIV therapy, dryness occurs in 10–20% of patients and nasal congestion in 20–50% [1]. The risk increases when using a nasal mask. To reduce the risk, we can ensure adequate hydration, choose the right mask, and use a humidifier. We can also add emollients.

4. Eye Complications and Conjunctivitis

Eye complications in critically ill patients are common. Ventilation exposes patients to a number of specific risk factors for the development of ocular complications. Increased air leakage can cause dry eyes, which can lead to conjunctivitis. Prevention of ocular complications is achieved by controlling leaks, tightening mask straps correctly, and using eye drops, i.e., artificial tears, as well as contacting and consulting the ophthalmologist.

5. Face Sore

The risk of erythema and skin ulceration increases with the duration of NIV use. Nasal pressure ulcers occur in 5–30% of patients who use NIV [10]. The development of skin lesions is a factor that can limit the tolerability of NIV therapy. Skin changes on the nose and the rest of the face are usually caused by the tightening of the belts and the increase in inspiratory pressure. The predisposition for the occurrence of these complications is often also related to the anatomy of the face and nose, the age of the patient, malnutrition, hypotension, and arteriosclerosis of the small vessels. To prevent these complications, we were able to correctly adjust the size and interface, check the mask and ligaments, optimize ventilatory support (slowly reduce the pressure), and, in many cases, use artificial skin dressings such as gel patches.

6. Leaks

Air leaks are common with noninvasive ventilation. Leaks depend on the interfaces, which are larger with a small face mask than with a larger mask. Large leaks reduce FiO2 and arterial oxygen saturation and increase ventilator self-triggering and exhaled rebreathing gas. They increase NIV failure. Leaks should therefore be carefully corrected during treatment. Leaks can be corrected by tightening the straps, which seal the mask. This increases the risk of discomfort and skin damage. Pressure-controlled ventilation causes fewer air leaks than volume-controlled ventilation.

7. Edema

Depending on which interface is used, the location of the edema will vary. When using helmets, it can occur in the tissue of the upper extremities [11]. To protect the patient from edema, we need to optimize the ventilatory support (i.e., slightly reduce the pressure) and sometimes change the mask [1].

In summary, to optimize patient care, NIV should be used by an experienced medical team that carefully selects patients according to available guidelines and appropriate clinical assessment, always considering the risk factors for NIV failure. Once NIV is started, patients should be closely monitored in the appropriate units until stabilization. Attention should be paid not only to vital signs and blood gas analysis results, but also to comfort, leakage, and coordination between patient and ventilator. The correct choice of device, appropriate management of ventilatory support, a qualified medical team, and careful clinical and instrumental monitoring are crucial to minimize the risk of complications during NIV.

References

1. Carron M, Freo U, BaHammam AS, Dellweg D, Guarracino F, Cosentini R, Feltracco P, Vianello A, Ori C, Esquinas A. Complications of non-invasive ventilation techniques: a comprehensive qualitative review of randomized trials. Br J Anaesth. 2013;110(6):896–914.
2. Huang GC, McSparron JI, Balk EM, et al. Procedural instruction in invasive bedside procedures: a systematic review and meta-analysis of effective teaching approaches. BMJ Qual Saf. 2016;25(4):281–94.
3. Lazovic B, Dmitrovic R, Simonovic I, Esqoinas A, Mina B, Zack S. Unusual complications of non-invasive mechanical ventilation (NIV) and high-flow nasal cannula (HFNC): a systematic review. Tuberk Toraks. 2022;70(2):197–202. English.
4. International consensus conferences in intensive care medicine: ventilator-associated lung injury in ARDS. This official conference report was cosponsored by the American Thoracic Society, The European Society of Intensive Care Medicine, and The Societé de Réanimation de Langue Française, and was approved by the ATS Board of Directors. Am J Respir Crit Care Med. 1999;160(6):2118–24.
5. Brower RG, Lanken PN, MacIntyre N, Matthay MA, Morris A, Ancukiewicz M, Schoenfeld D, Thompson BT. National Heart, Lung, and Blood Institute ARDS clinical trials network. Higher versus lower positive end-expiratory pressures in patients with the acute respiratory distress syndrome. N Engl J Med. 2004;351(4):327–36.
6. Hess DR. Noninvasive positive-pressure ventilation and ventilator-associated pneumonia. Respir Care. 2005;50(7):924–9. discussion 929–31.
7. Wiener-Kronish JP, Dorr HI. Ventilator-associated pneumonia: problems with diagnosis and therapy. Best Pract Res Clin Anaesthesiol. 2008;22:437–49.
8. Valipour A, Schneider F, Kössler W, Saliba S, Burghuber OC. Heart rate variability and spontaneous baroreflex sequences in supine healthy volunteers subjected to nasal positive airway pressure. J Appl Physiol. 2005;99(6):2137–43. https://doi.org/10.1152/japplphysiol.00003.2005. Epub 2005 Jul 7.
9. Hawker F, Breen D, Torzillo P, Herkes R. Randomized prospective trial of noninvasive positive pressure ventilation in acute respiratory failure. Am J Respir Crit Care Med. 1996;153(3):1188–9.
10. Celikel T, Sungur M, Ceyhan B, Karakurt S. Comparison of noninvasive positive pressure ventilation with standard medical therapy in hypercapnic acute respiratory failure. Chest. 1998;114(6):1636–42.
11. Antonelli M, Pennisi MA, Pelosi P, Gregoretti C, Squadrone V, Rocco M, Cecchini L, Chiumello D, Severgnini P, Proietti R, Navalesi P, Conti G. Noninvasive positive pressure ventilation using a helmet in patients with acute exacerbation of chronic obstructive pulmonary disease: a feasibility study. Anesthesiology. 2004;100(1):16–24.

Non-Invasive Ventilation: High-Risk Aerosol-Generating Procedure

22

Kishore Kumar, Manigandan Venkatesan, Kumari Sulochana, and Antonio M. Esquinas

22.1 Introduction

Noninvasive ventilation (NIV) is defined as the delivery of artificial ventilation to the lungs without requiring endotracheal intubation. Outside the operating theatre, negative-pressure noninvasive ventilation techniques were the common method of delivering mechanical ventilatory support during the first half of the twentieth century. However, in the year 1960, invasive positive pressure ventilation surpassed the negative pressure ventilation due to improved airway patency. Over the last decade, the re-emergence of NIV has provided ventilatory assistance with more ease, comfort, and safety [1]. NIV has become quite an essential and common component in both the Intensive Care Unit (ICU) and Emergency Department (ED) [2]. It is believed that NIV generates aerosols and droplets that may carry respiratory pathogens. Aerosols are airborne particles, either solid or liquid, up to 100 μm in diameter that remain suspended in the air significantly longer than the larger droplets, which settle more quickly under the influence of gravity [3]. Noninvasive respiratory support (NIRS) has seen growing use in ED and critical care settings for various conditions such as acute hypoxemic respiratory failure, pneumonia, and asthma [4, 5].

K. Kumar (✉)
Department of Respiratory Therapy, College of Pharmacy and Applied and Medical Science, Dar Al Uloom University, Riyadh, Saudi Arabia

M. Venkatesan
Department of Medicine, University of Texas Health Science Centre, San Antonio, TX, USA

K. Sulochana
Division of Respiratory Therapy, Critical Care Medicine, Bharti Hospital and Research Centre, Pune, India

A. M. Esquinas
Intensive Care Unit, Hospital Morales Meseguer, Murcia, Spain

© The Author(s), under exclusive license to Springer Nature Switzerland AG 2025
K. Panda et al. (eds.), *Noninvasive Ventilatory Approaches in Interventional Procedures*, Noninvasive Ventilation. The Essentials,
https://doi.org/10.1007/978-3-032-05328-2_22

NIV techniques are classified as aerosol-generating procedures (AGPs), a designation of particular importance given that respiratory infections like COVID-19 and tuberculosis are primarily transmitted via respiratory droplets [6]. As patients undergo respiratory care procedures, especially NIRS, healthcare workers face a risk of exposure to infectious particles, often due to aerosol generation [7]. In this chapter, we will explore the classification of aerosol-generating procedures, the risk associated with aerosol-generating procedures, and mitigation strategies for aerosol generation in NIV.

22.2 Classification as an Aerosol-Generating Procedure

Medical procedures that generate aerosols beyond those produced naturally by patients through breathing, coughing, sneezing, or talking are referred to as aerosol-generating procedures (AGPs) [8]. NIV procedures, such as bi-level positive airway pressure (BiPAP), continuous positive airway pressure (CPAP), and high-frequency oxygen ventilation (HFOV), are aerosol-generating procedures that mechanically generate and disperse aerosols and those that prompt the patient to produce aerosols and increase the risk of transmission of infection among healthcare workers [9, 10]. The term “aerosol” is a collection of solid, liquid, or both particles suspended in a carrier gas such as air [11, 12]. The particle size of the airborne droplets is classified by its size based on diameter, specifically in micrometers (μm). The droplet is nebulous and has been established based on its diameters ranging widely, >5, >10, or >100 μm [13]. Under normal atmospheric pressure, the airborne particle size is smaller than 100 μm [14]. While grouping aerosols by their size aids in understanding dispersal patterns, it is crucial to categorize them based on their deposition sites within the respiratory tract [15]. Aerosol dispersal patterns and deposition vary between small and large droplets. Aerosol particles <20 μm in size can create droplet nuclei and reach the lower respiratory tract, while those >20 μm are more likely to contact the eyes or mouth and accumulate in the upper respiratory tract. Droplet and droplet nuclei measurements can be performed using various methods, including microscopic observation, optical particle counting, aerodynamic particle counting, interferometric imaging, and laser aerosol particle spectrophotometry [16]. Measuring the behavior and movement of aerosols and their particles is quite challenging. In solids, every particle shares the same velocity and acceleration vector as the entire object. However, since aerosols are fluids, their particles do not share unique vectors as they do in solids. To simplify measurement in this context, the concept of “fluid parcel” is often applied, which represents the whole fluid [17]. The following table (Table 22.1) lists the top 10 procedure groups most identified as aerosol-generating procedures based on frequency across various source literatures. These procedures have a high potential for generating aerosols and, therefore, may pose a risk for airborne transmission. These interventions are considered aerosol-dispersing techniques when they spread exhaled bioaerosols from an infected person over a wide range of procedures, such as high flow nasal cannula (HFNC) and noninvasive ventilation (NIV). These interventions do not increase the amount of

Table 22.1 Top 10 aerosol-generating procedures

Procedure	Description
Intubation and extubation	Insertion and removal of the airway tube
Airway suctioning	Removal of secretions from the airway
Bronchoscopy	Endoscopic examination of the airways
Noninvasive ventilation	Respiratory support without intubation
Aerosol therapy (nebulization)	Medication delivery through aerosols
Cardiopulmonary resuscitation	Chest compression and ventilation
Sputum induction	Procedure to produce sputum for testing
Tracheostomy-related procedures	Surgical opening of the airway in the neck
Manual ventilation	Assisted ventilation
Autopsy	Postmortem examination

bioaerosols produced. The effects of spreading viruses containing bioaerosols depend on the viral load, particle size, and the flow and range of their movement [18].

22.3 Hazards and Transmission of Aerosol Generation from NIV

Coughing and sneezing are critical airway reflexes that can expel mucus particles up to a 9-meter distance. Research has indicated that over a 3-h flight, approximately 80% of the passengers could spread the infection from a single coughing individual [2]. When pathogens are present, these particles can infect nearby individuals and animals, significantly facilitating the transmission of airborne infections [19]. A key study suggesting that NIV carries a high risk of infection assessed particle dispersion using an experimental study in which smoke was introduced into a mannequin's lung during NIV. Smoke plumes released from the vented mask were photographed to assess particle dispersion. Many experts contend that NIV masks may provide a barrier preventing the release of secretions that would otherwise spread during coughing, sneezing, or speaking. Furthermore, there is a lack of controlled data comparing particle dispersion in individuals using NIV versus those who do not [9]. A recent study found that using standard face masks for NIV in patients with infectious diseases could lead to considerable exposure to infectious organisms within 1 meter from the patient's exhaled air. The spread of infected respiratory droplets may be intensified by increased mask leakage and worsened by higher inspiratory pressure levels [19]. A wide range of NIV masks are being used in intensive care units (ICUs), such as nasal masks, oronasal masks, helmets, or full-face masks. The following are potential sources of the leaks that permit aerosol dispersion during ventilation: (a) the mouth by using a nasal mask, (b) the region where the mask and face come into contact, and (c) masks with a purposeful leak port [20]. A helmet interface has been introduced in Europe for delivering NIV. Many patients find helmets more comfortable than facemasks. It is suggested that using a helmet interface for NIV, especially in negative-pressure rooms equipped with high-efficiency particulate air (HEPA), could help reduce the spread of infected respiratory droplets.

22.4 Strategies to Minimize Risk for Noninvasive Ventilation (NIV)

NIV, such as CPAP and BiPAP, is associated with a low transmission risk. The following strategies are used to prevent the risk of aerosol transmission from NIV including the following [21]:

1. Using a procedural mask or face tent scavenger.
2. Selecting an appropriate interface, such as a non-vented mask or helmet with an air cushion around the neck.
3. Configuring the mechanical ventilator by using a dual-limb ventilator with a filter at the expiratory port.
4. Using a single-limb ventilator with a filter placed at the expiratory port or between the masks.
5. A heat moisture exchange (HME) filter should be used between the mask and exhalation port to prevent transmission from any intentional leaks.

To reduce the risk of airborne pathogen spread, it is recommended to use a helmet with an air supply when available [22]. Recent research indicates that incorporating a neck cushion significantly minimizes the dispersal of aerosols [23]. NIV serves as a valuable alternative to invasive ventilation, particularly in the ICU and emergency care. However, due to its classification as an aerosol-generating procedure, it presents a notable infection control challenge. The increased potential for aerosol and droplet dispersion when using high inspiratory pressures or a standard mask with leak-prone designs can elevate the risk of transmitting respiratory infections to healthcare workers. A balanced approach that considers both patient benefits and healthcare provider safety is essential to successfully implementing NIV in infectious disease cases. The development of new interface designs and further research on particle dispersion in clinical settings are needed to optimize NIV use while minimizing the risk of transmission.

References

1. Mehta S, Hill NS. Noninvasive ventilation. Am J Respir Crit Care Med. 2001;163(2):540–77.
2. Esquinas AM, Pravinkumar SE, Scala R, Gay P, Soroksky A, Girault C, Han F, Hui DS, Papadakos PJ, Ambrosino N. Noninvasive mechanical ventilation in high-risk pulmonary infections: a clinical review. Eur Respir J. 2014;23(134):427–38.
3. Zhang MX, Lilien TA, van Etten-Jamaludin FS, Fraenkel CJ, Bonn D, Vlaar AP, Löndahl J, Klompas M, Bem RA. Generation of aerosols by noninvasive respiratory support modalities: a systematic review and meta-analysis. JAMA Netw Open. 2023;6(10):e2337258.

4. Kempker JA, Abril MK, Chen Y, Kramer MR, Waller LA, Martin GS. The epidemiology of respiratory failure in the United States 2002–2017: a serial cross-sectional study. Crit Care Explor. 2020;2(6):e0128.
5. Antonelli M, Conti G, Moro ML, Esquinas A, Gonzalez-Diaz G, Confalonieri M, Pelaia P, Principi T, Gregoretti C, Beltrame F, Pennisi M. Predictors of failure of noninvasive positive pressure ventilation in patients with acute hypoxemic respiratory failure: a multi-center study. Intensive Care Med. 2001;27:1718–28.
6. Kallet RH. Noninvasive ventilation in acute care: controversies and emerging concepts. Respir Care. 2009;54(2):259–63.
7. Klompas M, Baker MA, Rhee C, Tucker R, Fiumara K, Griesbach D, Bennett-Rizzo C, Salmasian H, Wang R, Wheeler N, Gallagher GR. A SARS-CoV-2 cluster in an acute care hospital. Ann Intern Med. 2021;174(6):794–802.
8. Davies A, Thomson G, Walker J, Bennett A. A review of the risks and disease transmission associated with aerosol generating medical procedures. J Infect Prev. 2009;10(4):122–6.
9. Fowler RA, Guest CB, Lapinsky SE, Sibbald WJ, Louie M, Tang P, Simor AE, Stewart TE. Transmission of severe acute respiratory syndrome during intubation and mechanical ventilation. Am J Respir Crit Care Med. 2004;169(11):1198–202.
10. Christian MD, Loutfy M, McDonald LC, Martinez KF, Ofner M, Wong T, Wallington T, Gold WL, Mederski B, Green K, Low DE. Possible SARS coronavirus transmission during cardiopulmonary resuscitation. Emerg Infect Dis. 2004;10(2):287.
11. Lohmann U, Lüönd F, Mahrt F. An introduction to clouds: from the microscale to climate. Cambridge University Press; 2016.
12. Jackson T, Deibert D, Wyatt G, Durand-Moreau Q, Adisesh A, Khunti K, Khunti S, Smith S, Chan XH, Ross L, Roberts N. Classification of aerosol-generating procedures: a rapid systematic review. BMJ Open Respir Res. 2020;7(1):e000730.
13. Xie X, Li Y, Chwang AT, Ho PL, Seto WH. How far droplets can move in indoor environments–revisiting the wells evaporation–falling curve. Indoor Air. 2007;17(3):211.
14. Kohanski MA, Lo LJ, Waring MS. Review of indoor aerosol generation, transport, and control in the context of COVID-19. Int Forum Allergy Rhinol. 2020;10(10):1173–9.
15. Thomas RJ. Particle size and pathogenicity in the respiratory tract. Virulence. 2013;4(8):847–58.
16. Esquinas AM, editor. Noninvasive mechanical ventilation in high risk infections, mass casualty and pandemics. Springer; 2023.
17. Nizam B, Utku T. NIV models to assess air and particle dispersion. In: Noninvasive mechanical ventilation in high risk infections, mass casualty and pandemics, vol. 5. Cham: Springer International Publishing; 2023. p. 135–44.
18. Dhand R, Li J. Coughs and sneezes: their role in transmission of respiratory viral infections, including SARS-CoV-2. Am J Respir Crit Care Med. 2020;202(5):651–9.
19. Hui DS, Chow BK, Ng SS, Chu LC, Hall SD, Gin T, Sung JJ, Chan MT. Exhaled air dispersion distances during noninvasive ventilation via different Respironics face masks. Chest. 2009;136(4):998–1005.
20. Pirzada AR, Aleissi SA, Almeneessier AS, BaHammam AS. Management of aerosol during noninvasive ventilation for patients with sleep-disordered breathing: important messages during the COVID-19 pandemic. Sleep Vigil. 2020;4:89–94.
21. Li J, Alolaiwat A, Fink JB, Dhand R. Aerosol-generating procedures and virus transmission. Respir Care. 2022;67(8):1022–42.
22. Gómez CC, Rodríguez ÓP, Torné ML, Santaolalla CE, Jiménez JF, Fernandez JG, Perales JM, Heili-Frades SB, Monreal MF, de Andres Nilsson JM, Arias EL. Clinical consensus recommendations regarding non-invasive respiratory support in the adult patient with acute respiratory failure secondary to SARS-CoV-2 infection. Med Intensiva (Engl Ed). 2020;44(7):429–38.
23. Whittle JS, Pavlov I, Sacchetti AD, Atwood C, Rosenberg MS. Respiratory support for adult patients with COVID-19. J Am Coll Emerg Physicians Open. 2020;1(2):95–101.

Part VII

Methodology of NIV during Clinical Procedures

Difficult Airway Scenarios: Preoxygenation, Devices, and Methodology

23

Isacco Curto, Greta Zunino, Silvia De Rosa, and Denise Battaglini

23.1 Introduction

Airway management involves a systematic approach to examining, planning, and employing various medical techniques and technologies to maintain or restore a safe and effective conduit for oxygenation and ventilation. These procedures are particularly indicated for patients experiencing airway obstruction or respiratory insufficiency. Proper and safe airway management is vital in anesthesiology and critical care to ensure patient safety [1].

Noninvasive ventilatory methods play a crucial role in providing adequate oxygenation and ventilation while minimizing the need for surgical interventions in challenging airway scenarios. Preoxygenation is a critical step in this process, as it enhances the oxygen reserve in the lungs prior to airway management. A range of technologies and approaches can be utilized to facilitate noninvasive breathing in

I. Curto
Anesthesia and Intensive Care, Santa Chiara Regional Hospital, APSS, Trento, Italy
e-mail: isacco.curto@bl.omceo.it

G. Zunino
Department of Surgical Sciences and Integrated Diagnostics, University of Genoa, Genoa, Italy

S. De Rosa
Anesthesia and Intensive Care, Santa Chiara Regional Hospital, APSS, Trento, Italy

Centre for Medical Sciences, CISMed, University of Trento, Trento, Italy

D. Battaglini (✉)
Department of Surgical Sciences and Integrated Diagnostics, University of Genoa, Genoa, Italy

Anesthesia and Intensive Care, IRCCS Ospedale Policlinicfo San Martino, Genoa, Italy
e-mail: denise.battaglini@unige.it

© The Author(s), under exclusive license to Springer Nature Switzerland AG 2025

K. Panda et al. (eds.), *Noninvasive Ventilatory Approaches in Interventional Procedures*, Noninvasive Ventilation. The Essentials,
https://doi.org/10.1007/978-3-032-05328-2_23

these situations. Patients in the intensive care unit (ICU) are at a higher risk for difficult airways compared to those in the operating room (OR) due to reduced oxygen reserve, individual patient characteristics (e.g., edema, trauma), and ICU-specific factors (e.g., limited access to the airway, suboptimal lighting) [2].

Noninvasive ventilation (NIV) is routinely employed in the management of acute respiratory failure (ARF) under specific clinical circumstances. Beyond the established benefits of reducing or delaying the need for invasive mechanical ventilation, recent data suggest that it may also be advantageous during the process of endotracheal intubation. NIV plays a pivotal role in modern preoxygenation practices, particularly in patients with complex airway needs or reduced functional reserves. By employing techniques such as continuous positive airway pressure (CPAP) and bilevel positive airway pressure (BiPAP), NIV optimizes oxygenation and enhances safety during airway management. However, among high-flow devices used for preoxygenation in difficult airway scenarios, high-flow oxygen therapy is gaining popularity [3].

The CPAP technique is frequently utilized for preoxygenation in challenging airway situations. CPAP delivers a continuous supply of continuous end-expiratory positive pressure, preventing airway collapse and improving oxygenation. It is particularly beneficial for patients with obstructive sleep apnea or underlying pulmonary conditions [4].

BiPAP may also be employed for non-invasive ventilation in difficult airway scenarios. BiPAP provides two distinct pressures for inspiration and expiration, thereby assisting patients experiencing respiratory distress. It is commonly used for patients suffering from ARF or chronic obstructive pulmonary disease (COPD) [4].

In addition to these devices, high-flow nasal oxygen (HFNO) has gained prominence in recent years. HFNO delivers heated and humidified oxygen at high flow rates, providing oxygenation and low positive pressure to the airways. This method improves oxygenation and reduces the work of breathing, making it especially useful for individuals with ARF requiring supplemental oxygen [5].

This chapter aims to identify when and how to utilize a noninvasive ventilation strategy for a difficult airway. It will summarize the evidence regarding the importance of preoxygenation and the maintenance of oxygenation during airway management, as well as outline strategies to address both predicted and unpredicted difficult airways.

23.2 Definition of a Difficult Airway

Although not standardized, the definition of a difficult airway encompasses challenging or failed intubations, as well as potential difficulties arising during various phases of the intubation process and subsequent mechanical ventilation (MV). In 2022 the American Society of Anesthesiologists (ASA) defined a difficult airway as a scenario in which a clinician trained in airway management encounters one or more of the following situations: (1) difficult facemask ventilation, (2) difficult laryngoscopy, (3) difficult supraglottic airway ventilation, (4) difficult or failed tracheal intubation, (5) difficult or failed tracheal extubation, (6) difficult or failed invasive airway access, and (7) inadequate ventilation [6]. This comprehensive definition assists the airway management team in planning each step of the intubation process, optimizing factors that contribute to success, and preventing potentially harmful complications.

The unanticipated difficult airway presents a significant challenge; however, the "unanticipated" aspect can be mitigated through thorough examination of the patient's history and characteristics. Guidelines provide clinicians with practical, well-structured recommendations, beginning with a comprehensive evaluation of the patient's airway [7], along with detailed strategies for managing both anticipated and unanticipated difficult airways. The literature emphasizes the necessity for airway management personnel to be well-prepared and adequately trained to prevent delays and complications, particularly in emergency situations [6]. Numerous schematic and cognitive tools have been developed to aid in this preparation [5–7]. Awareness of the human factor in airway management is increasing; the NAP4 report indicated that human factors may have contributed to 40% of major complications, with human error being a significant factor in 25% of these cases [2]. It is evident that human factors must be considered to ensure successful airway management [8].

A difficult airway may be unanticipated, arising during airway management maneuvers and potentially escalating into a real emergency characterized by the risk of a "cannot intubate, cannot oxygenate" (CICO) scenario, which can lead to hypoxic-ischemic brain injury and even death [1].

Preoperative clinical history and physical examination are essential for identifying potential difficulties in airway management before general anesthesia. Key factors include patient demographics, medical history, and physical features (Table 23.1), which can be assessed using scoring systems like the Wilson score (Fig. 23.1) and STOP-Bang score (Fig. 23.2).

Imaging techniques such as cervical X-rays and computed tomography (CT) scans aid in evaluating anatomical abnormalities, with ultrasound offering real-time assessment without radiation. Although transnasal flexible endoscopic laryngoscopy (TFEL) shows promise, its supporting evidence is limited. The history of prior difficult intubation is a strong predictor of future challenges, with the upper lip bite test being the most effective bedside assessment. A Wilson score of 2 or higher suggests a higher risk of difficult intubation [7].

The literature indicates that a single, robust airway assessment tool does not exist; therefore, the optimal approach involves a combination of tests and evaluations. Comprehensive airway assessment is critical for every patient undergoing general anesthesia and/or sedation, as it informs the selection of medications, equipment, and techniques appropriate for each patient and procedure [9].

Table 23.1 Physical features associated with possible complex airway management

Prominent incisors, moustaches, and a beard	Examine the patient.
Cervical spine mobility and extension of the lateral atlantoaxial joint	Ask the patient to move his/her head forward and backward to bend the neck. When backward, lift the face upward to evaluate the extension of the lateral atlantoaxial joint.
Mandibular movement	Perform the upper lip bite test: ask the patient to bite the upper lip with the lower incisors as much as he/she can. Classes II and III can be difficult to intubate.
Mandibular retrognathia and protrusion	Retrognathia: mandible shorter than 9 cm. Protrusion, when limited, is associated with a difficult airway.
Modified Mallampati test	In the sitting position, ask the patient to open the mouth and observe the size of the tongue and the pharynx and their relationship. Grades III or IV are associated with a difficult airway.
Neck circumference	Measure with a flexible ruler. If >40 cm mask ventilation, laryngoscopy, and endotracheal intubation can be difficult.
Thyromental distance	Measure the distance between the mandibular mental process and the thyroid cartilage notch/suprasternal fossa with the patient's head backward as far as he/she can: <4–7 cm.
Hyo-mental distance	Measure the distance between the mental prominence and the hyoid bone: <3–5 cm.
Thyromental height	Measure the distance between the anterior borders of the mentum and the thyroid cartilage, positioning the patient supine: ≤50 cm.

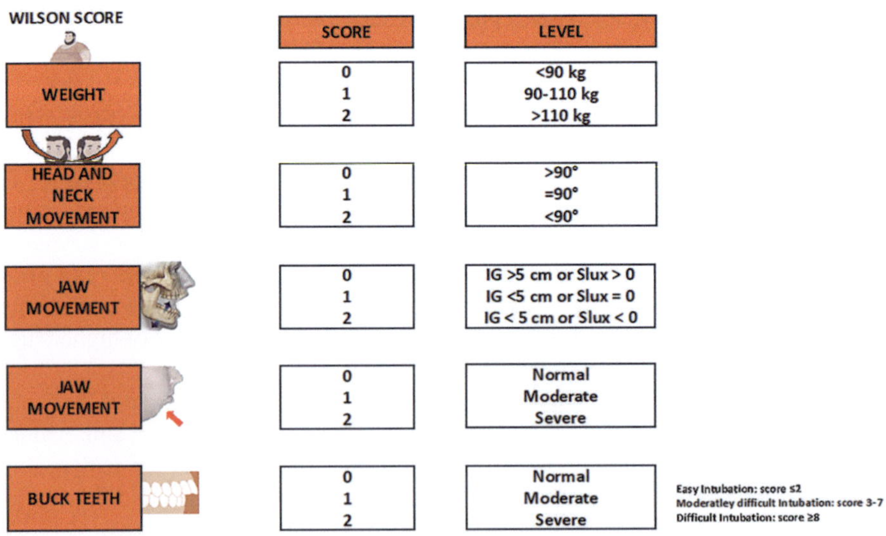

Fig. 23.1 Wilson score

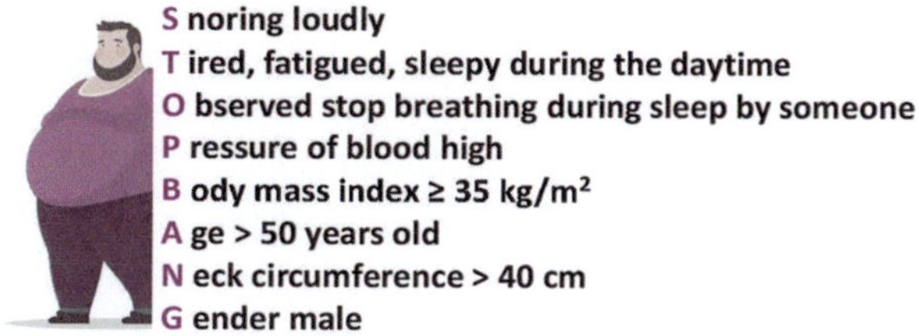

Fig. 23.2 STOP-Band Score. High risk of obstructive sleep apnea if yes from 5 to 8; intermediate, if yes from 3 to 4; low risk, if yes from 0 to 2

23.3 The Importance of Maintaining Oxygenation During Airway Management

Given that difficult ventilation and airway management can be unpredictable, preoxygenation is recommended for all patients undergoing deep sedation prior to endotracheal intubation [7, 9]. The primary goal of preoxygenation is to enhance the oxygen reserve and delay desaturation during the apneic phase, thereby extending the time available for laryngoscopy and intubation [7, 9]. In healthy patients breathing room air, desaturation (defined as peripheral oxygen saturation (SpO2), falling below 88–90%) typically occurs within 1–2 min; however, preoxygenation can prolong this to approximately 8 min [7, 10].

The safe apnea time refers to the interval between the cessation of breathing or ventilation and the onset of desaturation [10]. Preoxygenation aims to increase the fraction of alveolar oxygen (FAO2) and, consequently, elevate oxygen levels in the arterial, tissue, and venous compartments [10]. This process also facilitates the washout of alveolar nitrogen (N_2), known as denitrogenation, with target objectives of achieving an end-tidal O_2 concentration of 90% and an end-tidal N_2 concentration of 5% [9].

Patients undergoing preoxygenation should ideally be positioned in a 20° head-up position rather than in a completely supine position. Studies have demonstrated that this positioning prolongs the apneic period before SpO2 falls below 95%. For immobilized patients, the reverse Trendelenburg position may be a suitable alternative [10].

A significant factor contributing to the success of preoxygenation is the selection of the appropriate device, particularly the facemask. Factors such as facial hair (beards or mustaches), edentulous status, advanced age, sunken cheeks, and the presence of a gastric tube can compromise the seal between the mask and the patient's face. These considerations, along with the appropriate size of the mask, are essential to optimize the effectiveness of the breathing circuit employed [9, 10].

Various techniques for preoxygenation have been described. One method involves the patient taking eight deep breaths at an oxygen flow of 10 L/min over 60 s. This approach achieves arterial oxygen tension (PaO2) comparable to that attained through 3 min of tidal volume breathing at an oxygen flow of 5 L/min (PaO2 = 369 ± 69 mmHg) [9, 10]. However, utilizing a flow rate of 10 L/min instead of 5 L/min has only a minimal positive effect on reducing nitrogen rebreathing [9].

In spontaneous breathing using a fraction of inspired oxygen (FiO2) of 1 for 3 min, the initial denitrogenation is advantageous and helps achieve an FAO2 of 95%. However, in the presence of circuit leaks, these benefits diminish due to a decrease in FiO2 within the circuit [11].

The vital capacity technique is particularly useful for patients who may not cooperate fully. This maneuver begins with a forced expiration, followed by four or five deep breaths, ensuring that the inspiratory oxygen flow exceeds the peak inspiratory flow. Notably, spontaneous breathing in pure oxygen yields higher PaO2 values (397 ± 48 mmHg vs. 293 ± 86 mmHg) and prolongs the duration of apnea without desaturation [11].

23.4 Role of NIV in Preoxygenation

NIV is increasingly recognized as an essential component of preoxygenation strategies for managing difficult airways. It provides several advantages:

- *Enhanced oxygenation*: NIV prevents alveolar collapse and improves oxygen exchange. This is particularly beneficial in patients with obstructive sleep apnea, obesity, or underlying pulmonary conditions.
- *Prolonged safe apnea time*: By improving functional residual capacity (FRC), NIV extends the duration before desaturation occurs during the apneic phase of airway management.
- *Reduction in work of breathing*: NIV reduces the patient's respiratory effort, making it easier to achieve optimal oxygenation.

Advanced preoxygenation techniques have been evaluated for their efficacy. The application of positive end-expiratory pressure (PEEP) in spontaneously breathing patients has been shown to prolong the time until desaturation occurs [9]. Additionally, pressure support ventilation (PSV) has been found to enhance the fraction of expired oxygen (FeO2) in a group of healthy volunteers receiving preoxygenation, compared to spontaneous breathing at an FiO2 of 1. This improvement is likely due to a higher rate of denitrogenation and better mask adherence to the face [11].

The transnasal humidified rapid insufflation ventilatory exchange (THRIVE) system utilizes a nasal high-flow cannula that delivers oxygen at rates up to 70 L/min, generating a CPAP of 7 cm H_2O. This method not only improves oxygenation but also reduces carbon dioxide (CO_2) levels by flushing the dead space. When THRIVE is maintained during the induction of anesthesia and neuromuscular blockade, it extends the duration of safe apnea and mitigates CO_2 accumulation [9].

Finally, while often overlooked, apneic oxygenation (AO) is crucial for gaining safe time during airway management. To maximize the effectiveness of AO, optimal preoxygenation should be achieved, and airway patency must be maintained [9]. The effectiveness of AO is also influenced by the predicted functional residual capacity to body weight ratio (FRC/BW): patients with an FRC/BW below

37 ± 9 mL/kg can tolerate AO for no longer than 5 min, whereas those with a higher FRC/BW may sustain AO for up to 15 min [12]. AO can be administered using a nasopharyngeal or oropharyngeal cannula at an oxygen flow of 15 L/min, through a needle inserted into the cricothyroid membrane, or with the THRIVE system [7, 9].

Three systematic reviews have investigated the efficacy of apneic oxygenation (AO). Silva et al. found that AO during emergency intubation increased peri-intubation SpO2 and success rates for first-attempt intubation while reducing the incidence of hypoxemia [13]. In the emergency department setting, AO was associated with reduced hypoxemia during intubation maneuvers and significantly lower rates of critical desaturation [14]. White et al. reported substantial benefits of AO on SpO2 in elective surgical patients, obese patients, and those undergoing emergency intubation without respiratory failure [15]. Consequently, all high-risk patients should receive oxygen via nasal cannula (up to 15 L/min) in addition to standard preoxygenation and facemask ventilation during intubation efforts [7].

However, preoxygenation carries certain risks: (1) Unrecognized esophageal intubation may be delayed in detection, as hypoxemia and desaturation can occur minutes later in preoxygenated patients. Monitoring end-tidal CO_2 (EtCO2) immediately after intubation can help identify this issue earlier than relying solely on SpO2 monitoring [16]. (2) In patients undergoing general anesthesia in a supine position, suppression of spontaneous breathing can lead to a reduction in FRC and potential airway closure or collapse in dependent lung regions, resulting in compression and absorption atelectasis. In these areas, where alveolar ventilation is insufficient, nitrogen (N_2) remains in the alveolar space while oxygen (O_2) is absorbed, leading to further complications. Preoxygenation facilitates the replacement of N_2 with O_2, raising blood oxygen levels but also potentially accelerating absorption atelectasis in the dependent lung areas after the cessation of spontaneous breathing [9].

Several studies indicate that using decremental levels of FiO2 during preoxygenation can reduce lung atelectasis without compromising the time to arterial desaturation [17, 18]. Additionally, Cressey et al. demonstrated that applying 5 cm H_2O of CPAP during preoxygenation and 6 cm H_2O of PEEP during mask ventilation can prevent atelectasis [19]. Preoxygenation is also beneficial prior to reversing neuromuscular blockade and during extubation, supporting the patient as they transition from mechanical to spontaneous breathing [9].

23.5 Optimizing NIV in Difficult Airways Scenario

Certain patient populations require special consideration during preoxygenation. Pregnant patients, for instance, exhibit a reduced functional residual capacity (FRC) and increased oxygen consumption (VO2), making them prone to rapid desaturation during the apneic phase. Preoxygenation using eight deep breaths to achieve a FeO2 of 90% has been identified as an optimal technique for this group [11].

In patients with obesity (body mass index (BMI) >40 kg/m^2), pulmonary abnormalities are closely linked to their BMI. These patients typically present with low FRC, elevated VO2, and ventilation/perfusion (V/Q) ratio heterogeneity, resulting in faster desaturation (SpO2 <90%) prior to anesthesia and complete muscle relaxation compared to nonobese individuals. For example, desaturation occurs after an average of 2.7 min in mobile obese patients, whereas it takes about 6 min in those with normal body weight [9, 11]. Additionally, the high prevalence of obstructive sleep apnea in this population increases the risk of difficult mask ventilation and intubation [9].

Preoxygenation in a 25° head-up position, utilizing eight deep breaths or CPAP for 3 min, has been shown to enhance PaO2 and prolong the safe apnea time compared to a supine position. Applying a pressure support ventilation (PSV) of 5 cm H_2O alongside a CPAP level of 5 cm H_2O further improves PaO2 and prevents desaturation compared to spontaneous breathing [11]. It is also advisable to administer oxygen via nasal cannula or an oropharyngeal catheter during the apneic phase [9].

Patients with chronic obstructive pulmonary disease (COPD) present with lower FRC, V/Q mismatch, and higher VO2 [9]. A brief interruption of spontaneous breathing can lead to significant desaturation, making preoxygenation essential. The duration of tidal volume breathing necessary for effective preoxygenation can be monitored using FeO2, potentially lasting up to 5 min [11].

Elderly patients often experience respiratory muscle weakness, alterations in lung parenchyma (resulting in reduced elastic recoil), and diminished lung volumes, which contribute to V/Q mismatch and reduced pulmonary reserve. As a result, these patients benefit more from 3 min of tidal volume breathing compared to other preoxygenation techniques [9].

In emergency settings, preoxygenation is recommended, with hypoxemic PSV techniques demonstrating superiority over 3 min of tidal breathing. These techniques ensure higher SpO2 levels prior to intubation and result in lower arterial desaturation rates [11].

23.6 Preoxygenation and Apneic Oxygenation (AO)

Preoxygenation and AO offer substantial safety benefits and should be applied to all patients. Specifically, AO should be maintained throughout intubation attempts. NIV enhances these strategies by reducing alveolar collapse, improving oxygenation, and extending safe apnea times. The induction of general anesthesia should be tailored to the individual patient, with consideration for the added benefits of NIV. Neuromuscular blockade facilitates intubation and face mask ventilation; in cases of difficulty, further attempts should only be made once complete neuromuscular blockade is achieved [4, 7]. NIV (e.g., using the nasal interface) and HFNO during apneic phases have shown superior results in maintaining oxygenation and reducing desaturation risks.

23.7 Choice of Laryngoscopy

The decision between direct or video laryngoscopy depends on the anesthetist's experience and training, with video laryngoscopy increasingly preferred by some practitioners. According to DAS guidelines, the insertion of the laryngoscope into the oral cavity constitutes an intubation attempt, and clinicians should track the number of attempts, as each carries inherent risks. If difficulties arise, calling for assistance is essential, regardless of the operator's experience [2, 4, 7].

23.8 Improving Intubation Success

Subsequent intubation attempts should involve modifications that may enhance success, including changes in patient positioning, intubation devices, blades, introducers, and pharmacological adjustments. The laryngoscopy view can be improved with backward, upward, and rightward pressure (BURP) on the thyroid cartilage. A bougie can facilitate tracheal intubation, although blind insertion can cause trauma. Once the bougie is placed in the trachea, passing the endotracheal tube over it under direct or video guidance increases the likelihood of successful intubation; external cricoid pressure should be released during this process [6].

23.9 Limit on Attempts

The number of intubation attempts should be limited to three, with a fourth attempt reserved for the most experienced anesthesiologist [4, 7]. Successful placement of the endotracheal tube must be confirmed with capnography [2, 4, 7].

23.10 Failure to Intubate

If all attempts, including the fourth, fail, the situation is deemed a failed intubation. The focus should then shift to maintaining oxygenation via a supraglottic airway device (SAD). Second-generation SADs are preferred for airway control and oxygenation. Ideally, the chosen SAD should facilitate initial placement, maintain high seal pressure, separate the gastrointestinal from the respiratory tract, and permit intubation through the device. Placement of the SAD should also be limited to three attempts to prevent airway trauma [4, 7].

If SAD placement is successful, time can be utilized to consider various options, such as waking the patient, intubating through the SAD, or proceeding with SAD use without tracheal intubation, including options for front of the neck approach (FONA). If SAD placement fails, or if oxygenation via SAD is inadequate, the priority shifts to oxygenation via face mask ventilation [20–23].

23.11 Management of Oxygenation

If adequate oxygenation is achieved, the patient should be awakened after neuromuscular blockade reversal. If oxygenation is not possible, complete neuromuscular blockade should be ensured to maximize face mask ventilation success (the two-person technique is advisable). If ventilation fails, CICO must be declared, and front of neck access (FONA) should be performed [2, 4, 7, 26].

23.12 Cannot Intubate, Cannot Oxygenate (CICO) Scenario and the Front of Neck Access

Failed intubation, SAD placement, and ineffective mask ventilation can lead to severe complications, including hypoxic brain damage and death, if not promptly addressed. This critical situation, referred to as CICO, necessitates immediate declaration of its urgency to ensure all team members swiftly transition to the FONA plan [2, 6].

The DAS guidelines emphasize that successful management of CICO relies on continuous training and retraining in both technical and nontechnical skills, including decision-making, planning, preparation, and practical techniques. Research indicates that cognitive and practical abilities can decline under stress, highlighting the importance of regular practice [6].

An effective approach to FONA is the scalpel cricothyroidotomy (SC), a procedure that all anesthetists should be proficient in and regularly trained to perform.

SC is the most effective emergency technique for securing an airway. Various methods exist for this procedure, but none demonstrate clear superiority, as they share common elements: extending the neck, identifying the cricothyroid membrane, and inserting a cuffed tracheal tube [6, 25].

Before performing FONA, the patient should receive complete neuromuscular blockade and 100% FiO2. Positioning to enhance neck extension is crucial, which can be achieved by placing a pillow under the shoulders or lifting the patient, facilitating the "laryngeal handshake." This technique involves using the non-dominant hand to locate the hyoid and thyroid laminae, stabilizing the larynx with the fingers, and finding the cricothyroid membrane with the second finger.

Preparation involves gathering essential equipment: a number 10 scalpel blade, an angled tip bougie, and a 6.0-mm cuffed tube. The operator positions the non-dominant hand on the larynx to identify landmarks while the dominant hand performs the incision. After locating the cricothyroid membrane, a transverse stab incision is made, and the blade is turned 90° to maintain a vertical approach [6, 25].

Once the incision is made, the operator swaps hands, keeping the scalpel vertical and pulling towards themselves to open the incision. The bougie is gently introduced into the trachea, with the characteristic clicks indicating contact with tracheal rings. After removing the scalpel, the cuffed tube is guided into the trachea using the bougie, which is then removed. Cuff inflation and correct tube placement are confirmed via capnography [6, 26].

If the laryngeal landmarks are not palpable, a midline vertical incision (8–10 cm) can be made, with blunt dissection to locate the cricothyroid membrane before proceeding with the scalpel technique.

The narrow-bore (<4 mm) cannula technique presents notable limitations, primarily relying on a high-pressure system for ventilation, which carries risks such as barotrauma, kinking, and mispositioning of the cannula. Although it has been included in prior guidelines due to its familiarity among anesthetists, its use in a CICO scenario should be restricted to clinicians who routinely practice this technique [6, 26].

In contrast, wide-bore cannula techniques, particularly those utilizing a guidewire and designed kits, are less invasive than surgical approaches and resemble central venous line insertions. However, these techniques are not recommended in emergency situations due to their complexity under pressure [6, 26].

Furthermore, the use of a non-Seldinger wide-bore cannula with a trocar lacks robust evidence supporting its effectiveness in emergencies, as there are insufficient studies on its performance in such contexts [6, 26].

When dealing with unexpected airway challenges, the extubation process must be approached with equal diligence as intubation. Adhering to the "at-risk" algorithm outlined in the Difficult Airway Society (DAS) extubation guidelines is crucial, particularly if the patient requires intensive care support [24].

HFNO has gained significant attention in the literature for its role in preventing reintubation following extubation. Studies indicate that HFNO effectively provides a higher FiO2 and improves patient comfort by delivering humidified, heated oxygen at rates up to 70 L/min. This high flow can help maintain adequate oxygenation and reduce the work of breathing in patients with respiratory distress. Furthermore, HFNO can mitigate the risk of airway obstruction and improve overall respiratory mechanics, thus lowering the likelihood of reintubation. Evidence suggests that the use of HFNO post-extubation is particularly beneficial in high-risk populations, such as those with COPD or obesity, where traditional oxygen therapy may not suffice. Consequently, incorporating HFNO into post-extubation protocols may enhance patient outcomes and reduce the incidence of complications associated with reintubation [27].

23.13 Conclusions

Difficult airway management poses significant challenges for clinicians. Comprehensive preoperative assessment of patients is essential, encompassing clinical history, anatomical features, and imaging studies. The literature emphasizes that ensuring adequate oxygenation is paramount, often more critical than the specific techniques employed during airway management. The incorporation of NIV into preoxygenation protocols represents a significant advancement in airway management. By enhancing oxygenation, reducing the work of breathing, and prolonging safe apnea time, NIV provides clinicians with a powerful tool to manage difficult airway scenarios effectively. Future research should focus on optimizing NIV techniques and integrating them with other advanced preoxygenation strategies to improve patient outcomes.

Key Messages
Airway management is essential for ensuring safe and effective oxygenation and ventilation, particularly in patients with airway obstruction or respiratory insufficiency. This chapter discusses the significance of a systematic approach to airway management in anesthesiology and critical care, emphasizing noninvasive ventilatory methods that minimize the need for invasive interventions. Preoxygenation is highlighted as a crucial step to enhance oxygen reserves before airway management, especially in ICU patients at risk for difficult airways. The role of NIV, including CPAP and BiPAP, is explored in the context of acute respiratory failure and endotracheal intubation. Additionally, HFNO is presented as an emerging method for providing supplemental oxygen and reducing respiratory effort. This chapter aims to outline strategies for utilizing noninvasive ventilation in challenging airway scenarios, summarizing evidence on the importance of preoxygenation and oxygen maintenance during airway management, while addressing both predicted and unexpected difficult airways.

References

1. Xia M, Ma W, Zuo M, et al. Expert consensus on difficult airway assessment. Hepatobiliary Surg Nutr. 2023. https://doi.org/10.21037/hbsn-23-46.
2. Higgs A, McGrath BA, Goddard C, Rangasami J, Suntharalingam G, Gale R, Cook TM. Guidelines for the management of tracheal intubation in critically ill adults. Br J Anaesth. 2018;120:323–52.
3. Rochwerg B, Brochard L, Elliott MW. Official ERS/ATS clinical practice guidelines: noninvasive ventilation for acute respiratory failure. Eur Respir J. 2017;50:1602426.
4. Carrié C. Early non-invasive ventilation and high-flow nasal oxygen therapy for preventing endotracheal intubation in hypoxemic blunt chest trauma patients: the OptiTHO randomized trial. Crit Care. 2023;27:163.
5. Al-Husinat LI, et al. High-flow oxygen therapy in the perioperative setting and procedural sedation: a review of current evidence. J Clin Med. 2023;12(20):6685.
6. Apfelbaum JL, Hagberg CA, Connis RT, et al. American Society of Anesthesiologists practice guidelines for management of the difficult airway. Anesthesiology. 2022;136:31–81.
7. Detsky ME, Jivraj N. Will this patient be difficult to intubate? The rational clinical examination systematic review. Anesthesiology | JAMA | JAMA Netw. https://jamanetwork.com/journals/jama/article-abstract/2724031. Accessed 20 Jun 2023.
8. Gleeson S, Groom P, Mercer S. Human factors in complex airway management. BJA Educ. 2016;16:191–7.
9. Crawley S, Dalton A. Predicting the difficult airway. BJA Educ. 2015;15:253–7.
10. Azam Danish M. Preoxygenation and anesthesia: a detailed review. Cureus. 2021;13:e13240.
11. Bouroche G, Bourgain JL. Preoxygenation and general anesthesia: a review. Minerva Anestesiol. 2015;81:910–20.
12. Fraioli RL, Sheffer LA, Steffenson JL. Pulmonary and cardiovascular effects of apneic oxygenation in man. Anesthesiology. 1973;39:588–96.

13. e Silva LOJ, Cabrera D, Barrionuevo P, Johnson RL, Erwin PJ, Murad MH, Bellolio MF. Effectiveness of apneic oxygenation during intubation: a systematic review and meta-analysis. Ann Emerg Med. 2017;70:483–94.e11.
14. Binks MJ, Holyoak RS, Melhuish TM, Vlok R, Bond E, White LD. Apneic oxygenation during intubation in the emergency department and during retrieval: a systematic review and meta-analysis. Am J Emerg Med. 2017;35:1542–6.
15. White LD, Melhuish TM, White LK, Wallace LA. Apnoeic oxygenation during intubation: a systematic review and meta-analysis. Anaesth Intensive Care. 2017;45:21–7.
16. Chrimes N, Higgs A, Hagberg CA, et al. Preventing unrecognized oesophageal intubation: a consensus guideline from the project for universal management of airways and international airway societies*. Anaesthesia. 2022;77:1395–415.
17. Rothen HU, Sporre B, Engberg G, Wegenius G, Reber A, Hedenstierna G. Prevention of atelectasis during general anaesthesia. Lancet. 1995;345:1387–91.
18. Joyce CJ, Williams AB. Kinetics of absorption atelectasis during anesthesia: a mathematical model. J Appl Physiol. 1999;86:1116–25.
19. Cressey DM, Berthoud MC, Reilly CS. Effectiveness of continuous positive airway pressure to enhance pre-oxygenation in morbidly obese women. Anaesthesia. 2001;56:680–4.
20. Petrini F, Accorsi A, Adrario E, et al. Recommendations for airway control and difficult airway management. Minerva Anestesiol. 2005;71:617.
21. Vora J, Leslie D, Stacey M. Awake tracheal intubation. BJA Educ. 2022;22:298–305.
22. Klein AA, Meek T, Allcock E, et al. Recommendations for standards of monitoring during anaesthesia and recovery 2021. Anaesthesia. 2021;76:1212–23.
23. Desai N, Ratnayake G, Onwochei DN, El-Boghdadly K, Ahmad I. Airway devices for awake tracheal intubation in adults: a systematic review and network meta-analysis. Br J Anaesth. 2021;127:636–47.
24. Difficult Airway Society Extubation Guidelines Group, Popat M, Mitchell V, Dravid R, Patel A, Swampillai C, Higgs A. Difficult airway society guidelines for the management of tracheal extubation. Anaesthesia. 2012;67:318–40.
25. Duan Q, et al. Scalpel cricothyrotomy versus punctured cricothyrotomy in the context of the CICO crisis. A systematic review and meta-analysis. Anaesth Crit Care Pain Med. 2023;42(4):101211.
26. McKenna P, et al. Cricothyrotomy. Treasure Island: StatPearls Publishing; 2023.
27. Oczkowski S, et al. ERS clinical practice guidelines: high-flow nasal cannula in acute respiratory failure. Eur Respir J. 2022;59(4):2101574.

The Use of Noninvasive Ventilation in Regional Anesthesiology

24

Wojciech Gola and Szymon Bialka

24.1 Regional Anesthesiology: Meaning and Use

Regional anesthesiology techniques are increasingly used as the primary method of anesthesia or as a component of analgesia not only in trauma and orthopedic surgery but also in the growing number of indications in abdominal surgery, urology, thoracic surgery, and vascular surgery. Techniques of plexus and nerve blocks, fascial blocks, and central blockade have also become more commonly used in intensive care units in critically ill patients who require an optimum form of analgesia (patients after surgeries, trauma patients, or subjects with chronic pain). By administering perineural or intrathecal local anesthesia, we reversibly block nociceptive afferentation, which has an influence on the effective control of pain ailments. Such blockades can be used in the form of administration of one dose of the drug ("single shot") or as continuous blockades (administration of local anesthesia through an implanted catheter) in order to extend the analgesia for the following days [1]. The use of regional anesthesiology is associated with many advantages. One of the most significant benefits is the excellent control of postoperative acute pain as well as the efficient therapy of certain chronic pain syndromes. Successful pain therapy contributes to a decreased need for opioid analgesics, and, consequently, it reduces the complications and adverse reactions resulting from their systemic administration, such as respiratory depression, opioid-induced hyperalgesia, nausea, and vomiting. The next important advantage of the use of regional anesthesiology methods is the

W. Gola
Faculty of Medicine, Jan Kochanowski University, Kielce, Poland

Department of Anaesthesia and Intensive Care, Saint Lucas Hospital, Konskie, Poland

S. Bialka (✉)
Department of Anaesthesiology and Intensive Care, Faculty of Medical Sciences in Zabrze, Medical University of Silesia, Katowice, Poland

© The Author(s), under exclusive license to Springer Nature Switzerland AG 2025

K. Panda et al. (eds.), *Noninvasive Ventilatory Approaches in Interventional Procedures*, Noninvasive Ventilation. The Essentials,
https://doi.org/10.1007/978-3-032-05328-2_24

option to avoid instrumentation of the respiratory tract when it is necessary to perform an operative procedure and the reduced postoperative pulmonary complications. It is of great importance in the case of patients with comorbidities of the respiratory system, such as chronic obstructive pulmonary disease, chronic respiratory failure with an active or recent respiratory infection, and pathologic obesity with concomitant sleep apnea or obesity hypoventilation syndrome. The true renaissance of regional anesthesiology methods took place during the COVID-19 pandemic, where the possibility of their use would postpone the need for instrumentation of the respiratory tract multiple times as well as reduce the exposure to contagious aerosol, ensuring increased safety of the medical personnel and the patient. Many scientific societies issued recommendations for the use of regional anesthesiology methods, whenever possible, as the method of choice during the COVID-19 pandemic [2, 3]. The situation can also be extrapolated to all patients with comorbidities within the scope of the respiratory system. Other advantages of the use of blockades of peripheral nerves include the patient's hemodynamic stability during the surgery (it results from eliminating or reducing doses of anesthetic medications exhibiting a depressive impact on the cardiovascular system) as well as greater satisfaction of patient. In the case of critically ill patients staying at the intensive care unit, the use of regional anesthesiology techniques, apart from better pain control, influences the reduction of the amount of drugs used in analgosedation, makes the rehabilitation more efficient, and leads to early mobilization of the patient.

24.2 The Use of Regional Anesthesiology Combined with Noninvasive Ventilation

In many situations, the use of regional anesthesiology techniques combined with noninvasive ventilation provides the opportunity to safely perform surgeries within the scope of trauma and orthopedic surgery, general surgery, or vascular surgery [4, 5]. It mostly refers to patients with concomitant respiratory failure or an active infection of the respiratory system. The simultaneous use of plexus and peripheral blocks or central blockades and noninvasive ventilation provides the opportunity to avoid the need for intubation of a patient with concomitant or growing respiratory failure. Thus, it allows avoiding prolonged mechanical ventilation when there is a need for surgery. According to the literature, the combination of noninvasive ventilation with regional methods of anesthesia in patients with severe obstructive pulmonary disorders decreases the alveolar hypoventilation by improving the functionality of the diaphragm and better mobilization of the rib cage wall [6, 7]. This leads to enhanced ventilation in the involved sections of the lungs and, at the same time, results in a better proportion of ventilation to perfusion. The next group of patients, in the case of which the use of noninvasive ventilation in the perioperative period combined with regional anesthesiology techniques significantly reduces the number of respiratory complications during the perioperative period, includes patients with extreme obesity and concomitant obesity hypoventilation syndrome or sleep apnea [8]. Furthermore, there are data available for the effective application of noninvasive ventilation combined with regional anesthesiology techniques in low-invasive surgeries in patients with neuromuscular disorders, including myasthenia [9, 10]. Techniques of regional anesthesiology (most often subarachnoid anesthesia) constitute the golden standard for Caesarean section; it allows reducing the number of respiratory complications in that group of female patients as well as lowering the perioperative mortality rate. General anesthesia in the said group of female patients is associated with almost 20 times the increase in difficulties connected with intubation compared to the general population, as well as with a high risk of aspiration of gastric content during the instrumentation of the respiratory tract. Many data and studies indicate that the additional use of noninvasive ventilation during the perioperative period in the group of pregnant women with a concomitant respiratory disease, pulmonary edema in the course of eclampsia or preeclampsia, or a neuromuscular disease efficiently optimizes the respiratory parameters, reducing the risk of instrumentation of the respiratory tract [11–13].

The most common procedures in which one can use regional anesthesiology techniques as the primary element of anesthesia include procedures within the scope of trauma and orthopedic surgery performed in the region of the upper and lower limbs (fracture repositioning, joint reconstructive surgery, arthroscopy), general surgery procedures (amputations, hernioplasty), or vascular surgeries (endarterectomy of, e.g., neck veins, peripheral endarterectomy, intra-aortic repair procedures, peripheral vascular bypass grafting) [14]. In the case of the use of certain regional anesthesiology techniques, such as brachial plexus block from between the scalene muscles or block from the supraclavicular access, additional use of noninvasive ventilation might be at times extremely helpful. The abovementioned blocks are connected with the temporary block of the phrenic nerve, which, in the case of some groups of patients (obesity, COPD), can result in intensified symptoms of respiratory failure, the need for intubation, and prolonged ventilation in the perioperative period. The frequency of temporary block of the phrenic nerve and paralysis of the diaphragm after the block of the brachial plexus from between the scalene muscles reaches 100% in case of standard doses of a local anesthetic. In the case of a block from the supraclavicular access, the said frequency is high as well and can amount to 60%. In the abovementioned situations, the use of breathing support employing noninvasive mechanical ventilation can reduce the need for instrumentation of the respiratory tract and prolonged invasive mechanical ventilation.

In many cases, the use of regional anesthesiology techniques also requires the application of additional deep sedation. It is most often associated with the reduced range of anesthesia or the patient's request in order to improve their comfort for the time of the procedure. The use of deep sedation can intensify hypoventilation and, thus, lead to the development of postoperative respiratory complications. In such cases, the use of preventive noninvasive ventilation might be favorable by reducing the risk of hypoventilation and the need for instrumentation of the respiratory tract.

24.3 Side Effects of NIV During Regional Anesthesiology

Despite many advantages, the use of NIV bears the risk of patient-ventilator asynchrony, gastric insufflation, unfavorable hemodynamic effect (although less intensified than during invasive ventilation), and patient discomfort (mask mismatch, pain caused by pressure of the straps, air leak around the mask, noise, eye irritation). However, thanks to intraoperative use of sedatives (adjusted in terms of the administered dose), it is possible to significantly minimize the risk of adverse reactions to NIV.

24.4 Special Indications for NIV During Regional Anesthesiology

The use of central blockades can greatly influence respiratory function through reduced strength of respiratory muscles, weaker response of the respiratory system to the changes in blood gas parameters, reduced flexibility of the rib cage wall, the supine position (resulting in lower functional residual capacity (FRC)), or the development of relative hypovolemia. These factors can negate the potential advantages resulting from the use of regional anesthesia and, thus, avoid intraoperative endotracheal intubation and invasive mechanical ventilation. Thanks to the use of NIV and, at the same time, the reduced respiratory work, improved alveolar recruitment with preserved tidal volume (resulting in a better gas exchange), reduction of initial load and afterload of the left ventricle, and avoidance of complications connected with invasive mechanical ventilation, the application of regional anesthesiology along with intraoperative use of NIV can be favorable for specific patient groups. These include patients with COPD, restrictive diseases of the rib cage wall, or neuromuscular disorders. NIV improves the adjustment of ventilation to the perfusion in the lung and lowers the strain on the respiratory muscles. The said advantages are particularly important in the case of patients suffering from restrictive or obstructive lung diseases during surgery with the use of central blockade techniques. Such blockades impair the expiratory reserves of the lungs, increasing the risk of atelectasis and exacerbation of alveolar hypoventilation with a higher disproportion between ventilation and perfusion.

24.5 Conclusion

In recent years, the role of noninvasive ventilation and its use in perioperative care of patients subjected to surgeries and in intensive care units has become more important. By combining regional anesthesiology techniques with noninvasive ventilation, in many cases, it is possible to safely perform the surgery, reduce pulmonary complications, including alveolar hypoventilation, and avoid instrumentation of the respiratory tract as well as prolonged invasive ventilation in the postoperative period. NIV can be broadly used at any moment of operative treatment. However, it is used in the postoperative period after surgery. Nevertheless, the increasing number of reports indicates that the efficiency of its intraoperative application in patients with COPD, sleep apnea, or morbid obesity.

To summarize, the use of NIV combined with regional anesthesiology should be considered in the case of patients with predispositions for the development or exacerbation of respiratory failure, after a careful assessment of the patient's clinical condition and having confirmed that the advantages of NIV will be greater than its potential risks.

References

1. ASRA/ESRA COVID-19 Guidance for Regional Anesthesia March 31, 2020. https://www.asra.com/docs/default-source/guidelines-articles/covid-guidance-ra_r6_final.pdf?sfvrsn=2de410cc_4.
2. Lima RME, Reis LA, Thyrso de Lara FS, Dias LC, Matsumoto M, Mizubuti GB, Hamaji A, Cabral LW, LADST M, LHNE L. Recommendations for local-regional anesthesia during the COVID-19 pandemic. Braz J Anesthesiol. 2020;70(2):159–64. https://doi.org/10.1016/j.bjane.2020.06.002. Epub 2020 Jun 10. PMID: 32834193; PMCID: PMC7286225.
3. Lie SA, Wong SW, Wong LT, Wong TGL, Chong SY. Practical considerations for performing regional anesthesia: lessons learned from the COVID-19 pandemic. Considérations pratiques pour laréalisation de l'anesthésie régionale: les leçons tirées de la pandémie de COVID-19. Can J Anaesth. 2020;67(7):885–92. https://doi.org/10.1007/s12630-020-01637-0.
4. Kopp SL, Børglum J, Buvanendran A, et al. Anesthesia and analgesia practice pathway options for total knee arthroplasty: an evidence-based review by the American and European Societies of Regional Anesthesia and Pain Medicine. Reg Anesth Pain Med. 2017;42(6):683–97. https://doi.org/10.1097/AAP.0000000000000673.
5. Hutton M, Brull R, Macfarlane AJR. Regional anaesthesia and outcomes. BJA Educ. 2018;18(2):52–6. https://doi.org/10.1016/j.bjae.2017.10.002. Epub 2017 Nov 27. PMID: 33456810; PMCID: PMC7807931.
6. Tran DQ, Elgueta MF, Aliste J, Finlayson RJ. Diaphragm-sparing nerve blocks for shoulder surgery. Reg Anesth Pain Med. 2017;42(1):32–8. https://doi.org/10.1097/AAP.0000000000000529.
7. Aliste J, Bravo D, Layera S, Finlayson RJ, Tran DQ. Hemidiaphragmatic paralysis after supraclavicular block: more questions than answers. Reg Anesth Pain Med. 2019;44:901. https://doi.org/10.1136/rapm-2019-100463.
8. Leech CJ, Baba R, Dhar M. Spinal anaesthesia and non-invasive positive pressure ventilation for hip surgery in an obese patient with advanced chronic obstructive pulmonary disease. Br J Anaesth. 2007;98(6):763–5. https://doi.org/10.1093/bja/aem093.
9. Ferrandière M, Hazouard E, Ayoub J, et al. Non-invasive ventilation corrects alveolar hypoventilation during spinal anesthesia. Can J Anesth. 2006;53:404–8. https://doi.org/10.1007/BF03022508.
10. Hübler M, Litz R, Albrecht D. Combination of balanced and regional anaesthesia for minimally invasive surgery in a patient with myasthenia gravis. Eur J Anaesthesiol. 2000;17(5):325–8. https://doi.org/10.1046/j.1365-2346.2000.00671.x.
11. Erdogan G, Okyay DZ, Yurtlu S, et al. Non-invasive mechanical ventilation with spinal anesthesia for cesarean delivery. Int J Obstet Anesth. 2010;19:438–40.
12. Yuan N, El-Sayed YY, Ruoss SJ, Riley E, Enns GM, Robinson TE. Successful pregnancy and cesarean delivery via noninvasive ventilation in mitochondrial myopathy. J Perinatol. 2009;29(2):166–7. https://doi.org/10.1038/jp.2008.178.

13. Mushambi MC, Kinsella SM, Popat M, Swales H, Ramaswamy KK, Winton AL, Quinn AC, Obstetric Anaesthetists' Association; Difficult Airway Society. Obstetric Anaesthetists' Association and Difficult Airway Society guidelines for the management of difficult and failed tracheal intubation in obstetrics. Anaesthesia. 2015;70(11):1286–306. https://doi.org/10.1111/anae.13260. PMID: 26449292; PMCID: PMC4606761.
14. Cabrini L, Nobile L, Plumari VP, et al. Intraoperative prophylactic and therapeutic non-invasive ventilation: a systematic review. Br J Anaesth. 2014;112(4):638–47. https://doi.org/10.1093/bja/aet465.

NIV Procedures in Upper Airway Surgery 25

Michał Simlot, Jarosław Markowski, Krzysztof Niemczuk, Monika Szymańska-Czerwińska, and Jarosław Paluch

25.1 Introduction

Noninvasive mechanical ventilation (NIV) plays a crucial role in the treatment of respiratory diseases, offering significant benefits to patients suffering from acute and chronic respiratory failure [1, 2]. By using masks or other sealing devices, NIV enables breathing support without the need for tracheal intubation. This approach reduces the risk of complications associated with invasive methods, such as ventilator-associated infections or airway injuries [3, 4].

25.2 History and Development

The first attempts to use noninvasive ventilation date back to the 1920s when iron lungs were introduced to treat patients with poliomyelitis. However, modern NIV began to develop dynamically only in the 1980s and 1990s, with technological advancements and a better understanding of the physiological mechanisms of breathing [5, 6].

M. Simlot (✉) · J. Markowski
Department of Laryngology, Medical University of Silesia, Faculty of Medical Sciences in Katowice, Katowice, Poland
e-mail: jmarkowski@sum.edu.pl

K. Niemczuk · M. Szymańska-Czerwińska
Institute of Genetics and Animal Biotechnology of the Polish Academy of Sciences, Jastrzębiec, Poland
e-mail: k.niemczuk@igbzpan.pl; m.szymanska-czerwinska@igbzpan.pl

J. Paluch
Department of Laryngology, Medical University of Silesia, Faculty of Medical Sciences in Katowice, Katowice, Poland

Institute of Genetics and Animal Biotechnology of the Polish Academy of Sciences, Jastrzębiec, Poland
e-mail: jpaluch@sum.edu.pl

© The Author(s), under exclusive license to Springer Nature Switzerland AG 2025

K. Panda et al. (eds.), *Noninvasive Ventilatory Approaches in Interventional Procedures*, Noninvasive Ventilation. The Essentials,
https://doi.org/10.1007/978-3-032-05328-2_25

25.3 Mechanisms of Action

NIV works by applying positive pressure to the airways, which facilitates lung ventilation. The two main modes of operation are as follows:

1. *CPAP (continuous positive airway pressure)* involves maintaining constant pressure in the airways throughout the entire breathing cycle. It is mainly used in the treatment of obstructive sleep apnea and pulmonary edema [7, 8].
2. *BiPAP (Bilevel Positive Airway Pressure)* offers two pressure levels: higher during inhalation and lower during exhalation. It is used in cases where the patient requires support during both inhalation and exhalation, such as in chronic obstructive pulmonary disease (COPD) [9, 10].

25.4 Clinical Applications

NIV is used in various medical conditions, including the following:

- *Acute respiratory failure*—In COPD, NIV can significantly reduce the need for intubation [6, 7].
- *Obstructive sleep apnea*—CPAP is considered the gold standard in treating this condition [11].
- *Pulmonary edema*—NIV helps quickly alleviates dyspnea and improves blood oxygenation [12].
- *Respiratory muscle weakness*—In amyotrophic lateral sclerosis (ALS), for example, NIV supports breathing in patients with weakened respiratory muscles [13, 14].

25.5 Benefits and Limitations

Benefits

- *Reduced risk of infection*—The lack of a need for intubation reduces the risk of respiratory tract infections [1, 2].
- *Patient comfort*—NIV is generally better tolerated by patients compared to invasive ventilation [5].
- *Speed and ease of application*—NIV can be quickly implemented in various clinical settings [3].

Limitations

- *Improper mask fit*—It can lead to air leaks and reduced ventilation efficiency [9].
- *Requires patient cooperation*—The patient must be conscious and able to tolerate the mask, which can be problematic in severe respiratory failure [6].
- *Not suitable for patients with hemodynamic instability*—such as those with severe arrhythmia or cardiogenic shock [4].

25.6 Jet Ventilation

25.6.1 Method Description

Jet ventilation (JV) is a mechanical ventilation technique that uses short, high-pressure bursts of air or gas mixtures to ventilate the lungs [11, 12]. Unlike traditional mechanical ventilation, which delivers air using a constant flow, JV introduces small volumes of air at high pressure for short periods [13].

25.6.2 Mechanisms of Action

Jet ventilation is a mechanical ventilation technique that uses small, rapid jets of gas introduced into the patient's airways. Unlike traditional ventilation methods, where air or gas mixtures are delivered in larger volumes at slower speeds, this method uses higher pressures to deliver smaller amounts of gas in a short time [14]. This allows for effective gas exchange with minimal chest movement [15].

High-pressure devices are used in jet ventilation, which generate gas streams entering the airways through a thin catheter or a special laryngoscope equipped with air channels [16]. There are two main types of jet ventilation:

1. *High-frequency jet ventilation (HFJV)*—uses very fast, small-volume gas jets (often over 100 breaths per minute), providing exceptionally stable gas exchange and minimizing the risk of barotrauma [12, 13].
2. *Intermittent jet ventilation (IJV)*—characterized by less frequent but larger-volume gas jets [14, 15].

25.6.3 Application in Otolaryngology

Jet ventilation has found particular use in otolaryngology, especially during surgical procedures in the upper airway. It is the preferred method for several reasons:

1. *Safety and precision*: In surgeries involving the larynx, trachea, or pharynx, jet ventilation allows the surgeon better access to the operative field without the hindrance of intubation tubes [11, 16]. Traditional ventilation methods require intubation, which can limit visibility and operative space.
2. *Stability of the operative field*: Minimal chest movement and the lack of large gas volumes introduced into the lungs reduce the shifting of anatomical structures, which is crucial during precise procedures, such as laryngeal microsurgery [12, 13].
3. *Reduced risk of injury*: The use of jet ventilation decreases the risk of damage to the delicate structures of the larynx and trachea compared to traditional intubation [14, 15]. This is especially important in patients with difficult airways or existing pathological changes [16].

25.6.4 Examples of Application

1. *Laryngeal surgery*: Jet ventilation is widely used in laryngeal surgery, including the removal of polyps, tumors (Figs. 25.1, 25.2, 25.3, and 25.4), or other lesions [11, 12]. This method allows continuous operation with constant access to the airways, minimizing the need to interrupt the procedure to maintain airway patency.
2. *Therapeutic bronchoscopy*: In bronchoscopy procedures requiring advanced instrumentation and long operation times, jet ventilation provides continuous ventilation without the need to withdraw instruments [13, 14].
3. *Laser procedures in the airways*: Jet ventilation reduces the risk of explosion, which can occur due to the contact of traditional gases with the laser beam [15, 16]. The small amount of gas used in this method is less prone to ignition compared to full volumes of air or oxygen.

25.7 Examples to Use Jet Ventilation

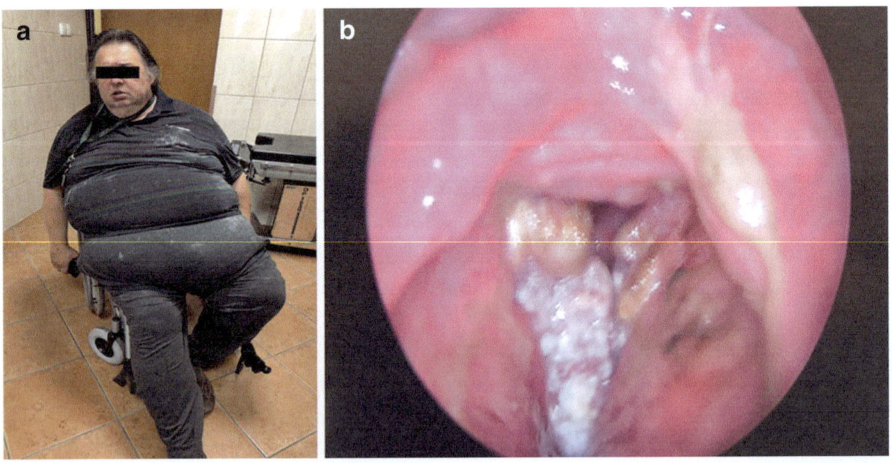

Fig. 25.1 Patient with laryngeal tumor: (**a**) general condition—body weight of more than 200 kg and multimorbidity. (**b**) local condition—advanced tumor of the larynx, significantly narrowing the glottic staple. *(Image material from Department of Laryngology, Medical University of Silesia, Katowice)*

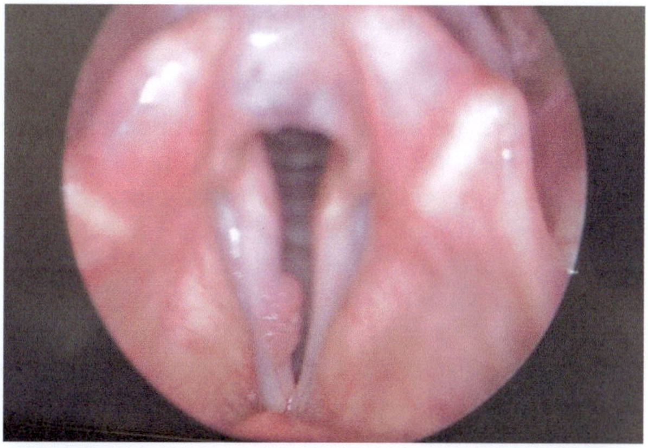

Fig. 25.2 Tumor with papillomatous appearance with strongly developed pathological vascularization—high risk of bleeding from the tumor during intubation. *(Image material from Department of Laryngology, Medical University of Silesia, Katowice)*

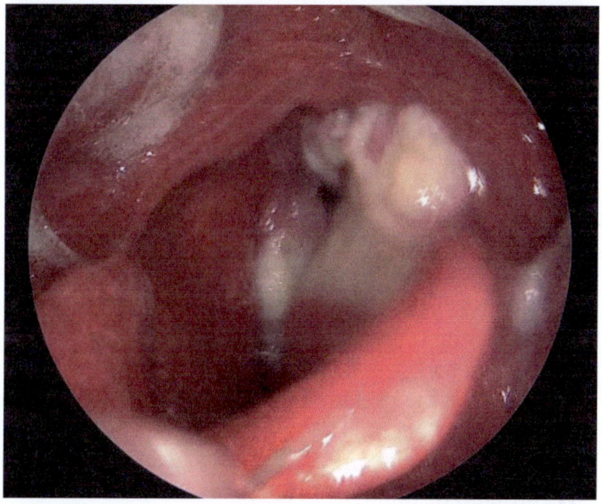

Fig. 25.3 Carcinoma of the left vocal fold: a massive tumor closing the laryngeal lumen—intubation impossible. *(Image material from Department of Laryngology, Medical University of Silesia, Katowice)*

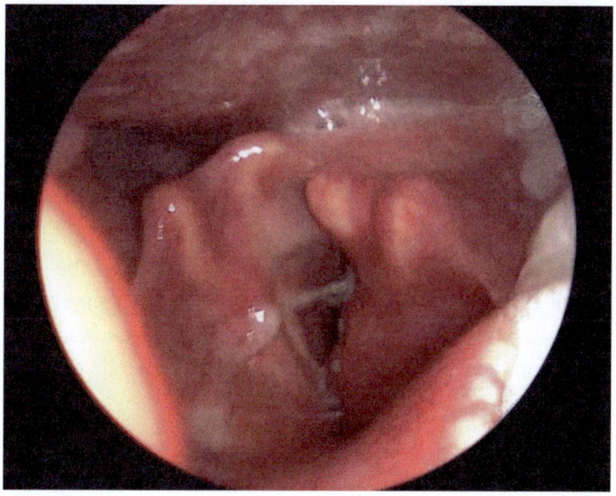

Fig. 25.4 Carcinoma of the left vocal fold: a massive tumor closing the laryngeal lumen—intubation impossible. *(Image material from Department of Laryngology, Medical University of Silesia, Katowice)*

25.8 Advantages and Limitations

Advantages

- *Better access to the operative field*: The absence or minimal size of the intubation tube allows for free operation [11, 12].
- *Less chest movement*: This facilitates precise surgeries [13, 14].
- *Reduced airway trauma*: The risk of mechanical and thermal damage is lower [15, 16].

Limitations

- *Requires advanced monitoring*: Jet ventilation requires precise monitoring of blood gases to avoid complications associated with hyperventilation or hypoventilation [12, 13].
- *Risk of barotrauma*: Improper setting of ventilation parameters can lead to lung injuries due to excessive pressure [14, 15].
- *Requires experienced personnel*: Conducting jet ventilation requires experience and specialized anesthesiology knowledge [16].

25.9 Clinical Applications

JV is particularly useful in situations where traditional mechanical ventilation may be difficult, inappropriate, or impossible. Examples of clinical applications include the following:

- *Airway surgery*—JV allows surgeons better access to the airways without obstructing the operative field, which is especially important during endoscopic procedures [11].
- *Patients with difficult airway access*—JV can be used in cases where intubation is difficult or impossible [15].
- *Treatment of acute respiratory conditions*—JV can be used as an auxiliary method in treating severe respiratory failure [12].

25.10 Benefits and Limitations

Benefits

- *Precise control of ventilation*—JV allows for accurate control of the amount of air delivered, which is especially important in delicate surgical procedures [13].
- *Minimal interference in the operative field*—the small catheters used in JV allow for better access to the airways during surgery [16].
- *Rapid response to changing conditions*—Pulsatile air delivery allows for quick adaptation to the changing ventilatory needs of the patient [14].

Limitations

- *Requires specialized equipment*—JV requires the use of specialized devices and catheters, which may be a limitation in some medical facilities [12].
- *Risk of barotrauma*—The high pressures used in JV can increase the risk of lung injury [13].
- *Need for experienced personnel*—JV requires qualified personnel familiar with the technique and capable of responding to potential complications [11].

25.11 Summary

Noninvasive mechanical ventilation is an alternative to intubation when intubation is not possible, increasing patient safety and reducing the risk of complications [5, 6]. Its applications range from ventilation during surgical procedures to acute to chronic respiratory diseases [1, 7]. Jet ventilation, on the other hand, is a precise method also used in otolaryngology, allowing safe and effective surgery for patients with difficult airway access [15, 16].

Bibliography

1. Ambrosino N, Vagheggini G. Noninvasive positive pressure ventilation in the acute care setting: where are we? Eur Respir J. 2008;31(4):874–86.
2. Brochard L. Noninvasive ventilation for acute respiratory failure. JAMA. 2000;284(18):2376–8.
3. Davidson AC, Banham S, Elliott M, Kennedy D, Gelder C, Glossop A, Church AC, Creagh-Brown BC, Thornton V. BTS/ICS guideline for the ventilatory management of acute hypercapnic respiratory failure in adults. Thorax. 2016;71(2):ii1–35.
4. Elliott MW, Confalonieri M, Nava S. Where to perform noninvasive ventilation? Eur Respir J. 2002;19(6):1159–66.
5. Mehta S, Hill NS. Noninvasive ventilation. Am J Respir Crit Care Med. 2001;163(2):540–77.
6. Nava S, Hill N. Non-invasive ventilation in acute respiratory failure. Lancet. 2009;374(9685):250–9.
7. Struik FM, Sprooten RTM, Kerstjens HAM, Bladder G, Zijnen M, Wijkstra PJ, Duiverman ML. Nocturnal non-invasive ventilation in COPD patients with prolonged hypercapnia after ventilatory support for acute respiratory failure: a randomised, controlled, parallel-group study. Thorax. 2014;69(9):826–34.
8. Windisch W. Noninvasive positive pressure ventilation in COPD. Crit Care Clin. 2008;24(3):527–38.
9. Wysocki M, Tric L. Noninvasive ventilation in acute respiratory failure. Eur Respir J. 1998;11(4):823–30.
10. Vitacca M, Clini E, Ambrosino N. Non-invasive mechanical ventilation in acute respiratory failure. Monaldi Arch Chest Dis. 2000;55(1):21–7.
11. Tobias JD. Applications of jet ventilation in children. Paediatr Anaesth. 2000;10(1):49–57.
12. Galvis AG, Holmes JH. Jet ventilation: anesthetic and technical considerations. Int Anesthesiol Clin. 2008;46(2):113–26.
13. Ratner EF, Lightdale JR. High-frequency jet ventilation. Curr Opin Anaesthesiol. 2006;19(4):355–60.

14. Gottlieb A, Mann C. High-frequency ventilation techniques. Best Pract Res Clin Anaesthesiol. 2004;18(4):641–57.
15. Patel A, Nouraei SA. Transnasal humidified rapid-insufflation ventilatory exchange (THRIVE): a physiological method of increasing apnoea time in patients with difficult airways. Anaesthesia. 2015;70(3):323–9.
16. Mirza S, Page C. The laryngeal mask airway in ENT surgery: an evaluation of its use in 105 patients undergoing microlaryngoscopy and rigid bronchoscopy. Clin Otolaryngol Allied Sci. 2004;29(4):337–41.

NIV Procedures in Electroconvulsive Therapy

26

Yukihide Koyama and Antonio M. Esquinas

26.1 Introduction

Electroconvulsive therapy (ECT) is an established treatment intervention for severe psychiatric diseases such as depression, schizophrenia, bipolar disorder, and Parkinson's disease. The indication of ECT has been broadened since Ceriletti and colleagues introduced it to the clinical settings as the specified treatment intervention for schizophrenia in Italy in 1938 [1]. Recently, more patients with severe depression and other mental diseases have undergone ECT because of its broadened indication and better outcomes. Regarding the characteristics of depressive individuals, previous reports have described a significant positive relationship between depression and obesity as commonly co-occurring medical conditions [2, 3]. Furthermore, the rate of obese individuals worldwide has recently almost tripled compared to 1975 [4]. Specifically, the rate of morbidly obese individuals (BMI >40 kg/m^2) among individuals with obesity has been increasing rapidly [5]. That is, the number of morbidly obese patients requiring ECT has been increasing worldwide.

Anesthetic management of ECT has been almost uniform across the world since the 1950s. Conventionally, preoxygenation with 100% oxygen is applied in a supine position with a facemask, and subsequently, oxygenation is maintained with manual mask ventilation throughout the procedure except for the period between the ECT stimulation and the termination of the seizure. That means an absolute apnea period exists during ECT under conventional management. Although airway management, specifically mask ventilation, is the most crucial maneuver in conventional ECT

Y. Koyama (✉)
Department of Anesthesia, Nippon Koukan Hospital, Kawasaki, Kanagawa Prefecture, Japan

A. M. Esquinas (✉)
Unidad de Cuidado Intensivo, Hospital Morales Meseguer, Murcia, Spain

© The Author(s), under exclusive license to Springer Nature Switzerland AG 2025

K. Panda et al. (eds.), *Noninvasive Ventilatory Approaches in Interventional Procedures*, Noninvasive Ventilation. The Essentials,
https://doi.org/10.1007/978-3-032-05328-2_26

management, it can often be difficult regardless of being obese or nonobese [6–9]. In addition, hypoxic episodes during ECT are not uncommon in obese individuals, and obesity is one of the independent risk factors of oxygen desaturation during ECT [7, 10]. Rapid decrease in oxygen saturation during apnea in obese individuals compared with nonobese individuals [11] is attributed to their unique physiological features such as decreased respiratory compliance, increased airway resistance, reduced functional residual capacity (FRC), high closing-capacity-to-FRC ratio, increased metabolic demand, and greater oxygen consumption [12]. Consequently, considering the considerable possibility of difficult mask ventilation and subsequent hypoxic episode, respiratory management strategies to prevent hypoxia, especially in morbidly obese individuals, are the most critical for conventional ECT management. Mechanical ventilation using a supraglottic airway device during the entire ECT in obese individuals has already been established as a preventive measure to avoid the apnea period and subsequent hypoxia and maintain appropriate oxygenation and CO_2 tension [7, 12]. On the other hand, as the preventive measures of oxygen desaturation in this population, the significance of noninvasive ventilation (NIV) has drawn attention [12]. NIV is the application of oxygen supply (ventilation support) via a face mask and, therefore, eliminates the need for tracheal intubation, including continuous positive airway pressure (CPAP), pressure support ventilation (PSV), noninvasive bi-level positive airway pressure (BiPAP), and high-flow nasal cannula (HFNC) oxygenation or humidified rapid-insufflation ventilatory exchange (THRIVE). NIV achieves comparative physiological benefits to conventional mechanical ventilation with tracheal intubation by reducing the work of breathing and improving gas exchange. These NIV techniques have been regarded as beneficial for the prevention of oxygen desaturation, especially in individuals with morbid obesity and respiratory impairment [13–17]. Furthermore, some reports described that the use of HFNC oxygenation/THRIVE during the entire ECT procedure without mask ventilation could be an alternative to the conventional method using face mask ventilation in nonobese individuals, suggesting some merits for severely depressive individuals [18, 19]. In addition to maintaining appropriate oxygenation, appropriate CO_2 tension is also crucial in ECT anesthesia because hypocapnia immediately before electrical stimulation is necessary to ensure adequate seizure duration and subsequent better outcomes of the therapy [20]. Based on previous studies, NIVs can help as supportive measures for conventional ECT and novel techniques to accomplish the entire ECT without conventional maneuvers using manual mask ventilation.

In this chapter, we describe the efficacy of NIVs on ECT from two viewpoints: supportive techniques for conventional ECT management and novel techniques to accomplish the entire ECT without mask ventilation. Specifically, we describe the significance of preventing hypoxia and maintaining appropriate oxygenation during ECT, effective anesthetic methods to avoid oxygen desaturation in patients with morbid obesity and respiratory impairment using NIVs, and the novel ECT management with the application of HFNC oxygenation for the entire ECT in nonobese individuals.

26.2 ECT for Obese Individuals

Hypoxia often occurs during ECT, especially in morbidly obese patients. Various strategies for preventing hypoxia are currently available during ECT, including patient positioning (head-up position), enhancing apneic oxygenation, and the use of NIVs such as conventional low-flow nasal cannula oxygenation and noninvasive positive pressure ventilation (NPPV) such as CPAP, PSV, and BiPAP, and HFNC oxygenation. To ensure appropriate oxygenation in individuals with morbid obesity and respiratory impairment during ECT, in addition to NIV, the head-up position and enhancing apneic oxygenation during and after preoxygenation should be considered.

26.3 Patient Positioning

Patient positioning is one of the most crucial measures to prevent hypoxia, especially in obese patients during ECT, before applying NIV. Obese individuals have reduced FRC, resulting in reduced oxygen reserves [21], suggesting that a rapid decrease in oxygen saturation during apnea in morbidly obese patients [11] is due to the unique physiological features of this population. Head-up positioning of a patient increases FRC due to the descent of the diaphragm and reduced pulmonary blood volume, leading to increased oxygen reserves and subsequent improvement of oxygenation, specifically in this population. In a previous report, preoxygenation in a head-up position was reported to be more effective than in the supine position to prevent oxygen desaturation in morbidly obese patients during ECT [7]. Accordingly, a head-up position called a ramp position (Fig. 26.1) should be considered to increase FRC and oxygen reserves in preventing hypoxia in patients with morbid obesity and respiratory impairment during ECT.

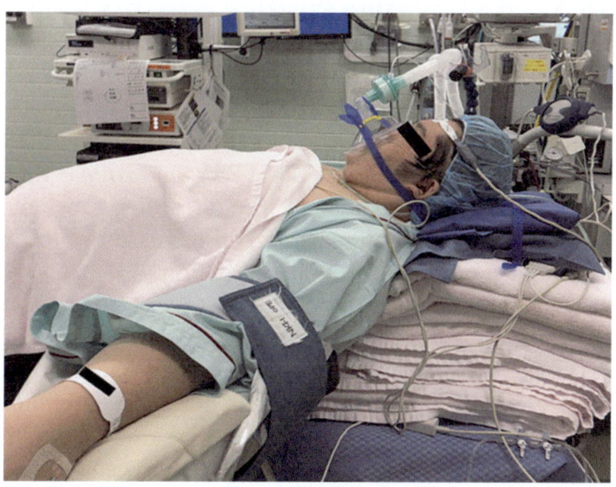

Fig. 26.1 Ramp position in a morbidly obese patient (Written informed consent was obtained from the patient for the presentation of the photo)

Next, we propose some helpful NIV techniques during ECT to maintain appropriate oxygenation and promote CO_2 washout that is necessary to ensure ideal seizure duration and better outcomes.

26.4 Enhancement of Apneic Oxygenation

Enhancing apneic oxygenation is one of the most fundamental measures for respiratory management to promote better oxygenation, delivering oxygen to the alveoli, even while the individual's lungs are not ventilated. The underlying mechanism of apneic oxygenation is due to the gas flow difference between oxygen (from the alveoli to the blood at a rate of 250 mL/min) and CO_2 (from the blood to the alveoli at a rate of 20 mL/min), creating the pressure difference and gas movement from the pharynx to the alveoli [22]. This phenomenon significantly improves oxygenation, extends the safe apnea period, and thus makes a significant impact on respiratory management in vulnerable patients, especially with morbid obesity and respiratory insufficiency. Enhancing apneic oxygenation is crucial for conventional ECT management to extend the safe apnea period and improve oxygenation because the apnea period exists between the electrical stimulus and the termination of seizure with conventional management. Some techniques to enhance apneic oxygenation after induction of anesthesia have been reported, including conventional low-flow nasal cannula oxygenation via a nasopharyngeal catheter and standard nasal cannula prongs, and HFNC oxygenation. Oxygen insufflation to the upper airway at low and high-flow rates immediately after conventional preoxygenation in a head-up position significantly improves oxygen saturation and delays the onset of desaturation in morbidly obese patients [16, 17]. Accordingly, these techniques of oxygen insufflation can also be applied to conventional ECT management to ensure a safe apnea period.

26.5 Noninvasive Positive Pressure Ventilation (NPPV) During Preoxygenation

To our knowledge, no report has described the efficacy of NPPV on ECT management. NPPV is the application of mechanical ventilation without tracheal intubation, including continuous CPAP, PSV, and BiPAP. Similar to the effects of invasive mechanical ventilation, NPPV can also offer beneficial physiological effects, such as respiratory muscle unloading, an increase in FRC, gas exchange improvement, and augmentation of alveolar ventilation [23]. Thus, considering the physiological effects of NPPV, it can work as a strategy for respiratory management and help improve oxygenation, prevent hypoxia during the apnea period, and promote CO_2 washout in patients, especially with morbid obesity and respiratory impairment undergoing ECT. NPPV is currently the most commonly used respiratory treatment to help critically ill patients recover from acute respiratory failure [23–25]. Regarding the efficacy of NPPV on preoxygenation in morbidly obese individuals compared with conventional preoxygenation, preoxygenation with NPPV, such as low-pressure CPAP and PSV, contributed to better oxygenation and prevented oxygen desaturation successfully during anesthetic induction in morbidly obese individuals [13]. Furthermore, preoxygenation with BiPAP before induction of anesthesia significantly improved oxygenation and promoted CO_2 washout in bariatric patients [14]. These reports suggest that preoxygenation with NPPV can also help improve oxygenation, prevent desaturation, and promote CO_2 washout during ECT in this population. However, NPPV requires the patient's optimal cooperation and understanding for successful respiratory management because fitting the face mask tightly on the patient's face is mandatory. Therefore, NPPV may not be ideal for some mentally ill patients requiring ECT. We should consider the indication of NPPV for ECT in each case. However, with optimal cooperation and understanding, preoxygenation with NPPV can help promote better oxygenation and CO_2 washout to ensure better outcomes in patients with morbid obesity and respiratory impairment undergoing ECT. In general, NPPV can seldom help support respiratory function after spontaneous breathing completely disappears, which differs from the features of HFNC oxygenation. The efficacy of NPPV may be limited to the preoxygenation period. However, NPPV for the preoxygenation period during ECT appears beneficial in those populations with optimal cooperation and understanding.

26.6 HFNC Oxygenation/THRIVE

NPPV has been the primary choice to support vulnerable patients with respiratory impairment. However, it is not always applicable due to the patient's tolerance limitation, including critical mental illness requiring ECT because of the requirement of a tightly fitting facemask. HFNC oxygenation has recently been introduced as a novel measure to improve oxygenation in patients with respiratory insufficiency in clinical settings [26]. HFNC oxygenation represents a recent breakthrough in the field of apneic oxygenation, enhancing both oxygenation and CO_2 washout, compared with conventional low-flow nasal oxygenation [27]. In contrast to NPPV, HFNC oxygenation does not require a patient's tolerance, which could be significantly advantageous for mentally ill patients. In general, the apparatus of HFNC oxygenation is composed of an air/oxygen blender, an active heated humidifier, a single heated circuit, and a specified nasal cannula. At the air/oxygen blender, the inspiratory fraction of oxygen (FiO_2) can range from 0.21 to 1.0 in a flow of up to 60 to 70 L/min [26]. This apparatus can provide a high flow of heated and humidified gas to patients, which is considered to have some advantages on respiratory function, such as better CO_2 washout in anatomical dead space, providing positive end-expiratory pressure, a stable fraction of inspired oxygen, and appropriate humidification without discomfort [26].

Previous reports described the efficacy of HFNC oxygenation on the entire ECT management without conventional management using mask ventilation in nonobese individuals [18, 19]. Zhu et al. reported that HFNC oxygenation during the entire ECT could be an alternative to conventional ECT management using mask ventilation. No differences were found in the lowest intra-operative SpO_2, seizure duration, breathing recovery time, conscious recovery time, and the incidence of adverse events during ECT between the HFNC oxygenation throughout the procedure and the conventional ECT management groups in nonobese patients. However, they did not examine CO_2 levels throughout the procedure [18]. Jonker et al. [19] also reported no difference in seizure duration during ECT between the HFNC oxygenation throughout the procedure and the conventional mask ventilation groups. In addition, no oxygen desaturations were also found in the HFNC oxygenation group, and patient comfort showed no difference compared to the conventional ECT management group. In their study [19], they turned down the oxygen flow rate to 0 L/min to avoid any chance of an outbreak of fire from 10 s before electric stimulation to its end. Furthermore, in contrast to Zhu's study, they measured transcutaneous CO_2 constantly during the procedure. Transcutaneous CO_2 gradually increased during the procedure in the HFNC group. The maximum CO_2 level in the patients of the HFNC group was 76 mmHg [18]. Considering no differences in seizure duration between the two groups in the two studies, in nonobese individuals, HFNC oxygenation throughout the procedure can be an alternative to conventional ECT management in terms of therapeutic effect. However, some cases with HFNC oxygenation showed critical CO_2 retention, suggesting the possibility that long-term prognosis would be uncertain in this novel ECT management. Further studies are warranted to investigate the long-term outcomes in patients undergoing ECT using this innovative technique.

In morbidly obese populations, Ricottilli et al. [17] demonstrated that HFNC oxygenation in a ramp position before and during anesthesia induction significantly prolonged the safe apnea period compared to the conventional method. Accordingly, preoxygenation with HFNC in a ramp position could help prevent oxygen desaturation during ECT in patients with morbid obesity. To our knowledge, however, there are no reports investigating the efficacy of HFNC oxygenation for the entire ECT in this population. In contrast to nonobese individuals, although the efficiency of HFNC preoxygenation in morbidly obese patients to enhance apneic oxygenation and subsequently prolong the safe apnea period was described [17], the efficacy and safety of the application of HFNC oxygenation for the entire ECT management in this population remain uncertain. Furthermore, Mukherjee et al. [28] pointed out the possibility that the application of HFNC oxygenation interrupts the earlier detection of CO_2 retention and airway obstruction compared to mask ventilation in morbidly obese individuals. In this regard, we should meticulously pay attention to its application to obese individuals undergoing ECT, not to miss signs of CO2 retention and airway obstruction. Meanwhile, one case report described the application of HFNC oxygenation for the entire ECT management in a pregnant patient with severe depression was successful without any adverse events [29]. Considering the similar physiological features of expectant mothers, we believe further studies are also warranted to determine if the application of HFNC oxygenation for the entire ECT management benefits obese individuals from a future perspective.

References

1. Linington A, Harris B. Fifty years of electroconvulsive therapy. BMJ. 1988;297:1354–5.
2. Mannan M, Mamun A, Doi S, Clavarino A. Prospective associations between depression and obesity for adolescent males and females- a systematic review and meta-analysis of longitudinal studies. PLoS One. 2016;11:e0157240.
3. Hidese S, Asano S, Saito K, Sasayama D, Kunugi H. Association of depression with body mass index classification, metabolic disease, and lifestyle: a web-based survey involving 11,876 Japanese people. J Psychiatr Res. 2018;102:23–8.
4. World Health Organization (WHO). Available at: https://www.who.int/news-room/fact-sheets/detail/obesity-and-overweight. Accessed 31 Jan 2023.
5. Sturm R, Hattori A. Morbid obesity rates continue to rise rapidly in the United States. Int J Obes. 2013;37:889–91.
6. Goldfarb JW, Bittner EA, George E, Welch C, Schmidt U. Successful management of a morbidly obese patient for electroconvulsive therapy with elective tracheostomy. J Clin Anesth. 2011;23:241–3.
7. Koyama Y, Nishioka H, Ibaraki T, Ozawa A, Kamoshida N, Akihisa Y, Andoh T. Successful anesthetic management of morbidly obese patients during electroconvulsive therapy with the ProSeal laryngeal mask airway in a head-up position: a report of 2 cases. J ECT. 2017;33:e30–1.
8. Gautam P, Gaul TK, Luthra N. Prediction of difficult mask ventilation. Eur J Anaesthesiol. 2005;22:638–40.
9. Rose DK, Cohen MM. The airway: problems and predictions in 18,500 patients. Can J Anaesth. 1994;41:372–83.
10. Surve R, Bansal S, Sriganesh K, Subbakrishna DK, Thirthalli J, Umamaheswara Rao GS. Incidence and risk factors for oxygen desaturation during recovery from modified electroconvulsive therapy: a prospective observational study. J Anaesthesiol Clin Pharmacol. 2015;31:99–103.
11. Tanoubi I, Drolet P, Donati F. Optimizing preoxygenation in adults. Can J Anaesth. 2009;56:449–66.
12. Koyama Y, Tsuzaki K, Suzuki T, Ozaki M, Saito S. Prevention of oxygen desaturation in morbidly obese patients during electroconvulsive therapy: a narrative review. J ECT. 2020;36:161–7.
13. Harbut P, Gozdzik W, Stjernfält E, Marsk R, Hesselvik JF. Continuous positive airway pressure/pressure supports pre-oxygenation of morbidly obese patients. Acta Anaesthesiol Scand. 2014;58:675–80.
14. El-Khatib MF, Kanazi G, Baraka AS. Noninvasive bilevel positive airway pressure for preoxygenation of the critically ill morbidly obese patient. Can J Anaesth. 2007;54:744–7.
15. Moon TS, Tai K, Kim A, Gonzales MX, Lu R, Pak T, Smith K, Chen JL, Minhajuddin AT, Nnamani N, Fox PE, Ogunnaike B. Apneic oxygenation during prolonged laryngoscopy in obese patients: a randomized, double-blinded, controlled trial of nasal cannula oxygen administration. Obes Surg. 2019;29:3992–9.
16. Baraka AS, Taha SK, Siddik-Sayyid SM, Kanazi GE, El-Khatib MF, Dagher CM, Chehade JM, Abdallah FW, Hajj RE. Supplementation of pre-oxygenation in morbidly obese patients using nasopharyngeal oxygen insufflation. Anaesthesia. 2007;62:769–73.
17. Ricottilli F, Ickx B, Van Obbergh L. High-flow nasal cannula preoxygenation in obese patients undergoing general anesthesia: a randomised controlled trial. Br J Anaesth. 2019;123:e443–4. (Abstracts from the Difficult Airway Society meeting, Edinburgh, November 28–30, 2018).
18. Zhu Y, Kang Y, Wei J, Hu J, Wang C, Wang S. Effect of high-flow nasal cannula versus conventional facemask ventilation for patients undergoing modified electroconvulsive therapy: a randomised controlled, noninferiority trial. Eur J Anaesthesiol. 2019;36:309–10.
19. Jonker Y, Rutten DJ, van Exel ER, Stek ML, de Bruin PE, Huitink JM. Transnasal humidified rapid-insufflation ventilatory exchange during electroconvulsive therapy: a feasibility study. J ECT. 2019;35:110–4.

20. Chater SN, Simpson KH. Effect of passive hyperventilation on seizure duration in patients undergoing electroconvulsive therapy. Br J Anaesth. 1988;60:70–3.
21. Altermatt FR, Muñoz HR, Delfino AE, Cortínez LI. Pre-oxygenation in the obese patient: effects of position on tolerance to apnoea. Br J Anaesth. 2005;95:706–9.
22. Shah U, Wong J, Wong DT, Chung F. Preoxygenation and intraoperative ventilation strategies in obese patients: a comprehensive review. Curr Opin Anaesthesiol. 2016;29:109–18.
23. Scala R, Pisani L. Noninvasive ventilation in acute respiratory failure: which recipe for success? Eur Respir Rev. 2018;27:180029.
24. Koyama Y, Kohno M, Tsuzaki K, Kamiyama K, Morimoto Y. Bilevel positive airway pressure therapy in a patient with myotonic dystrophy and postoperative respiratory failure: a case report. Saudi J Anaesth. 2020;14:241–3.
25. Koyama Y, Tsuzaki K, Shimizu H, Kuroda J, Shimizu S. Successful bilevel positive airway pressure therapy in a patient with amyotrophic lateral sclerosis after emergency laparotomy: a case report. Saudi J Anaesth. 2020;14:538–40.
26. Nishimura M. High-flow nasal cannula oxygen therapy in adults. J Intensive Care. 2015;3:15.
27. Lyons C, Callaghan M. Uses and mechanisms of apnoeic oxygenation: a narrative review. Anaesthesia. 2019;74:497–507.
28. Mukherjee P, Mandal M, Esquinas AM. Preoxygenation in super morbid obesity in emergency laparotomy: a new frontier? Saudi J Anaesth. 2023;17:296–7.
29. Vaithialingam B, Bansal S, Ramesh VJ, Muthuchellappan R. Trans-nasal humidified rapid insufflation ventilatory exchange (THRIVE) ventilation during electroconvulsive therapy (ECT) for a pregnant patient- a novel technique. Asian J Psychiatr. 2022;70:103023.

NIV Procedures in Awake Thoracic Surgery Non-intubated Video-Assisted Thoracoscopic Surgery

27

İsmail Sarbay and Akif Turna

27.1 Introduction

Video-assisted thoracic surgery (VATS), alongside robotic-assisted procedures, has significantly reduced the morbidity associated with traditional open thoracotomies. The concept of non-intubated VATS (NI-VATS) challenges long-standing surgical and anesthetic conventions, aiming to reduce perioperative stress and enhance patient recovery [1].

Traditionally, thoracic surgeries have relied on general anesthesia and endotracheal intubation to secure the airway and maintain ventilation, but these can lead to complications like postoperative nausea, respiratory infections, and prolonged recovery. Intubation itself carries risks such as airway trauma and vocal cord damage [2].

NI-VATS leverages regional anesthesia, sedation, and advanced airway management to avoid intubation and mechanical ventilation, aligning with enhanced recovery after surgery (ERAS) principles [3]. This approach preserves the patient's spontaneous breathing, avoiding hemodynamic fluctuations associated with general anesthesia [4].

Early thoracoscopic examinations under local anesthesia date back to the mid-twentieth century. Nezu and colleagues reported the first cases in 1997 using local anesthesia to perform minor pulmonary resections in an awake patient [5]. Technological advancements have further propelled the adoption of NI-VATS, and

İ. Sarbay
Sinop Atatürk State Hospital, Sinop, Turkey

A. Turna (✉)
Department of Thoracic Surgery, Istanbul University-Cerrahpaşa, Cerrahpaşa Medical Faculty, Istanbul, Turkey
e-mail: aturna@iuc.edu.tr

© The Author(s), under exclusive license to Springer Nature Switzerland AG 2025

K. Panda et al. (eds.), *Noninvasive Ventilatory Approaches in Interventional Procedures*, Noninvasive Ventilation. The Essentials,
https://doi.org/10.1007/978-3-032-05328-2_27

in 2007, the first non-intubated major thoracic procedures including lobectomy, chest wall resection, and thymectomy were reported [6]. Subsequent studies have consistently reported favorable outcomes in terms of safety, efficacy, and patient satisfaction [7].

27.2 Historical Context and Evolution

The journey towards NI-VATS is rooted in the evolution of thoracic surgery and anesthesia. Early twentieth-century thoracic surgery was predominantly performed using open thoracotomy under general anesthesia, which was associated with significant postoperative pain, prolonged hospital stays, and higher morbidity [8]. The mid-twentieth century saw the introduction of thoracic epidural anesthesia, allowing for pain control and muscle relaxation without deep general anesthesia [9]. The advent of VATS in the late 1980s marked a significant milestone, leveraging video technology for thoracic procedures through small incisions. Initially used for diagnostic purposes, VATS evolved to include major lung resections, esophageal surgery, and mediastinal procedures [10].

The early twenty-first century witnessed the push towards non-intubated techniques, driven by the desire to reduce physiological stress and complications associated with general anesthesia [1]. Key advancements in regional anesthesia, sedation protocols, and airway management played crucial roles. Technological advancements like high-definition video cameras and specialized thoracoscopic instruments have facilitated the transition to less-invasive techniques [11]. Advanced airway management devices, including LMAs and bronchial blockers, have enabled safer ventilation strategies during non-intubated procedures [12]. Ongoing research continues to optimize techniques, expand indications, and explore integrations with ERAS protocols and robotic-assisted surgery [13, 14].

27.3 Indications and Patient Selection

NI-VATS is suitable for specific thoracic procedures but requires careful patient selection to ensure safety and optimize outcomes. It is appropriate for small pulmonary nodule resections, lung biopsies, pleurodesis, pleural biopsies, spontaneous pneumothorax management, sympathectomy, localized lung resections, segmentectomies, wedge resections, and certain mediastinal procedures [15]. Successful implementation of NI-VATS relies on careful patient selection. Criteria include absence of significant comorbidities, adequate baseline pulmonary function, suitable anatomical location and size of the lesion, and patient cooperation [16, 17].

Absolute contraindications include conditions like severe obstructive sleep apnea or difficult airway anatomy, which can compromise airway patency or pose significant risks during sedation or regional anesthesia [18]. A comprehensive preoperative evaluation should include medical history, physical examination, diagnostic imaging, pulmonary function tests, and an anesthesiology consultation. Patient cooperation is essential; preoperative counseling and psychological assessment can help identify suitable candidates [19, 20].

27.4 Anesthetic Techniques and Patient Management

NI-VATS requires a well-coordinated anesthetic approach to ensure patient comfort and safety while maintaining spontaneous ventilation. A thorough preoperative assessment, including patient counseling to alleviate anxiety, is essential [21].

Sedation involves short-acting agents like midazolam, propofol, and dexmedetomidine; the latter is favored for its sedative and analgesic properties without significant respiratory depression. Effective analgesia is crucial, using regional anesthesia techniques like thoracic epidural anesthesia (TEA) or paravertebral block (PVB), along with local infiltration and intercostal nerve blocks [22–24].

Airway management strategies include using LMAs, nasal high-flow oxygen therapy, and jet ventilation to maintain a patent airway and adequate gas exchange without intubation. Intraoperative monitoring includes ECG, pulse oximetry, capnography, noninvasive blood pressure, and periodic ABG analysis [25]. Intraoperative management focuses on patient positioning, managing hypoxia, and maintaining hemodynamic stability [26]. Postoperative care focuses on pain control, avoiding opioid agents, early mobilization, monitoring for complications, and discharge planning [27, 28].

27.5 Surgical Technique

Preparation and setup for NI-VATS include detailed preoperative planning, with close collaboration between surgeons and anesthesiologists to tailor the surgical and anesthetic plan. The patient is positioned in a lateral decubitus position, a sterile field is established, and surgical instruments and video equipment are organized [16, 29].

The procedure involves small incisions for thoracoscope and instrument insertion, thoracoscopic examination, lung isolation, precise surgical resection using specialized instruments, hemostasis, and closure [30]. Technical considerations include the use of phrenic nerve blocks or carbon dioxide insufflation to improve surgical conditions, maintaining spontaneous ventilation, handling intraoperative hypoxia, managing patient movement, and optimizing surgical ergonomics [31].

Surgeon expertise and experience play a critical role in the successful execution of NI-VATS. Given the unique challenges posed by maintaining spontaneous ventilation and the need for precise instrument handling within a confined thoracic cavity, specialized training is essential. Surgeons must be adept at thoracoscopic techniques and familiar with the specific dynamics of non-intubated procedures [18]. Ongoing education and simulation training can further enhance skill development, ultimately contributing to improved patient outcomes.

27.6 Benefits and Outcomes

NI-VATS offers numerous advantages over traditional methods, including reduced perioperative stress, preserved spontaneous ventilation, decreased postoperative pain, shorter hospital stays, and enhanced recovery after surgery (ERAS) compliance [32]. Clinical outcomes demonstrate the safety and feasibility of NI-VATS, with studies reporting lower postoperative complications, comparable oncological outcomes, higher patient satisfaction, and cost-effectiveness [33].

Beyond the immediate perioperative benefits, NI-VATS has been associated with improved long-term outcomes and quality of life. Patients often report sustained improvements in respiratory function and overall physical well-being, which contribute to a quicker return to normal activities [34]. The minimally invasive nature of NI-VATS not only reduces the physical toll of surgery but also minimizes the psychological impact, leading to higher overall patient satisfaction in the long term [35].

The economic benefits of NI-VATS extend beyond individual patient outcomes, offering significant advantages to healthcare systems as a whole. By reducing the need for extensive postoperative care and shortening hospital stays, NI-VATS can help lower overall healthcare costs [16, 32]. This is particularly relevant in value-based healthcare models that prioritize cost-effective care without compromising quality.

27.7 Challenges and Limitations

The success of NI-VATS is closely tied to the availability of advanced technology, such as high-definition video systems, specialized thoracoscopic instruments, and sophisticated airway management devices [18]. Successful NI-VATS requires expertise, coordination between the surgical and anesthesiology teams, comprehensive training programs to overcome the learning curve, and advanced equipment [21, 34].

Patient cooperation and psychological readiness are crucial for the success of NI-VATS, as patients may remain awake and aware during the procedure. Anxiety, claustrophobia, or discomfort can lead to patient movement, compromising the surgical field and increasing the risk of complications [32]. Preoperative counseling and psychological support are therefore essential components of the patient management strategy, helping to ensure that patients are well-prepared and able to tolerate the procedure without undue stress [21].

Potential risks of NI-VATS include patient movement, intraoperative hypoxia (can be mitigated by optimizing patient positioning and using high-flow oxygen therapy), and airway management challenges in case of conversion to intubation. These risks and the limited applicability of this technique for complex surgeries underscore the need for careful patient selection and preoperative planning [19, 32].

Prisciandaro and colleagues performed an exploratory systematic review and meta-analysis, and they found that NI-VATS lobectomies for resectable NSCLC seem to have comparable perioperative and postoperative outcomes to the traditional intubated VATS approach [35]. The long-term benefits for patients with lung cancer need to be carefully assessed.

27.8 Future Directions

The field of NI-VATS is rapidly evolving, with ongoing research and innovations aimed at refining techniques and expanding its applications [15]. Key areas of focus include the development of advanced anesthetic methods and the integration of robotic-assisted surgery to further reduce invasiveness and enhance surgical precision [13, 17, 37].

Future research is exploring the feasibility of applying NI-VATS to more complex thoracic procedures, such as extensive mediastinal surgeries, and expanding its use in high-risk patient populations. Additionally, the combination of NI-VATS with enhanced recovery after surgery (ERAS) protocols is being studied to improve patient outcomes [3, 36].

Multicenter clinical trials are crucial for gathering robust data across diverse populations, which will help establish evidence-based guidelines and drive the broader adoption of NI-VATS [2, 16]. Ultimately, these advancements have the potential to transform thoracic surgery, offering patients a safer, less invasive, and more comfortable surgical experience.

27.9 Conclusion

NI-VATS represents a significant advancement in thoracic surgery, offering numerous benefits over traditional intubated approaches. By preserving spontaneous ventilation and avoiding the risks associated with general anesthesia and intubation, NI-VATS enhances patient safety, reduces postoperative pain, shortens hospital stays, and aligns with enhanced recovery protocols.

The successful implementation of NI-VATS hinges on careful patient selection, precise and tailored anesthetic techniques, and the collaborative expertise of both surgical and anesthesiology teams. As the procedure evolves, ongoing research and innovation will be crucial to expanding its indications, optimizing patient outcomes, and overcoming current limitations.

Looking to the future, the integration of advanced technologies, such as robotic-assisted surgery, and the development of comprehensive training programs will be essential in driving the broader adoption of NI-VATS. Ultimately, NI-VATS has the potential to transform thoracic surgery, offering patients a safer, less invasive, and more comfortable surgical experience, setting a new standard in the field.

References

1. Chen J-S, Cheng Y-J, Hung M-H, et al. Nonintubated thoracoscopic lobectomy for lung cancer. Ann Surg. 2011;254:1038–43.
2. Zhang X-X, Song C-T, Gao Z, et al. A comparison of non-intubated video-assisted thoracic surgery with spontaneous ventilation and intubated video-assisted thoracic surgery: a meta-analysis based on 14 randomized controlled trials. J Thorac Dis. 2021;13:1624–40.
3. Cai L-S, Hou B, Jin H, et al. Clinical evaluation of the rapid recovery of patients who underwent video-assisted thoracoscopic lung surgery under non-intubated anesthesia. Ann Transl Med. 2021;9:1783.
4. Mugnaini G, Viggiano D, Fontanari P, et al. Awake uniportal VATS sublobar lung resections in high-comorbidity patients: single-center early post-operative outcomes. Front Surg. 2023;10:1120414.
5. Nezu K, Kushibe K, Tojo T, et al. Thoracoscopic wedge resection of blebs under local anesthesia with sedation for treatment of a spontaneous pneumothorax. Chest. 1997;111:230–5.
6. Al-Abdullatief M, Wahood A, Al-Shirawi N, et al. Awake anaesthesia for major thoracic surgical procedures: an observational study. Eur J Cardiothorac Surg. 2007;32:346–50.
7. Wen Y, Liang H, Qiu G, et al. Non-intubated spontaneous ventilation in video-assisted thoracoscopic surgery: a meta-analysis. Eur J Cardiothorac Surg. 2020;57:428–37.
8. Seely AJE, Ivanovic J, Threader J, et al. Systematic classification of morbidity and mortality after thoracic surgery. Ann Thorac Surg. 2010;90:936–42. discussion 942
9. Slinger PD, Campos JH. Anesthesia for thoracic surgery. In: Miller's Anesthesia Elsevier; 2010:1819–1887.
10. McKenna RJ Jr, Houck W, Fuller CB. Video-assisted thoracic surgery lobectomy: experience with 1,100 cases. Ann Thorac Surg. 2006;81:421–5. discussion 425–6
11. Li S, Zhong Y, Chen Z, et al. Non-intubated thoracic surgery: an Asian perspective. Video Assist Thorac Surg. 2021;6:24.
12. Kiss G, Castillo M. Nonintubated anesthesia in thoracic surgery: general issues. Ann Transl Med. 2015;3:110.
13. Wang R, Gonzalez-Rivas D, Wang C, et al. Non-intubated uniportal robotic-assisted thoracic surgery: the future of thoracic surgery? Ann Cardiothorac Surg. 2023;12:49–51.
14. Kösek V, Al Masri E, Redwan B. Recent advances in non-intubated robotic-assisted thoracic surgery (NiRATS) for tracheal/airway resection and reconstruction. Ann Transl Med. 2021;9:1510.
15. Yanik F. Current overview of awake, non-intubated, video-assisted thoracic surgery. Wideochir Inne Tech Malo Inwazyjne. 2023;18:445–52.
16. Kocatürk C, Kutluk AC, Usluer O, et al. Comparison of awake and intubated video-assisted thoracoscopic surgery in the diagnosis of pleural diseases: a prospective multicenter randomized trial. Turk Gogus Kalp Damar Cerrahisi Derg. 2019;27:550–6.
17. Anile M, Vannucci J, Ferrante F, et al. Non-intubated thoracic surgery: standpoints and perspectives. Front Surg. 2022;9:937633.
18. Kiss G, Castillo M. Non-intubated anesthesia in thoracic surgery-technical issues. Ann Transl Med. 2015;3:109.
19. Chiang X-H, Lin M-W. Converting to intubation during non-intubated thoracic surgery: incidence, indication, technique, and prevention. Front Surg. 2021;8:769850.
20. Mudannayake R, Martinez G, Bello I, et al. Non-intubated thoracic surgery: a physiological approach. Arch Bronconeumol. 2023;59:699–701.
21. Irons JF, Martinez G. Anaesthetic considerations for non-intubated thoracic surgery. J Visc Surg. 2016;2:61.
22. Park SY. Non-intubated thoracic surgery under thoracic epidural anesthesia. Korean J Anesthesiol. 2017;70:235–6.

23. Deng H-Y, Zhu Z-J, Wang Y-C, et al. Non-intubated video-assisted thoracoscopic surgery under loco-regional anaesthesia for thoracic surgery: a meta-analysis. Interact Cardiovasc Thorac Surg. 2016;23:31–40.
24. Alagoz A, Findik G, Sazak H, et al. Non-intubated video-assisted thoracoscopic surgery under combination of erector spinae plane block and thoracic paravertebral block. BMC Anesthesiol. 2022;22:99.
25. Rosboch GL, Lyberis P, Ceraolo E, et al. The anesthesiologist's perspective regarding non-intubated thoracic surgery: a scoping review. Front Surg. 2022;9:868287.
26. Fabo C, Oszlanyi A, Lantos J, et al. Non-intubated thoracoscopic surgery-tips and tricks from anesthesiological aspects: a mini review. Front Surg. 2021;8:818456.
27. Furák J, Barta Z, Lantos J, et al. Better intraoperative cardiopulmonary stability and similar postoperative results of spontaneous ventilation combined with intubation than non-intubated thoracic surgery. Gen Thorac Cardiovasc Surg. 2022;70:559–65.
28. Ke H-H, Liou J-Y, Teng W-N, et al. Opioid-sparing anesthesia with dexmedetomidine provides stable hemodynamic and short hospital stay in non-intubated video-assisted thoracoscopic surgery: a propensity score matching cohort study. BMC Anesthesiol. 2023;23:110.
29. Grott M, Eichhorn M, Eichhorn F, et al. Thoracic surgery in the non-intubated spontaneously breathing patient. Respir Res. 2022;23:379.
30. Ambrogi V, Patirelis A, Tajè R. Non-intubated thoracic surgery: wedge resections for peripheral pulmonary nodules. Front Surg. 2022;9:853643.
31. Pathonsamit C, Tantraworasin A, Poopipatpab S, et al. Perioperative outcomes of non-intubated versus intubated video-assisted thoracoscopic surgery in different thoracic procedures: a propensity score-matched analysis. BMC Anesthesiol. 2022;22:154.
32. Janík M, Juhos P, Lučenič M, et al. Non-intubated thoracoscopic surgery-pros and cons. Front Surg. 2021;8:801718.
33. Liu J, Cui F, He J. Non-intubated video-assisted thoracoscopic surgery anatomical resections: a new perspective for treatment of lung cancer. Ann Transl Med. 2015;3:102.
34. Bin G, Wenjun L, Yu G, et al. Non-intubated video-assisted thoracoscopic surgery. *J Vis Exp*. Epub ahead of print May 26, 2023. https://doi.org/10.3791/65235.
35. Prisciandro E, Bertolaccini L, Sedda G, Spaggiari L. Non-intubated thoracoscopic lobectomies for lung cancer: an exploratory systematic review and meta-analysis. Inter Cardiovasc Thorac Surg. 2020;31:499–506.
36. Elsayed HH, Moharram AA. Tailored anaesthesia for thoracoscopic surgery promoting enhanced recovery: the state of the art. Anaesth Crit Care Pain Med. 2021;40:100846.
37. Gonzalez-Rivas D, Bonome C, Fieira E, et al. Non-intubated video-assisted thoracoscopic lung resections: the future of thoracic surgery? Eur J Cardiothorac Surg. 2016;49:721–31.

28 CPAP in Pleural Thoracentesis Procedure

Łukasz Minarowski, Katarzyna Guziejko,
and Robert M. Mróz

28.1 Introduction

Thoracocentesis is a widely used medical procedure in which a hollow needle or small catheter is inserted into the pleural space between the lung and the chest wall to remove excess fluid or air. This procedure is commonly performed to manage pneumothorax, hemothorax, and pleural effusions [1]. While thoracocentesis is generally a safe and effective procedure, there are potential complications that can arise, including the risk of subclavian vessel injury due to improper chest tube placement [2]. Various techniques and devices have been developed to mitigate these risks and improve the safety and efficacy of thoracocentesis [1, 3].

One such technique may be continuous positive airway pressure during the procedure (CPAP).

Ł. Minarowski (✉)
Department of Lung Diseases and Tuberculosis, Medical University of Bialystok, Bialystok, Poland

Department of Respiratory Pathophysiology, Medical University of Bialystok, Bialystok, Poland
e-mail: lukasz.minarowski@umb.edu.pl

K. Guziejko · R. M. Mróz
Department of Lung Diseases and Tuberculosis, Medical University of Bialystok, Bialystok, Poland
e-mail: katarzyna.guziejko@umb.edu.pl; robert.mroz@umb.edu.pl

© The Author(s), under exclusive license to Springer Nature Switzerland AG 2025

K. Panda et al. (eds.), *Noninvasive Ventilatory Approaches in Interventional Procedures*, Noninvasive Ventilation. The Essentials,
https://doi.org/10.1007/978-3-032-05328-2_28

28.2 Anatomy and Physiology of the Pleural Space

The pleural space is the potential between the visceral pleura (lung) and the parietal pleura (chest wall) [2]. In a healthy individual, this space contains a small amount of pleural fluid that acts as a lubricant to allow the smooth sliding of the lung against the chest wall during respiration. Various pathological conditions, such as malignancy, infection, or trauma, can accumulate excess fluid, air, or blood in the pleural space, resulting in pleural effusion, pneumothorax, or hemothorax, respectively [1].

Thoracocentesis is a procedure in which a hollow needle or small catheter is inserted into the pleural space to remove the excess fluid or air. This procedure can provide immediate symptom relief and help diagnose the underlying cause of the pleural effusion or pneumothorax [4].

28.2.1 Functions of the Pleura

The pleural space serves several essential functions, including the following:

- Facilitating the smooth sliding of the lung against the chest wall during respiration [5].
- Lubrication between the lung and chest wall [6].
- Absorption of pleural fluid to maintain a small amount of fluid in the pleural space [7].
- Preventing excessive fluid accumulation in the pleural space [8].
- Containing immune cells and mediators that defend against infection [9].

28.3 Thoracocentesis

Thoracic injuries account for a significant proportion of trauma-related deaths [2]. Tube thoracostomy, or chest tube placement, is commonly performed to drain the pleural space in pneumothorax, hemothorax, or pleural effusion cases. While thoracocentesis is generally safe and effective, it is not without risks. Potential complications include pneumothorax, hemothorax, infection, and subclavian vessel injury [2, 10]. Subclavian vessel injury is a rare but potentially life-threatening complication that can occur due to improper chest tube placement [11–13]. Routine use of lung ultrasound (LUS) during the procedure is recommended to decrease the risk of complications [13]. Complications of thoracocentesis include the following:

- Pneumothorax: 2–6% [14].
- Hemothorax: 1% [13].
- Re-expansion pulmonary oedema [15].
- Infection [13].
- Organ laceration (rare bleeding in patients with coagulopathy/thrombocytopenia).

- Chylothorax (especially in case of underlying malignancy) [16].
- Jugular vein rupture [13].
- Air embolism [13].

The percentage of each complication varies depending on the technique used and the operator's experience [13, 14, 17–20].

28.3.1 Pleural Effusion and Indications for Thoracentesis

Pleural effusion is an abnormal accumulation of fluid in the pleural space. There are various causes of pleural effusion, including heart failure, malignancy, infection, pulmonary embolism, and autoimmune disorders. Light's criteria are commonly used to differentiate the underlying aetiology of a pleural effusion based on the pleural fluid analysis.

Thoracentesis is indicated in the following situations: dyspnoea, respiratory failure, large pleural effusions, unexplained pleural effusions, or suspected malignant effusions [4, 21]. Therapeutically, thoracocentesis is performed to relieve symptoms associated with significant pleural effusions, such as dyspnoea and chest discomfort. It is typically indicated when the fluid volume is substantial enough to cause respiratory distress, with guidelines suggesting removal of between 500 and 1500 mL for symptomatic relief [22]. In empyema or complicated parapneumonic effusions, thoracocentesis can be diagnostic and therapeutic, allowing for the drainage of infected fluid [23]. Clinical contraindications for thoracocentesis include severe bleeding diathesis, pulmonary hypertension, and lack of a safe needle insertion site [24].

28.3.2 Techniques of Thoracocentesis

There are several techniques and equipment used for thoracocentesis, including the following:

Blind technique: Traditionally, thoracocentesis was performed using a blind technique, typically at the seventh to ninth intercostal spaces. This method involves palpating anatomical landmarks to locate the appropriate intercostal space for needle insertion [25]. However, this approach carries a higher risk of complications such as pneumothorax and injury to surrounding structures, particularly in patients with significant pleural effusions or anatomical abnormalities.

Ultrasound-guided technique: Ultrasound has revolutionised thoracocentesis, significantly improving its safety and efficacy. Ultrasound allows for real-time visualisation of the pleural space, enabling precise needle placement and reducing the likelihood of complications [26, 27]. Studies have shown that ultrasound guidance decreases the incidence of complications associated with thoracocentesis, making it a preferred method in clinical practice [28].

28.4 The Role of CPAP in Pleural Thoracentesis

Continuous positive airway pressure (CPAP) has been investigated as an adjunct to pleural thoracentesis to mitigate the risks of procedure-related complications. Lung re-expansion following fluid removal can lead to negative intrathoracic pressure, which may cause rapid lung expansion and subsequent pulmonary oedema, known as re-expansion pulmonary oedema (REPE, also quoted as RPO or RPE). The incidence of REPE is around 1%, and REPE-related mortality was reported as high as 21% [29]. Applying CPAP during this procedure can mitigate some complications associated with rapid changes in pleural pressure, thereby improving patient outcomes.

As stated in the guidelines for thoracentesis, the procedure should be performed using ultrasound guidance to minimise the risk of complications [6]. Additionally, CPAP has been proposed as a potential strategy to further enhance the safety of thoracocentesis, especially in mechanically ventilated patients at higher risk of respiratory compromise.

28.4.1 Mechanism of Action and Physiological Effects of CPAP

CPAP exerts several physiological effects that can be beneficial during thoracocentesis.

- CPAP increases intrathoracic pressure, counteracting the negative pressure created by fluid removal and preventing rapid lung expansion [30].
- CPAP improves oxygenation by increasing functional residual capacity and promoting alveolar recruitment [31].
- CPAP can reduce intrapulmonary shunt, improving ventilation-perfusion matching [32].
- CPAP has been linked to favourable autonomic responses, such as reduced sympathetic hyperactivity and improved heart rate variability [33].
- The modulation of the autonomic nervous system through CPAP may also enhance patient comfort [34].

These effects of CPAP may help prevent complications such as re-expansion of pulmonary oedema and hypoxemia during thoracocentesis.

28.4.2 Clinical Evidence and Research Studies

In a 1980 study of the impact of thoracentesis on pleural pressure (Ppl), Light et al. [1] defined a Ppl that reached −20 cm H_2O as a criterion for termination of the procedure [35]. The −20 cm H_2O cut-off was an arbitrary value based upon prior animal studies [36] linking such highly negative values to developing re-expansion pulmonary oedema. Grabczak et al. have described the value of real-time pleural manometry in REPE prevention [37].

The concept of risk of REPE when Ppl went below −20 cm H_2O was accepted for over 30 years. In a study of the implications of Ppl published in 2006, Feller-Kopman et al. referred to pressures lower than −20 cm H_2O during thoracentesis as "potentially dangerous" [38]. Thus, the recommended volume of evacuated fluid should not exceed 1000–1500 mL [29].

Later studies challenged this concept. The study conducted by Abouzgheib et al. investigated the impact of CPAP on pleural fluid pressures during thoracentesis due to various illnesses (80% malignancy, 4% CHF, and 16% unspecified effusion) [39]. In this prospective study, 49 patients who underwent thoracocentesis were randomly assigned to the CPAP or no-CPAP group at +5 cm H_2O; neither type of mask nor CPAP device was given. The manometer was zeroed for the site of entry into the pleural space. Gravity drainage of the pleural space was performed with serial end-expiratory pleural pressure (Ppl) measurements. Thoracentesis was aborted if a patient reported intolerable chest pain/discomfort or persistent cough. The initial Ppl was defined as the opening pleural pressure (PplO), and the final Ppl as the closing pleural pressure (PplC). The protocol did not include a routine post-thoracentesis chest X-ray. Volumes removed were comparable for the two groups (means of 1380 and 1396 mL for CPAP and control groups, respectively). Average PplO, PplC, and ΔPpl are listed in Table 28.1, as is the mean volume drained per centimetre water pressure for both groups. The average fluid removed per centimetre of water pressure was 117 mL for the CPAP versus 80 mL for the control group, caused by increased pleural compliance. Presumably, due to this increase in compliance, no patient in the CPAP group had a PplC below −20 cm H_2O. Finally, eight patients had final Ppl below −20 cm H_2O; none developed re-expansion pulmonary oedema [39].

Dos Santos et al., in a blinded study, randomly assigned 150 patients who had chest drainage into three groups: two sham CPAPs of 4 cm H_2O, one with respiratory and mobilisation techniques to hasten fluid drainage, and a third group with a

Table 28.1 The table presents mean values of total drained fluid, fluid volume per cm H_2O, and pleural pressure measurements (PplO, PplC, ΔPpl). Normality was tested using the two-sided Kolmogorov–Smirnov test. Group differences were analysed using the Welch two-sample t-test; significant differences are indicated with corresponding p-values and 95% confidence intervals. (Adopted from [39])

	CPAP ($n = 25$)	Control ($n = 24$)	Significance
Mean drainage, mL	1380	1396	n.a.
Mean drainage/cm H_2O, mL	117	80	$p = 0{,}023$ (95%CI 6.41–82.61)
Mean PplO (range), cm H_2O	3.76 (15 to −4)	0.7 (15 to −7)	n.a.
Mean PplC (range), cm H_2O	−8 (6 to −20)	−16.7 (−2 to −35)	n.a.
Mean ΔPpl (range), cm H_2O	11.8 (4 to 21)	17.4 (6 to 33)	n.a.

CPAP of 15 cm H_2O [40]. All techniques increased the volume of fluid drained and decreased respiratory distress during the procedure, with no incidence of REPE in either group.

In the most recent RCT of pleural manometry–guided thoracocentesis, Hassaballa et al., in a cohort of 110 patients with large malignant pleural effusion, showed that the risk of REPE is associated with the Ppl drop of 17 cm H_2O—the difference between mean opening and closing pressure in the non-symptomatic cluster minus its standard deviation; a cut-off value that had not any RPE symptom [41].

Ruwanpathirana et al. describe a procedure of thoracocentesis during BiPAP ventilation (IPAP = 18 cmH_2O, EPAP = 10 cm H_2O, FiO_2 = 0.7) [42]. The authors suggest that BiPAP ventilation led to higher Ppl, facilitating drainage.

Attout et al. report a case of an 80-year-old female patient with massive (4000 mL) intractable hepatic hydrothorax successfully treated with thoracocentesis and nasal CPAP [43]. This approach was proposed based on other cases published in Japan [44, 45].

Ng et al. present a case involving a patient who underwent pleural thoracocentesis for the management of a refractory chylothorax [46]. During the procedure, continuous positive airway pressure (CPAP) was employed to facilitate lung expansion and to ensure an effective seal. This case study highlights the potential efficacy of combining CPAP with talc pleurodesis as a treatment strategy for refractory chylothorax.

28.5 Summary

In summary, the application of continuous positive airway pressure (CPAP) during pleural thoracentesis has been shown to enhance clinical outcomes for adult patients with pleural effusion. Although additional research is warranted to validate these findings and to explore the optimal integration of CPAP with other therapeutic interventions for improved patient care, the results of this study offer valuable insights into the potential advantages of utilising CPAP during this procedure for patients with pleural effusions of diverse etiologies.

Acknowledgements According to the COPE position statement on AI tool use, the authors would like to acknowledge the use of various software tools to support the preparation of this manuscript. The text was translated, edited, and refined with artificial intelligence (AI) and language assistance programs. Specifically, DeepL was employed for translation, Grammarly for language and grammar correction, and Scite.ai for contextual literature searches. Mendeley was used for reference management, and Jenni.ai provided editorial assistance. It should be noted that the content of this manuscript was not generated solely by AI. Instead, AI tools were utilised to facilitate and improve the quality of translation, editing, and manuscript organisation, with all content reviewed and refined by the authors.

References

1. Kumar K, Basker S, Jeslin L, Chandrasekaran K, Matthias AM. Anaesthesia for pediatric video assisted thoracoscopic surgery. J Anaesthesiol Clin Pharmacol. 2011;27(1):12–6.
2. Patel R, Barlas K, Omonbude D, Patil P, Patil S. Subclavian vessel injury from chest-drain malposition in the treatment of a pneumothorax in the presence of a lateral third open clavicular fracture. Radiol Case Rep. 2022;17(9):3436–8.
3. Ghahramanifar M, Haghani M, Ghadimi Moghadam A, Haghani A, Ghadimi Moghadam AK. A new conveyable device for electro-drainage of thorax. J Biomed Phys Eng. 2018;8(4):453–6.
4. Sokolowski JW Jr, Burgher LW, Jones FL Jr, Patterson JR, Selecky PA. Guidelines for thoracentesis and needle biopsy of the pleura. This position paper of the American Thoracic Society was adopted by the ATS Board of directors in June 1988. Am Rev Respir Dis. 1989;140(1):257–8.
5. Burstiner L, Al Khalili Y. Anatomy, Thorax, Pleurae. In: StatPearls. Treasure Island: StatPearls Publishing; 2023.
6. O'Connor RE, Feldstein JS, Bouzoukis JK. Thoracentesis in the emergency department. J Emerg Med. 1985;2(6):433–42.
7. Friedberg JS, Kucharczuk JC. Pleura: anatomy, physiology, and disorders. Surgery. 2008:1551–70.
8. Lai-Fook SJ. Pleural mechanics and fluid exchange. Physiol Rev. 2004;84(2):385–410. https://doi.org/10.1152/physrev.00026.2003.
9. Weldon E, Williams J. Pleural disease in the emergency department. Emerg Med Clin North Am. 2012;30(2):475–99. https://doi.org/10.1016/j.emc.2011.10.012.
10. Quigley RL. Thoracentesis and chest tube drainage. Crit Care Clin. 1995;11(1):111–26.
11. Mao M, Hughes R, Papadimos TJ, Stawicki SP. Complications of chest tubes: a focused clinical synopsis. Curr Opin Pulm Med. 2015;21(4):376–86. https://doi.org/10.1097/MCP.0000000000000169.
12. Takanami I. Pulmonary artery perforation by a tube thoracostomy. Interact Cardiovasc Thorac Surg. 2005;4(5):473–4. https://doi.org/10.1510/icvts.2005.113357.
13. Cantey EP, Walter JM, Corbridge T, Barsuk JH. Complications of thoracentesis: incidence, risk factors, and strategies for prevention. Curr Opin Pulm Med. 2016;22(4):378–85. https://doi.org/10.1097/MCP.0000000000000285.
14. Yu H. Management of pleural effusion, empyema, and lung abscess. Semin Intervent Radiol. 2011;28(1):75–86. https://doi.org/10.1055/s-0031-1273942. PMID: 22379278; PMCID: PMC3140254
15. Sherman SC. Reexpansion pulmonary edema: a case report and review of the current literature. J Emerg Med. 2003;24(1):23–7. https://doi.org/10.1016/s0736-4679(02)00663-7.
16. Cook S, Ali S, Pracher F, Gautam A. Chylothorax complicating central venous access and thoracocentesis in an infant with parapneumonic empyema. J Paediatr Child Health. 2021;57(8):1331–3. https://doi.org/10.1111/jpc.15214.
17. Jones PW, Moyers JP, Rogers JT, Rodriguez RM, Lee YC, Light RW. Ultrasound-guided thoracentesis: is it a safer method? Chest. 2003;123(2):418–23. https://doi.org/10.1378/chest.123.2.418.
18. Łochowski MP, Kozak J. Video-assisted thoracic surgery complications. Wideochir Inne Tech Maloinwazyjne. 2014;9(4):495–500. https://doi.org/10.5114/wiitm.2014.44250.
19. Wise D, Davies G, Coats T, Lockey D, Hyde J, Good A. Emergency thoracotomy: "how to do it". Emerg Med J. 2005;22(1):22–4. https://doi.org/10.1136/emj.2003.012963.
20. Ault MJ, Rosen BT, Scher J, Feinglass J, Barsuk JH. Thoracentesis outcomes: a 12-year experience. Thorax. 2015;70(2):127–32. https://doi.org/10.1136/thoraxjnl-2014-206114.
21. Myatt R. Diagnosis and management of patients with pleural effusions. Nurs Stand. 2014;28(41):51–8. https://doi.org/10.7748/ns.28.41.51.e8849.

22. Asciak R, Bedawi EO, Bhatnagar R, et al. British Thoracic Society clinical statement on pleural procedures. Thorax. 2023;78(Suppl 3):s43–68. https://doi.org/10.1136/thorax-2022-219371.
23. Lang-Lazdunski L, Bille A, Lal R, et al. Pleurectomy/decortication is superior to extrapleural pneumonectomy in the multimodality management of patients with malignant pleural mesothelioma. J Thorac Oncol. 2012;7(4):737–43. https://doi.org/10.1097/JTO.0b013e31824ab6c5.
24. Thomsen TW, DeLaPena J, Setnik GS. Videos in clinical medicine. Thoracentesis N Engl J Med. 2006;355(15):e16. https://doi.org/10.1056/NEJMvcm053812.
25. Sigrist N. Thoracocentesis. In: Silverstein D, Hopper K, editors. Small animal critical care medicine. St. Louis, Missouri: Elsevier; 2015. p. 1029–31.
26. Fakoya FA, du Plessis M, Gbenimacho IB. Ultrasound and stethoscope as tools in medical education and practice: considerations for the archives. Adv Med Educ Pract. 2016;7:381–7. Published 2016 Jul 13. https://doi.org/10.2147/AMEP.S99740.
27. Dancel R, Schnobrich D, Puri N, et al. Recommendations on the use of ultrasound guidance for adult thoracentesis: a position statement of the Society of Hospital Medicine. J Hosp Med. 2018;13(2):126–35. https://doi.org/10.12788/jhm.2940.
28. Mukund A, Kumar Dp V, Condati NK, Bhadoria AS, Sarin SK. Efficacy and safety of ultrasound guided percutaneous glue embolisation in iatrogenic haemorrhagic complications of paracentesis and thoracocentesis in cirrhotic patients. Br J Radiol. 2018;91(1081):20170259. https://doi.org/10.1259/bjr.20170259.
29. Stawicki SP, Sarani B, Braslow BM. Reexpansion pulmonary edema. OPUS 12. Scientist. 2008;2(2):29–31.
30. Marshall A, Pittard M. Use of continuous positive airway pressure (CPAP) in the critically ill–physiological principles. Aust Crit Care. 1999;12(4):154–8. https://doi.org/10.1016/s1036-7314(99)70602-8.
31. Orta DA, Tucker NH 3rd, Green LE, Yergin BM, Olsen GN. Severe hypoxemia secondary to pulmonary embolisation treated successfully with the use of a CPAP (continuous positive airway pressure) mask. Chest. 1978;74(5):588–90. https://doi.org/10.1378/chest.74.5.588.
32. Kim YD, Ko S, Kim D, Lim H, Lee JH, Kim MH. The effects of incremental continuous positive airway pressure on arterial oxygenation and pulmonary shunt during one-lung ventilation. Korean J Anesthesiol. 2012;62(3):256–9. https://doi.org/10.4097/kjae.2012.62.3.256.
33. Shin JH, Song MJ, Kim JH. Acute Effect of positive airway pressure on heart rate variability in obstructive sleep apnea. J Clin Med. 2023;12(24):7606. Published 2023 Dec 10. https://doi.org/10.3390/jcm12247606.
34. Salsone M, Marelli S, Vescio B, et al. Usefulness of cardiac parasympathetic index in CPAP-treated patients with obstructive sleep apnea: a preliminary study. J Sleep Res. 2020;29(2):e12893. https://doi.org/10.1111/jsr.12893.
35. Light RW, Jenkinson SG, Minh VD, George RB. Observations on pleural fluid pressures as fluid is withdrawn during thoracentesis. Am Rev Respir Dis. 1980;121(5):799–804. https://doi.org/10.1164/arrd.1980.121.5.799.
36. Waqaruddin M, Bernstein A. Re-expansion pulmonary oedema. Thorax. 1975;30(1):54–60. https://doi.org/10.1136/thx.30.1.54.
37. Grabczak EM, Krenke R, Zielinska-Krawczyk M, Light RW. Pleural manometry in patients with pleural diseases – the usefulness in clinical practice. Respir Med. 2018;145:230–6. https://doi.org/10.1016/j.rmed.2018.01.014.
38. Feller-Kopman D, Berkowitz D, Boiselle P, Ernst A. Large-volume thoracentesis and the risk of reexpansion pulmonary edema. Ann Thorac Surg. 2007;84(5):1656–61. https://doi.org/10.1016/j.athoracsur.2007.06.038.

39. Abouzgheib W, Arya R, Cruz-Morel K, et al. The impact of continuous positive airway pressure upon pleural fluid pressures during thoracentesis. Respiration. 2019;98(1):55–9. https://doi.org/10.1159/000496610.
40. Dos Santos EDC, da Silva JS, de Assis Filho MTT, Vidal MB, Monte MC, Lunardi AC. Adding positive airway pressure to mobilisation and respiratory techniques hastens pleural drainage: a randomised trial. J Physiother. 2020;66(1):19–26. https://doi.org/10.1016/j.jphys.2019.11.006.
41. Hassaballa AS, Mostafa A, Hikal T, Elnori A, Elsayed HH. Pleural manometry during thoracocentesis in patients with malignant pleural effusion: a randomised controlled trial. Can J Respir Ther. 2023;59:33–44. Published 2023 Jan 20. https://doi.org/10.29390/cjrt-2022-047.
42. Ruwanpathirana PS, Karunatillake R, Jayasinghe S. Positive pressure-assisted pleural aspiration: a case report of a novel procedure and a review of literature. SAGE Open Med Case Rep. 2022;10:2050313X221122450. Published 2022 Sep 8. https://doi.org/10.1177/2050313X221122450.
43. Attout H, Samaan KJF, Bouhamla H, Amichi S, Dahmani K. Intractable hepatic hydrothorax: a successful outcome following CPAP treatment. Eur J Case Rep Intern Med. 2022;9(10):003610. Published 2022 Oct 10. https://doi.org/10.12890/2022_003610.
44. Saito R, Rai T, Saito H, et al. Nihon Shokakibyo Gakkai Zasshi. 2006;103(10):1146–51.
45. Yamamoto M, Miyashita M, Okamoto S, et al. Nippon Naika Gakkai Zasshi. 2015;104(3):590–2. https://doi.org/10.2169/naika.104.590.
46. Ng BH, Nik Abeed NN, Abdul Hamid MF, Soo CI, Low HJ, Ban AY. Resolution of refractory chylothorax with a combination of talc pleurodesis and CPAP. Respirol Case Rep. 2020;8(7):e00624. Published 2020 Jul 15. https://doi.org/10.1002/rcr2.624.

NIV Procedures in Gynecology and Obstetrics

29

Lily Liu, Jieun Bae, and Yi McWhorter

29.1 General Society Guidelines

General society guidelines endorse the use of noninvasive positive pressure ventilation (NIPPV) during the perioperative/periprocedural time for hypoxemic patients in general to reduce risks of atelectasis, pneumonia, prevent intubation, and mortality [1]. Table 29.1 Patients' vital signs are monitored continuously, and periodic arterial blood gas (ABG) sampling is recommended in its titration. NIPPV has also been recommended to be used in post-extubation failure after abdominal and cardiac surgery. Other patient populations who may benefit from such modality include patients received lung resection, solid organ transplant, and bronchoscopy. High-flow nasal cannula (HFNC) can be used if not tolerating other forms of noninvasive respiratory support techniques [1]. The guideline did not address ways to prevent possible complications from NIPPV or how and where to initiate it. In this chapter, we will discuss common pathophysiology associated with patients needing obstetrical and gynecological procedures as well as review current evidence in the application of NIPPV therapy.

L. Liu · J. Bae
Kirk Kerkorian School of Medicine at UNLV, Las Vegas, NV, USA
e-mail: liul7@unlv.nevada.edu; Baej13@unlv.nevada.edu

Y. McWhorter (✉)
Department of Critical Care Medicine, HCA Healthcare; Mountain View Hospital, Las Vegas, NV, USA
e-mail: Yi.McWhorter@hcahealthcare.com

© The Author(s), under exclusive license to Springer Nature Switzerland AG 2025

K. Panda et al. (eds.), *Noninvasive Ventilatory Approaches in Interventional Procedures*, Noninvasive Ventilation. The Essentials,
https://doi.org/10.1007/978-3-032-05328-2_29

Table 29.1 Noninvasive respiratory support in the hypoxaemic perioperative/periprocedural patient: A joint ESA/ESICM guideline [1]

Number	Recommendation	Grade
Recommendations for peri-operative/periprocedural hypoxaemic patients with acute respiratory failure.		
R1	In the peri-operative/periprocedural hypoxaemic patient, the use of either NIPPV or CPAP (based on local expertise) is preferred to COT to improve oxygenation.	1B
R2	In the postoperative hypoxaemic patient after cardiac surgery we suggest using NIPPV rather than CPAP to reduce the risk of atelectasis.	2C
R3	In the postoperative hypoxaemic patient after upper abdominal surgery, we suggest CPAP or NIPPV rather than COT to reduce the risk of hospital-acquired pneumonia and its associated complications.	2B
R4	In the peri-operative/periprocedural hypoxaemic patient, either NIPPV or CPAP is preferred over COT to prevent re-intubation.	2B
R5	In the peri-operative/periprocedural hypoxaemic patient, we suggest to use NIPPV rather than COT to resolve atelectasis.	2C
Which patients may benefit from the use of non-invasive respiratory support techniques for hypoxaemic patients with acute respiratory failure?		
R6	NIPPV or CPAP immediately post-extubation for hypoxaemic patients at risk of developing acute respiratory failure after abdominal surgery.	1B
R7	Either NIPPV or CPAP may be considered for prevention of further respiratory deterioration in hypoxaemic patients after cardiac surgery.	2C
R8	HFNC may be considered for hypoxaemic patients after cardiac surgery.	2C
R9	NIPPV may be considered for prevention of atelectasis in hypoxaemic patients after lung resection.	2C
R10	NIPPV in hypoxaemic patients after solid organ transplantation.	2B
R11	In the hypoxaemic patient requiring bronchoscopy, we suggest using non-invasive respiratory support techniques rather than COT.	2B
What minimal standards of haemodynamic and respiratory monitoring and what laboratory and radiological tests are required during the support period?		
R12	We suggest that peri-operative/periprocedural hypoxaemic patients undergoing NIPPV should be treated by clinicians with recognised competence and skill in airway management and ventilation of patients with lung injury.	2C
R13	We suggest that peri-operative/periprocedural patients treated with non-invasive respiratory support techniques be examined periodically for signs of respiratory distress, neurological deterioration and interface intolerance by a clinician with recognised competence and skill in airway management and ventilation of patients with lung injury.	2C

(continued)

Table 29.1 (continued)

Number	Recommendation	Grade
R14	We suggest that peri-operative/periprocedural hypoxaemic patients receiving NIPPV undergo continuous physiological monitoring including pulse oximetry, blood pressure measurement and electrocardiography. When a closed NIPPV device is being used, we suggest monitoring of flow and pressure ventilation waveforms.	2C
R15	In peri-operative/periprocedural hypoxaemic patients treated with a non-invasive respiratory support technique, we suggest periodic arterial blood gas sampling after the first hour of treatment, at least every 6 h during the first 24 h and then daily until the end of the treatment period.	2C
R16	We cannot provide a recommendation regarding the need for routine imaging. However, in the presence of clinical deterioration, chest imaging should be considered during NIPPV treatment in hypoxaemic peri-operative/periprocedural patients.	2C
What are the (ways to prevent) avoidable complications in patients receiving various types of non-invasive respiratory support?		
R17	Enteral nutrition and routine studies addressing prevention of complications and good practice should be a priority, as these topics require further research.	–
R18	We suggest using a HFNC rather than conventional oxygen therapy in the peri-operative/periprocedural hypoxaemic patient with low tolerance to other forms of non-invasive respiratory support techniques.	2B
How and where to initiate non-invasive respiratory support?		
R19	We recommend that future randomised studies address this query and therefore decided to refrain from issuing a recommendation on this topic.	–

COT conventional oxygen therapy, *CPAP* continuous positive airway pressure, *HFNC* high-flow nasal cannula, *NIPPV* non-invasive positive pressure ventilation

29.2 Obstetrics

29.2.1 Pulmonary: Sleep Disordered Breathing

Hormonal, upper airway, and physiological changes during pregnancy place women at risk for sleep disordered breathing (SDB) in pregnancy with profound maternal and fetal implications. The chronic alkalotic respiratory state during pregnancy was modulated by progesterone levels to facilitate fetal gas exchange through placental circulation. The marked increase in tidal volume by 45% and reduction in functional residual capacity (FRC) result in slightly reduced vital capacity (VC). Therefore, acute on chronic pulmonary disease during pregnancy may not be well tolerated by the mother. Women with known SDB prior to pregnancy generally experience worsening of symptoms during pregnancy. However, its diagnosis is challenging in the obstetric population with reported sensitivities of 36–39% and specificities of 68–77% using the Epworth Sleepiness Scale or the Berlin Questionnaire [2].

SDB not only complicates pregnancy, including gestational hypertension, gestational diabetes, and preeclampsia, but it also increases the risk of cardiovascular disease later in life [2]. Meta-analysis further demonstrated its risk for gestational hypertension, gestational diabetes, preeclampsia, Cesarean-section (C-section), postoperative wound complications, pulmonary edema, preterm birth, and NICU admission [3]. The proposed mechanisms for increased morbidity include chronic inflammation, an increase in oxidative stress, and sympathetic activation [2].

Application of continuous positive airway pressure (CPAP) is the treatment of choice for obstructive sleep apnea (OSA). While scientific evidence supports its use in the general population, it has mixed results in patient outcomes in the obstetric population, and its recommended use has been largely inconclusive, though it favors its use. Kalkhoff's study did not find CPAP for OSA decreasing composite adverse pregnancy outcomes or hospital costs in the sleep study. This study had limitations in small sample size, low CPAP prescription rates, and poor compliance [4]. In contrast, nasal CPAP may lead to a lowering of blood pressure in patients with preeclampsia when used to treat SDB associated with nasal flow limitation [5]. Subjects in the study by Guilleminault 2004 tolerated nasal CPAP as the treatment for SDB during pregnancy with improved outcome; however, it required close follow-up to titrate the level, in this case, increasing the prescribed pressure as pregnancy advances [6]. Favorable outcomes observed include spontaneous diuresis and optimal outcomes, especially when SDB is associated with pulmonary hypertension [7]. Two observational studies with women suspected of OSA found that CPAP treatment may mitigate the risk of severe OSA-related cardiovascular morbidity and mortality, such as stroke. This excessive risk was also found to be more prominent in younger women [8]. During antepartum care, co-management with a sleep medicine expert is recommended to facilitate ongoing assessment of CPAP prescription and titration, in addition to modifying risk factors such as maternal obesity [9].

29.2.2 Cardiovascular: Preeclampsia and Hypertensive Disorders

Preeclampsia is the leading cause of maternal death, severe maternal morbidity, maternal intensive care unit (ICU) admissions, C-section, and prematurity. It results in 70,000 maternal deaths and 500,000 fetal deaths worldwide every year [10]. A prospective cohort study found that patients who are at high risk for OSA, screened by the Berlin Questionnaire (BQ) during the second trimester, remained an independent risk factor for preeclampsia-eclampsia after adjusting for confounders. The limitations of this study included the use of BQ instead of polysomnography (PSG), and preexisting and newly diagnosed OSA were not differentiated [11].

Through a series of small studies, it is conflicting whether gestational hypertension or preeclampsia can be helped by adjunct CPAP treatment. Guilleminault studied whether early nasal CPAP, started during the first trimester, could mitigate the risk of preeclampsia through a pilot study. Based on full PSG, nasal CPAP was insufficient in preventing the occurrence of preeclampsia, early spontaneous abortion, or premature birth. The investigators identified prior preeclampsia and obesity as potential confounders in the causal relationship between OSA and preeclampsia, because nonobese patients with prior hypertension were able to maintain normal blood pressure with antihypertensive therapy and CPAP [12]. In a separate study, investigators found that partial upper airway obstruction during sleep may be eliminated with the use of nasal CPAP and decrease blood pressure in women with preeclampsia, thus extending the in utero time for the compromised fetus [13]. Similarly, another study found that inspiratory flow limitation due to OSA and oxygen desaturation were associated with a reduction in total fetal movements, and CPAP may be able to reverse the outcome in patients with preeclampsia [14]. CPAP also maintains cardiac output through reduction of peripheral vascular resistance in patients with preeclampsia, thus optimizing maternal and fetal outcome [15]. One recent systematic review supports the great benefits of CPAP use for SDB during pregnancy. However, the neonatal and fetal outcomes are unclear in this study [16].

29.2.3 Cardiovascular: Pulmonary Edema

The normal cardiovascular physiology of pregnancy involves a high flow-low resistance state with expansion of plasma volume and a decrease in peripheral vascular resistance to accommodate the gravid uterus. At term, cardiac output increases by 43% with a 17% increase in heart rate, 21% decrease in systemic vascular resistance, and 14% decrease in colloid oncotic pressure [17]. As a result, parturients are prone to develop cardiogenic pulmonary edema and hypoxemic respiratory failure. In addition, tocolytic therapy by beta-adrenergic agonists also predisposes pregnant patients to develop pulmonary edema. Proposed mechanisms are unique to the pregnant state and include its induced increase in antidiuretic hormone secretion, thus exacerbating the existing hypervolemic state. In addition, beta-agonists activate the renin-angiotensin system, which in turn could lead to salt and water retention. CPAP has been used in the obstetric population to successfully treat severe pulmonary edema induced by tocolytic therapy with beta-adrenergic agonist, thus reducing the need for invasive mechanical ventilation [18]. CPAP improves oxygenation by decreasing intrapulmonary shunting, ventilation-to-perfusion mismatch, and work of breathing [19].

29.2.4 Gestational Hypertension

In the part II study by Poyares, pregnant women with hypertension and chronic snoring were studied, and nasal CPAP was used during the first 8 weeks of pregnancy, combined with standard prenatal care led to better blood pressure control and an uncomplicated pregnancy [20]. Similarly, a slightly larger study by Stajic, the group treated with CPAP had significantly lower incidence of hypertensive syndrome, night oxygen saturation, and a lower Epworth Sleepiness Scale score, after a month of therapy. In this study, the respiratory event index was significantly associated with hypertension severity [21]. Another positive study was done in an obese cohort by Rice, who demonstrated that treatment of OSA with CPAP in pregnancy did reduce the hypertensive-related complications [22]. In contrast, Reid et al. found CPAP had decreased OSA severity without improvement in blood pressure or inflammatory markers. In a study by Wang et al., more severe form of OSA had significantly lower adverse pregnancy outcomes when treated with CPAP than pregnant women with mild to moderate OSA [23].

29.2.5 Gestational Diabetes

In a study examining maternal SDB and glucose metabolism in early gestation in overweight and obese women, SDB and insulin resistance exhibit dose-response association. This effect was not observed between respiratory event index severity and insulin secretion. Therefore, early SDB screening may improve glucose metabolic outcome [24]. The study done by Chirakalwasan et al. studied CPAP in obese pregnant patients with GDM and OSA. They found that 2 weeks of CPAP in females with GDM and OSA did not result in improved glucose levels, but insulin secretion and sensitivity improved in those who were compliant with CPAP. Pregnancy-related complications of preterm delivery, unplanned C-section, and NICU admission were observed among those with >2 weeks of CPAP use [25].

29.3 Gynecology

CPAP and mandibular advancement devices both reduced blood pressure and cortisol levels in postmenopausal women suffering from OSA, though sleep quality and mortality were not affected [26]. CPAP is considered the standard of treatment in menopausal women. Women, increased age, and being referred by a specialist were factors that led to non-adherence to CPAP therapy [27]. In an overall review, a review article by Medlin on OSA and the impact on surgical outcomes in gynecology, the authors advocated for screening strategies for women and treatment modalities specifically related to the female sex and surgical issues specifically related to gynecological procedures. Future investigations should be focused on anesthesia prescription, postoperative narcotic use, recovery room management, and discharge planning [28].

29.4 Special Considerations

In cases of women with severe congenital kyphoscoliosis, NIPPV can be used to mitigate pregnancy-related symptoms onset usually around the 20th week of gestation. A case of successful home and peripartum treatment has been described by Kahler using nasal intermittent positive pressure ventilation with bilevel positive airway pressure (BIPAP) [29].

In one case report in a parturient suspected of OHS, the author suspected that early diagnosis and institution of NIPPV could have prevented the need for mechanical ventilation, as it reduces airway obstruction in the short term and pulmonary mechanics, stimulates central respiratory response to hypercarbia, and reduces mortality in the long term [30].

During the peri-partum period, neuraxial anesthesia combined with BIPAP helped to successfully manage a parturient with idiopathic pulmonary hemosiderosis to minimize cardiopulmonary disturbances during labor [31].

In cases of high-risk pregnancy, such as twin pregnancy, CPAP has been advocated as an adjunct to antihypertensive medications to help manage OSA with pre-eclampsia to normalize blood pressure and reduce urinary protein [32].

Stourac described the successful use of home BiPAP for patients with secondary Ondine's curse, which can occur after a brainstem insult related to eclamptic seizure [33].

In recent years, CPAP has the potential to be used as a rescue device for respiratory failure to avoid invasive mechanical ventilation and iatrogenic preterm birth in parturients diagnosed with COVID-19 pneumonia. Helmet-CPAP was also proven to be feasible, safe, well-tolerated, and improved oxygenation in pregnant women with moderate-to-severe acute respiratory failure due to SARS-CoV-2 pneumonia [34].

Lastly, Iwama studied 213 relatively healthy patients undergoing lower extremity or abdominal gynecological surgery using BIPAP with combined epidural-propofol anesthesia in adults with ASA I, II, elective surgery below the lower abdomen surgery with no nasal obstruction or upper airway obstruction or gastro-esophageal pathology [35].

29.5 Conclusion

In conclusion, procedures in the obstetrics and gynecology specialty require clinicians to pay special attention to the pathophysiology that is unique to this patient population. In addition to medical management of chronic comorbidities, the application of NIPPV has shown a positive impact on maternal outcome, especially in patients with preexisting conditions that warrant such treatment. Though robust evidence is lacking in this group of patients, successes in NIPPV therapeutics hold promise in smaller trials, warranting its consideration as an adjunctive treatment when indicated.

29.6 Disclosures

Conflicts of Interest The above listed authors, Dr. McWhorter, Student Doctors Liu and Bae have no conflicts of interest to declare.

Funding This research was supported (in whole or in part) by HCA Healthcare and/or an HCA Healthcare affiliated entity. The views expressed in this publication represent those of the author(s) and do not necessarily represent the official views of HCA Healthcare or any of its affiliated entities.

References

1. Leone M, Einav S, Chiumello D, Constantin JM, De Robertis E, Abreu MG, Gregoretti C, Jaber S, Maggiore SM, Pelosi P, Sorbello M, Afshari A. Noninvasive respiratory support in the hypoxaemic peri-operative/periprocedural patient: a joint ESA/ESICM guideline. Eur J Anaesthesiol. 2020;37(4):265–79. https://doi.org/10.1097/EJA.0000000000001166. PMID: 32132408
2. Cain MA, Ricciuti J, Louis JM. Sleep-disordered breathing and future cardiovascular disease risk. Semin Perinatol. 2015;39(4):304–9. https://doi.org/10.1053/j.semperi.2015.05.010. Epub 2015 Jul 2. PMID: 26143090
3. Liu L, Su G, Wang S, Zhu B. The prevalence of obstructive sleep apnea and its association with pregnancy-related health outcomes: a systematic review and meta-analysis. Sleep Breath. 2019;23(2):399–412. https://doi.org/10.1007/s11325-018-1714-7. Epub 2018 Sep 25. PMID: 30255484
4. Kalkhoff SM, Lutgendorf MA, Morrison TC, Han T, Spence DL. A randomized controlled trial of sleep study surveillance with targeted autoregulated positive airway pressure therapy for obstructive sleep apnea in pregnancy. Am J Obstet Gynecol MFM. 2022;4(3):100571. https://doi.org/10.1016/j.ajogmf.2022.100571. Epub 2022 Jan 17. PMID: 35051670
5. Edwards N, Middleton PG, Blyton DM, Sullivan CE. Sleep disordered breathing and pregnancy. Thorax. 2002;57(6):555–8. https://doi.org/10.1136/thorax.57.6.555. PMID: 12037233; PMCID: PMC1746354
6. Guilleminault C, Kreutzer M, Chang JL. Pregnancy, sleep disordered breathing and treatment with nasal continuous positive airway pressure. Sleep Med. 2004;5(1):43–51. https://doi.org/10.1016/j.sleep.2003.07.001. PMID: 14725826
7. Lewis DF, Chesson AL, Edwards MS, Weeks JW, Adair CD. Obstructive sleep apnea during pregnancy resulting in pulmonary hypertension. South Med J. 1998;91(8):761–2. https://doi.org/10.1097/00007611-199808000-00013. PMID: 9715225
8. Campos-Rodriguez F, Martinez-Garcia MA, Reyes-Nuñez N, Caballero-Martinez I, Catalan-Serra P, Almeida-Gonzalez CV. Role of sleep apnea and continuous positive airway pressure therapy in the incidence of stroke or coronary heart disease in women. Am J Respir Crit Care Med. 2014;189(12):1544–50. https://doi.org/10.1164/rccm.201311-2012OC. PMID: 24673616
9. Simhan HN. Antepartum care of the obese patient. Clin Obstet Gynecol. 2016;59(1):148–57. https://doi.org/10.1097/GRF.0000000000000173. PMID: 26756260
10. Rana S, Lemoine E, Granger JP, Karumanchi SA. Preeclampsia: pathophysiology, challenges, and perspectives. Circ Res. 2019;124(7):1094–112. https://doi.org/10.1161/CIRCRESAHA.118.313276. Erratum in: Circ Res 2020 Jan 3;126(1):e8. PMID: 30920918
11. Jaimchariyatam N, Na-Rungsri K, Tungsanga S, Lertmaharit S, Lohsoonthorn V, Totienchai S. Obstructive sleep apnea as a risk factor for preeclampsia-eclampsia. Sleep Breath. 2019;23(2):687–93. https://doi.org/10.1007/s11325-018-1758-8. Epub 2018 Nov 27. PMID: 30484015
12. Guilleminault C, Palombini L, Poyares D, Takaoka S, Huynh NT, El-Sayed Y. Pre-eclampsia and nasal CPAP: part 1. Early intervention with nasal CPAP in pregnant women with risk-factors for pre-eclampsia: preliminary findings. Sleep Med. 2007;9(1):9–14. https://doi.org/10.1016/j.sleep.2007.04.020. Epub 2007 Jul 17. PMID: 17644420

13. Edwards N, Blyton DM, Kirjavainen T, Kesby GJ, Sullivan CE. Nasal continuous positive airway pressure reduces sleep-induced blood pressure increments in preeclampsia. Am J Respir Crit Care Med. 2000;162(1):252–7. https://doi.org/10.1164/ajrccm.162.1.9905006. Erratum in: Am J Respir Crit Care Med 2000 Dec;162(6):2358. PMID: 10903250
14. Blyton DM, Skilton MR, Edwards N, Hennessy A, Celermajer DS, Sullivan CE. Treatment of sleep disordered breathing reverses low fetal activity levels in preeclampsia. Sleep. 2013;36(1):15–21. https://doi.org/10.5665/sleep.2292. PMID: 23288967; PMCID: PMC3524539
15. Blyton DM, Sullivan CE, Edwards N. Reduced nocturnal cardiac output associated with preeclampsia is minimized with the use of nocturnal nasal CPAP. Sleep. 2004;27(1):79–84. https://doi.org/10.1093/sleep/27.1.79. PMID: 14998241
16. Migueis DP, Urel A, Dos Santos CC, Accetta A, Burla M. The cardiovascular, metabolic, fetal and neonatal effects of CPAP use in pregnant women: a systematic review. Sleep Sci. 2022;15(Spec 1):264–77. https://doi.org/10.5935/1984-0063.20210024. PMID: 35273777; PMCID: PMC8889985
17. Bernstein. Chestnut's obstetric anesthesia: principles and practice. 6th ed. Elsevier; 2019.
18. De La Chapelle A, Benoit S, Bouregba M, Durand-Reville M, Raucoules-Aimé M. The treatment of severe pulmonary edema induced by beta adrenergic agonist tocolytic therapy with continuous positive airway pressure delivered by face mask. Anesth Analg. 2002;94(6):1593–4. https://doi.org/10.1097/00000539-200206000-00042. PMID: 12032034
19. Mehta S, Hill NS. Noninvasive ventilation. Am J Respir Crit Care Med. 2001;163(2):540–77. https://doi.org/10.1164/ajrccm.163.2.9906116. PMID: 11179136
20. Poyares D, Guilleminault C, Hachul H, Fujita L, Takaoka S, Tufik S, Sass N. Pre-eclampsia and nasal CPAP: part 2. Hypertension during pregnancy, chronic snoring, and early nasal CPAP intervention. Sleep Med. 2007;9(1):15–21. https://doi.org/10.1016/j.sleep.2007.04.019. Epub 2007 Jul 20. PMID: 17644475
21. Stajić D, Ilić D, Vuković J, Baturan B, Ilić A, Milovančev A. The effect of continuous positive airway pressure treatment on hypertensive disorder in pregnant women with obstructive sleep apnea. Sleep Breath. 2022;26(1):297–305. https://doi.org/10.1007/s11325-021-02397-x. Epub 2021 May 22. PMID: 34021466
22. Rice AL, Bajaj S, Wiedmer AM, Jacobson N, Stanic AK, Antony KM, Bazalakova MH. Continuous positive airway pressure treatment of obstructive sleep apnea and hypertensive complications in high-risk pregnancy. Sleep Breath. 2022;27(2):621–9. https://doi.org/10.1007/s11325-022-02669-0. Epub ahead of print. PMID: 35750926; PMCID: PMC9789204
23. Wang X. Obstructive sleep apnoea in pregnant women with chronic hypertension: a retrospective study. Research Square. https://doi.org/10.21203/rs.3.rs-2158065/v1.
24. Sanapo L, Bublitz MH, Bai A, Mehta N, Messerlian GM, Catalano P, Bourjeily G. Association between sleep disordered breathing in early pregnancy and glucose metabolism. Sleep. 2022;45(4):zsab281. https://doi.org/10.1093/sleep/zsab281. PMID: 34999843; PMCID: PMC8996028
25. Chirakalwasan N, Amnakkittikul S, Wanitcharoenkul E, Charoensri S, Saetung S, Chanprasertyothin S, Chailurkit LO, Panburana P, Bumrungphuet S, Thakkinstian A, Reutrakul S. Continuous positive airway pressure therapy in gestational diabetes with obstructive sleep apnea: a randomized controlled trial. J Clin Sleep Med. 2018;14(3):327–36. https://doi.org/10.5664/jcsm.6972. PMID: 29458699; PMCID: PMC5837834
26. Silvestri R, Aricò I, Bonanni E, Bonsignore M, Caretto M, Caruso D, Di Perri MC, Galletta S, Lecca RM, Lombardi C, Maestri M, Miccoli M, Palagini L, Provini F, Puligheddu M, Savarese M, Spaggiari MC, Simoncini T. Italian Association of Sleep Medicine (AIMS) position statement and guideline on the treatment of menopausal sleep disorders. Maturitas. 2019;129:30–9. https://doi.org/10.1016/j.maturitas.2019.08.006. Epub 2019 Aug 15. PMID: 31547910
27. Tal JZ, Suh SA, Dowdle CL, Nowakowski S. Treatment of insomnia, insomnia symptoms, and obstructive sleep apnea during and after menopause: therapeutic approaches. Curr Psychiatr

Rev. 2015;11(1):63–83. https://doi.org/10.2174/1573400510666140929194848. PMID: 26478725; PMCID: PMC4607064

28. Medlin EE, Rice LW, Al-Niaimi A. Obstructive sleep apnea and the impact on surgical outcomes in gynecology. Obstet Gynecol Surv. 2018;73(4):242–50. https://doi.org/10.1097/OGX.0000000000000555. PMID: 29701869
29. Kähler CM, Högl B, Habeler R, Brezinka C, Hamacher J, Dienstl A, Prior C. Management of respiratory deterioration in a pregnant patient with severe kyphoscoliosis by non-invasive positive pressure ventilation. Wien Klin Wochenschr. 2002;114(19–20):874–7. PMID: 12503480.Togioka BM, McConville SS, Penchoen-Lind RM, Schenning KJ. Diagnosis and management of obesity hypoventilation syndrome during labor. Case Rep Anesthesiol. 2021 Aug 25;2021:8096212. https://doi.org/10.1155/2021/8096212. PMID: 34484837; PMCID: PMC8413020
30. Allen TK, George RB, Peterson-Layne C, Habib AS. Management of a parturient with an acute exacerbation of idiopathic pulmonary haemosiderosis and posterior spinal instrumentation. Br J Anaesth. 2008;100(2):235–9. https://doi.org/10.1093/bja/aem375. PMID: 18211996
31. Kim MS, Moon MJ, Lee YH, Chae KY, Ahn EH. Treatment of superimposed preeclampsia on chronic hypertension in a twin pregnancy with automatic continuous positive airway pressure: a case report. BMC Pulm Med. 2020;20(1):157. https://doi.org/10.1186/s12890-020-01196-6. PMID: 32493271; PMCID: PMC7268687
32. Štourač P, Hradilová T, Straževská E, Turčáni P, Štouračová A, Janků P, Skřičková J, Gál R. Eclampsia as a cause of secondary non-obstructive central sleep hypoventilation. Ceska Gynekol. 2015;80(1):16–9. PMID: 25723073
33. Reindorf M, Newman J, Ingle T. Successful use of CPAP in a pregnant patient with COVID-19 pneumonia. BMJ Case Rep. 2021;14(3):e238055. https://doi.org/10.1136/bcr-2020-238055. PMID: 33685910; PMCID: PMC7942271
34. Iwama H. Application of nasal bi-level positive airway pressure to respiratory support during combined epidural-propofol anesthesia. J Clin Anesth. 2002;14(1):24–33. https://doi.org/10.1016/s0952-8180(01)00348-8. PMID: 11880018

NIV Procedures: Fiberoptic Bronchoscopy (Lung Lavage)

30

Anna Danel and Szymon Skoczyński

30.1 Fiberoptic Bronchoscopy

Fiberoptic bronchoscopy is a valuable diagnostic tool in modern pulmonology. As technology advances, the role of flexible bronchoscopy (FOB) for both diagnostic and therapeutic indications is continually expanding. Pre-procedural planning of FOB is of tremendous value in both maximizing benefits and minimizing risks. Indications for FOB are often thought of in terms of diagnosis and therapy. Among the most common are lung cancer, airway obstruction, evaluation of suspected pulmonary infections, diagnostic process of interstitial lung disease, as well as removal of foreign bodies, airway clearance with bacteriological sampling, and hemoptysis management [1]. Moreover, despite advanced imaging modalities, bronchoscopy remains the only method to rule out endobronchial disease, effectively visualize and evaluate changes in the bronchial mucosa, and obtain diagnostic samples [2].

30.1.1 Contraindications and Complications

Absolute contraindications to FOB are limited to refractory hypoxemia, hemodynamic instability, life-threatening arrhythmias, lack of informed consent, inadequate equipment or facility, and an inexperienced operator [3]. The incidence of

A. Danel (✉)
Department of Lung Diseases and Tuberculosis, Faculty of Medical Sciences in Zabrze, Medical University of Silesia, Katowice, Poland

Doctoral School in Medical University of Silesia, Katowice, Poland

S. Skoczyński
Department of Lung Diseases and Tuberculosis, Faculty of Medical Sciences in Zabrze, Medical University of Silesia in Katowice, Zabrze, Poland

© The Author(s), under exclusive license to Springer Nature Switzerland AG 2025

K. Panda et al. (eds.), *Noninvasive Ventilatory Approaches in Interventional Procedures*, Noninvasive Ventilation. The Essentials,
https://doi.org/10.1007/978-3-032-05328-2_30

complications and overall mortality during bronchoscopy is low. Facciolongo et al. in their multicenter prospective study of 20,986 bronchoscopies estimated the complication rate at 1.1%, with the most commonly observed complications as follows: hemoptysis 0.45%, hypoxemia 0.12%, pneumothorax 0.1%, pulmonary edema 0.07%, and bronchospasm 0.04%. An extremely low mortality rate of 0.02% confirmed the high safety of this diagnostic and therapeutic method. As respiratory failure is one of the most serious FOB risk factors, performing this procedure in hypoxemic patients is considered hazardous. Nevertheless, in some patients, FOB is essential to make a diagnosis and start proper treatment. The majority of patients qualified for bronchoscopy initially suffer from gas exchange alterations due to interstitial lung diseases or airway diseases. Moreover, procedures performed during exams, such as suction leading to alveolar collapse due to the generation of negative airway pressure or even the presence of the bronchoscope narrowing the tracheal lumen by up to 10–15%, create a significant risk for acute respiratory failure. It was observed that during the FOB arterial partial pressure of oxygen decreases by 10–20 mmHg. Hypoxemia can cause subsequent complications such as arrhythmias in 11–40% of patients, but these cardiac rhythm disturbances are rarely clinically important [4].

30.2 Bronchoalveolar Lavage

Bronchoalveolar lavage (BAL) is a minimally invasive procedure used in the diagnostic process of various lung diseases, as well as for research purposes. Performing BAL allows to collection of samples of respiratory secretions from distal airspaces for the examination of cellular and noncellular constituents [5]. Despite the widespread use of BAL, there are still no standards for the BAL technique and protocols for processing and analyzing BAL fluid. Nevertheless, based on clinical practice, it is recommended that BAL should be carried out with FOB wedged in a specific segmental or subsegmental bronchus. In patients with interstitial lung diseases (ILD), the right middle lobe and lingula of the left upper lobe are the preferential areas because of their accessibility, while maintaining diagnostic sensitivity due to the diffuse nature of ILD [6]. However, nowadays most of these patients undergo HRCT before bronchoscopy, which allows BAL to be performed in more targeted areas that may yield more accurate cellular findings [5]. To retrieve a specimen, a sufficient volume of isotonic saline (usually 100–300 ml) has to be instilled [7]. Although BAL salvage <60% is considered not diagnostic in ILD, little is known about how to optimize technical aspects of the procedure, such as the type and magnitude of negative pressure to retrieve instilled fluid (the guidelines suggest that a negative suction pressure of less than 100 mm Hg should be used). However, the most important thing is to avoid airway collapse [8]. Therefore, to control the process and prevent unexpected bronchial closure, suction should be performed manually (see Fig. 30.1).

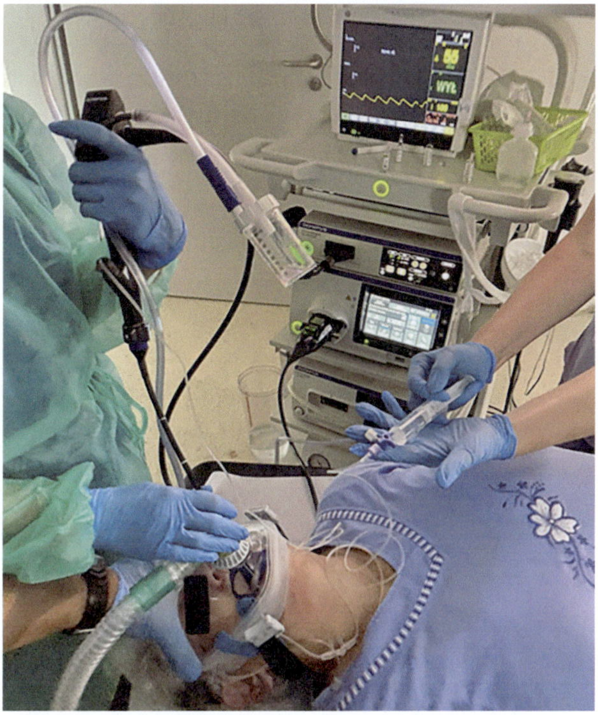

Fig. 30.1 Bronchoalveolar lavage (BAL) with administration of 0.9% NaCl and manual BAL suctioning during fiberoptic bronchoscopy. The procedure is assisted with noninvasive ventilation (NIV) with the use of a dedicated mask to increase BAL safety

30.2.1 Potential Factors Responsible for Decreased BAL Salvage

Predictors of poor BAL recovery are still missing. It is suspected that emphysema is the leading cause of insufficient BAL salvage. Other reasons for inadequate recovery may include sex, age, disease state, hemodynamic instability, bronchial collapse, the bronchus used for the procedure, coughing during the procedure, and pulmonary function [9, 10].

30.2.2 Diagnostic Value of BAL

The clinical utility of BAL analyses is particularly valuable in narrowing the differential diagnoses of ILD at the early stages of the disease when there is still no specific pattern in HRCT imaging [5]. BAL alone is a sensitive method to establish the diagnosis of respiratory infections caused by bacteria, mycobacteria, viruses, and other opportunistic infections of the lung in immunocompromised patients [11]. When it comes to diagnosing infectious diseases, the mini-BAL test, performed relatively often in intensive care units (ICUs), is also worth mentioning. A sterile, single-lumen, closed, telescoping catheter inserted through a tracheal tube is utilized for mini-BAL. The volume of inserted saline solution ranges from 20 to 150 ml, with 20 ml being the most commonly used amount. This volume is primarily for sampling the bronchial space and is not sufficient for alveolar sampling [12]. In general, increasing administered volume facilitates improved salvage but increases the risk of hypoxemia. As it is less invasive and less costly than BAL, it may be considered as an alternative diagnostic tool to bronchoscopic methods of respiratory sampling [13]. Cytological analysis may also allow to detect malignancies with an ambiguous picture in imaging studies [14]. In COPD, bronchoscopy with BAL is of particular importance in research on the pathomechanisms of the disease as well as on pharmacotherapy.

30.2.3 Contraindications for the Procedure

The American Thoracic Society stated that FOB should be avoided in hypoxemic patients with arterial partial pressure of oxygen <75 mmHg or blood saturation < 90% with supplemental oxygen [15]. It is especially important when FOB is performed with the BAL, as it prolongs the procedure and, more importantly, causes temporary local atelectasis and pulmonary shunt, which may result in respiratory failure exacerbation [16]. As severe hypoxemia is considered a contraindication for FOB and BAL, diseases characterized by rapidly progressing dyspnea remain a diagnostic challenge. Acute interstitial pneumonia (AIP) is one such disease entity. It is a rare, often fatal, idiopathic lung disease leading to respiratory failure occurring in patients without preexisting lung disease. Unlike in other interstitial diseases, the patient's condition deteriorates significantly over the course of days. For this reason, prompt differential diagnosis and initiation of treatment are crucial. Performing BAL in these patients allows to exclude an infectious cause of the disease, collagen vascular disorders, and capillaritis. Even though the diagnosis of AIP is made on the basis of the characteristic histological findings, the neutrophil predominance with occasional evidence of hemorrhage related to diffuse alveolar damage in the cytological analysis of the material obtained during BAL may suggest the diagnosis of this entity [17].

30.3 Noninvasive Ventilation

Noninvasive ventilation (NIV) refers to the administration of ventilatory support without the use of an invasive endotracheal airway. Air, usually with additional oxygen, is delivered via a face mask under positive pressure, which may decrease the need for endotracheal intubation (ETI) [18].

30.3.1 Indications

NIV is commonly used in emergency, ICU, and pulmonary and internal medicine wards for numerous indications [19]. The latest American Thoracic Society/European Respiratory Society guidelines from 2020 emphasize the role of NIV in the context of treatment of acute respiratory failure, especially in acute-on-chronic respiratory acidosis secondary to COPD exacerbation where pH $\leq$ 7.35, in cardiogenic pulmonary edema and as a prevention of ETI and mechanical ventilation [20]. NIV may also be beneficial in the treatment of various chronic respiratory diseases such as COPD with stable chronic hypercapnia, obesity hypoventilation syndrome, and sleep-related breathing disorders including obstructive sleep apnea. This method remains the gold standard treatment for chronic respiratory failure secondary to neuromuscular disorders, too.

30.3.2 NIV-Assisted FOB

NIV allows safe FOB in both diagnostic and therapeutic indications in patients with exacerbation of respiratory failure as well as in patients with severe chronic respiratory failure [4]. For the performance of bronchoscopy during NIV, it is essential to utilize an appropriate oronasal or full-face mask equipped with a dedicated port for the insertion of a bronchofiberscope. This mask should be snugly fitted to the patient's face and secured using Velcro straps covering the patient's head. In patients with severe hypoxemia, NIV is probably superior to conventional oxygen supplementation in preventing gas-exchange deterioration during FOB with better hemodynamic tolerance [21], but this has yet to be confirmed in prospective randomized controlled trials. FOB may also be performed in patients ventilated via ventilation Helmets. Hypoxemic patients, even in the ICU, can safely undergo diagnostic and therapeutic bronchoscopy with NIV support, mostly avoiding intubation and with low complication rates [22, 23]. According to numerous publications, NIV prevents the collapsing of the peripheral airways, reduces the risk of developing atelectasis, facilitates alveoli recruitment, increases vital capacity and lung susceptibility, and helps compensate for resistance and extra work of breathing created by the bronchoscope during the procedure [18, 20, 24, 25]. This is especially important when the FOB is performed with the BAL, as it makes the procedure longer and is at greater risk of secondary hypoxemia. To prevent desaturation, NICE guidelines suggest continuous positive airway pressure (CPAP) with oxygen support in patients with hypoxia undergoing bronchoscopy to prevent desaturation. However, there is still a lack of clear recommendations for NIV use in high-risk patients during FOB, with the description of qualification criteria and risk of complications [26]. Unfortunately, the studies conducted so far concerned small groups of patients, and there is an urgent need for prospective multicenter studies to define procedure-related risk, indications, contraindications, and NIV setting modalities to optimize the test conditions.

Proposition of NIV and/or CPAP settings for BAL performance are precisely described in the literature, but this still requires prospective verification [27, 28]. Based on our unpublished observations and a literature review, we may speculate that positive airway pressure devices like CPAP or NIV not only improve the safety of the procedure by preventing hypoxemia during FOB [22, 29–31] but also may increase BAL salvage volume in some patients [32]. We have experience of performing selective therapeutic lung lavage with NIV support in a patient with pulmonary alveolar proteinosis who did not consent to standard whole lung lavage treatment. The described method was a safe, effective, and resource-saving treatment option. Moreover, thanks to the application of positive end-expiratory pressure, which stabilized the alveolar space and decreased the risk of hypoxemia, the amount of recovered saline increased. Therefore, to obtain more reliable data on that topic, a prospective international multicenter randomized trial is underway (NCT05631132). It was designed to evaluate whether NIV or CPAP devices used during the FOB can increase the BAL salvage, improve its diagnostic value, and guarantee the safety of this procedure in groups of patients diagnosed with chronic obstructive pulmonary disease and ILD.

30.3.2.1 Case Study—FOB-NIV in Clinical Practice

Patients with chronic respiratory failure demand high diagnostic caution as the underlying lung disease may lead to the exhaustion of the patient's respiratory reserves and rapid clinical deterioration. In the days immediately preceding the preparation of this chapter, a patient from Ukraine came to our pulmonology department due to decompensation of chronic respiratory failure. Patient with a long-term history of lung disease, qualified for lung transplantation, without a specific diagnosis prior to our evaluation without prior pulmonologist input. Until the day of admission to the department, only steroid therapy has been used. According to the patient's history, the dyspnea has increased in recent weeks. On admission, hypoxemic respiratory failure with a PaO_2 of 55 mmHg and a PaO_2/FiO_2 ratio of 262 mmHg was observed in blood gas analysis without supplemental oxygen. High-resolution computed tomography (HRCT) of the lungs was ordered to assess the radiological pattern and the severity of the disease. During the transport to the computed tomography laboratory, the patient's clinical condition deteriorated, with a drop in oxygen saturation measured with a transcutaneous pulse oximeter to 60%. After a few minutes of passive oxygen therapy through a nasal cannula clinical condition was stabilized with an increase in oxygen saturation to normal levels ($SpO_2 = 96\%$). A biological test carried out under controlled conditions in the ward confirmed very poor pulmonary reserve in this patient. To prevent another decompensation, the HRCT imaging was performed with a high-flow nasal cannula oxygen supply system with good tolerance. The study revealed extensive ground-glass opacification superimposed on fixed interstitial changes of the type of fibrotic mesh. (See Fig. 30.2).

In order to optimize treatment and exclude an infectious disease background, FOB was performed with the collection of samples for tests, which excluded the presence of pathogens in the respiratory tract. To extend the diagnostics towards interstitial lung diseases, the decision to perform BAL was made. Due to the high risk of exacerbation of respiratory failure, it was decided to conduct an exam on NIV. No significant periprocedural complications were observed. The BAL recovery was diagnostic (133 ml/200 ml; >60%). In the following days, we were informed that a tissue-compatible donor was available, and the patient underwent a lung transplant.

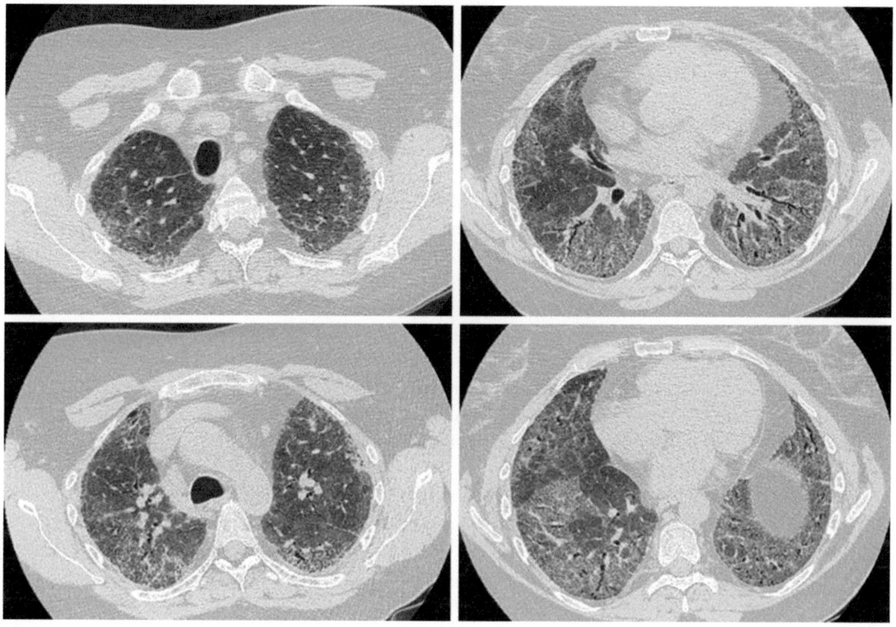

Fig. 30.2 HRCT of the lung, axial planes made at different heights. Extensive ground-glass opacification superimposed on reticular abnormalities

30.4 Summary

- Sufficient bronchoalveolar lavage is a valuable diagnostic tool for differentiating lung diseases; however, it may lead to complications such as hypoxemia.
- Noninvasive ventilation increases the safety of bronchoscopy and its accompanying procedures, such as bronchoalveolar lavage.
- Positive airway pressure devices like NIV and/or CPAP may improve sample salvage volume and diagnostic accuracy in certain patients.

References

1. Miller RJ, Casal RF, Lazarus DR, Ost DE, Eapen GA. Flexible bronchoscopy. Clin Chest Med. 2018;39(1):1–16.
2. Naidich D, Lee J, Garay S, McCauley D, Aranda C, Boyd A. Comparison of CT and fiberoptic bronchoscopy in the evaluation of bronchial disease. Am J Roentgenol. 1987;148(1):1–7.
3. Facciolongo N, Patelli M, Gasparini S, Lazzari Agli L, Salio M, Simonassi C, et al. Incidence of complications in bronchoscopy. Multicentre prospective study of 20,986 bronchoscopies. Monaldi Arch Chest Dis [Internet]. 2016. [cited 2024 Aug 31];71(1):8.
4. Esquinas A, Zuil M, Scala R, Chiner E. Broncoscopia durante la ventilación mecánica no invasiva: revisión de técnicas y procedimientos. Arch Bronconeumol. 2013;49(3):105–12.

5. Davidson KR, Ha DM, Schwarz MI, Chan ED. Bronchoalveolar lavage as a diagnostic procedure: a review of known cellular and molecular findings in various lung diseases. J Thorac Dis. 2020;12(9):4991–5019.
6. Baughman R. Technical aspects of Bronchoalveolar lavage: recommendations for a standard procedure. Semin Respir Crit Care Med. 2007;28(5):475–85.
7. Klech H. Technical recommendations and guidelines for bronchoalveolar lavage (BAL). Report of the European Society of Pneumology Task Group. Eur Respir J. 1989;2(6):561–85.
8. Meyer KC, Raghu G, Baughman RP, Brown KK, Costabel U, du Bois RM, et al. An official American Thoracic Society clinical practice guideline: the clinical utility of bronchoalveolar lavage cellular analysis in interstitial lung disease. Am J Respir Crit Care Med. 2012;185(9):1004–14.
9. Skoczyński S, Tobiczyk E, Minarowski Ł, Świerczyńska M, Mróz R, Barczyk A. Is it possible to predict whether BAL salvage is going to be diagnostic? Adv Resp Med. 2019;87(1):20–5.
10. Shikano K, Abe M, Shiko Y, Tsushima K, Yoshioka K, Ishiwata T, et al. What are the factors affecting the recovery rate of bronchoalveolar lavage fluid? Clin Resp J. 2022 Feb;16(2):142–51.
11. Rust M, Albera C, Carratu L, Danel C, lsraei-Biet D, Klech H, Rennard Sl, Robalo-Cordeiro AJA, Semenzato G, Velluti G, Worth H. The clinical use of BAL in patients with pulmonary infections. ERJ. 1990;3:954–61.
12. Erden V, Basaranoglu G, Beycan I, Delatioğlu H, Hamzaoglu NS. Reproducibility of mini-BAL culture results using 10 ml or 20 ml instilled fluid. Intensive Care Med. 2003;29(10):1856.
13. Tasbakan MS, Gurgun A, Basoglu OK, Ekren PK, Pullukcu H, Bacakoglu F. Comparison of Bronchoalveolar lavage and mini-Bronchoalveolar lavage in the diagnosis of pneumonia in immunocompromised patients. Respiration. 2011;81(3):229–35.
14. Poletti V, Chilosi M, Olivieri D. Diagnostic invasive procedures in diffuse infiltrative lung diseases. Respiration. 2004;71(2):107–19.
15. Goldstein RA, Rohatgi PK, Bergofsky EH, Block ER, Daniele RP, Dantzker DR, Davis GS, Hunninghake GW, King TE Jr, Metzger WJ, et al. Clinical role of Bronchoalveolar lavage in adults with pulmonary disease. Am Rev Respir Dis. 1990 Aug;142(2):481–6.
16. Pirozyński M, Sliwiński P, Zieliński J. Effect of different volumes of BAL fluid on arterial oxygen saturation. Eur Respir J. 1988 Dec;1(10):943–7.
17. Bonaccorsi A, Cancellieri A, Chilosi M, Trisolini R, Boaron M, Crimi N, et al. Acute interstitial pneumonia: report of a series. Eur Respir J. 2003 Jan;21(1):187–91.
18. Gupta S, Ramasubban S, Dixit S, Mishra R, Zirpe KG, Khilnani GC, et al. ISCCM guidelines for the use of non-invasive ventilation in acute respiratory failure in adult ICUs. Indian J Crit Care Med. 2020;24(S1):S61–81.
19. Elliott M, Nava S, Schonhofer B, editors. Non-invasive ventilation and weaning: principles and practice [Internet]. 0th ed. CRC Press; 2010. [cited 2024 Aug 31]
20. Rochwerg B, Brochard L, Elliott MW, Hess D, Hill NS, Nava S, et al. Official ERS/ATS clinical practice guidelines: noninvasive ventilation for acute respiratory failure. Eur Respir J. 2017 Aug;50(2):1602426.
21. Nong L, Liang W, Yu Y, Xi Y, Liu D, Zhang J, et al. Noninvasive ventilation support during fiberoptic bronchoscopy-guided nasotracheal intubation effectively prevents severe hypoxemia. J Crit Care. 2020 Apr;56:12–7.
22. Korkmaz Ekren P, Basarik Aydogan B, Gurgun A, Tasbakan MS, Bacakoglu F, Nava S. Can fiberoptic bronchoscopy be applied to critically ill patients treated with noninvasive ventilation for acute respiratory distress syndrome? Prospective observational study. BMC Pulm Med. 2016 Dec;16(1):89.
23. Agarwal R, Khan A, Aggarwal AN, Gupta D. Bronchoscopic lung biopsy using noninvasive Ventilatory support: case series and review of literature of NIV-assisted bronchoscopy. Respir Care. 2012 Nov;57(11):1927–36.
24. Lee P, Mathur PN. Safe to sedate for bronchoscopy despite respiratory failure. Respiration. 2010;79(4):276.

25. Alsous F, Amoateng-Adjepong Y, Manthous CA. Noninvasive ventilation: experience at a community teaching hospital. Intensive Care Med. 1999;25(5):458–63.
26. Du Rand IA, Blaikley J, Booton R, Chaudhuri N, Gupta V, Khalid S, et al. British Thoracic Society guideline for diagnostic flexible bronchoscopy in adults: accredited by NICE. Thorax. 2013 Aug;68(Suppl 1):i1–44.
27. Danel A, Tobiczyk E, Warcholiński A, Trzaska-Sobczak M, Swinarew A, Brożek G, et al. May noninvasive mechanical ventilation and/or continuous positive airway pressure increase the bronchoalveolar lavage salvage in patients with pulmonary diseases? Randomized clinical trial – study protocol. Adv Med Sci. 2023 Sep;68(2):482–90.
28. Oraczewska A, Cofta S, Warcholiński A, Trejnowska E, Brożek G, Swinarew A, et al. The use of non-invasive respiratory assistance to facilitate bronchofiberoscopy performance in patients with hypoxemic (type one) respiratory failure – study protocol. Adv Med Sci. 2023 Sep;68(2):474–81.
29. Skoczyński S, Minarowski Ł, Tobiczyk E, Oraczewska A, Glinka K, Ficek K, et al. Noninvasive ventilation-facilitated bronchofiberoscopy in patients with respiratory failure. In: Pokorski M, editor. Advances in pulmonary medicine: research and innovations [Internet]. Cham: Springer International Publishing; 2019. p. 53–64. [cited 2024 Aug 31] (Advances in Experimental Medicine and Biology; vol. 1160).
30. Skoczyński S, Ogonowski M, Tobiczyk E, Krzyżak D, Brożek G, Wierzbicka A, et al. Risk factors of complications during noninvasive mechanical ventilation -assisted flexible bronchoscopy. Adv Med Sci. 2021 Sep;66(2):246–53.
31. Scala R, Guidelli L. Clinical value of bronchoscopy in acute respiratory failure. Diagnostics. 2021;11(10):1755.
32. Skoczynski S, Wyskida K, Rzepka-Wrona P, Wyskida M, Uszok-Gawel E, Bartocha D, et al. Novel method of noninvasive ventilation supported therapeutic lavage in pulmonary alveolar proteinosis proves to relieve dyspnea, normalize pulmonary function test results and recover exercise capacity: a short communication. J Thorac Dis. 2018 Apr;10(4):2467–73.

31 Noninvasive Ventilation-Assisted Diagnostic and Therapeutic Procedures by Conventional and Interventional Flexible Bronchoscopy

Semra Bilaceroglu

Noninvasive ventilation (NIV) is generally used in the management of exacerbations of chronic obstructive pulmonary disease (COPD) as well as in the treatment of obstructive sleep apnea, obesity hypoventilation syndrome, and chronic respiratory failure in neuromuscular disease. NIV is any form of ventilatory support applied without endotracheal intubation and generally includes continuous positive airway pressure (CPAP) or bi-level positive airway pressure (BiPAP), besides other modes. Applied through a nasal or face mask, NIV can be used for improving postoperative hypoxemia, reducing pulmonary complications after thoracic, cardiac, or upper-abdominal surgery, facilitating weaning in intubated COPD patients, and reducing intubation rate in acute cardiogenic pulmonary edema and hypoxic respiratory failure in immunocompromised patients. The main purpose of using NIV during bronchoscopy in high-risk patients is to avoid intubation. Another indication is symptomatic expiratory central airway collapse, which can benefit from NIV [1–7].

Temporary alterations in gas exchange, hemodynamics, and lung mechanics secondary to the decrease in airway size can occur during bronchoscopy. Several studies and systematic reviews suggest that NIV during bronchoscopy can facilitate the diagnostic and therapeutic procedures by improving gas exchange in a hypoxemic patient [1, 6, 8–10].

In hypoxemic patients, options for managing diagnostic or therapeutic interventions have usually been intubation and bronchoscopy during invasive mechanical ventilation, surgical lung biopsy, or empirical treatment. Intubation and invasive

(I give my authorization for publishing my private e-mail address in the book.)

S. Bilaceroglu (✉)
University of Health Sciences-Turkiye, Izmir Faculty of Medicine, Izmir Dr. Suat Seren Training and Research Hospital for Thoracic Medicine and Surgery, Izmir, Turkiye

© The Author(s), under exclusive license to Springer Nature Switzerland AG 2025

K. Panda et al. (eds.), *Noninvasive Ventilatory Approaches in Interventional Procedures*, Noninvasive Ventilation. The Essentials,
https://doi.org/10.1007/978-3-032-05328-2_31

mechanical ventilation may lead to severe complications. Surgical lung biopsy, although with high sensitivity and specificity, cannot be performed in most of the critical cases. An empirical treatment can have potential toxicities, excessive costs, and the risk of not treating a reversible disease. Thus, alternative strategies, such as NIV, are needed in these critical cases [3, 5, 7–9].

This chapter focuses on the indications, contraindications, technique and complications of NIV-facilitated bronchoscopy, related risk factors and predictors of failure, and diagnostic and therapeutic procedures performed during conventional and interventional flexible bronchoscopy on NIV.

31.1 NIV During Bronchoscopy—Indications

31.1.1 Refractory Hypoxemia

In respiratory disorders, bronchoscopy can be difficult and risky. Flexible bronchoscopy can cause respiratory and cardiac complications by occupying 10–15% of the normal tracheal lumen, increasing the work of breathing, and decreasing partial arterial oxygen pressure (PaO_2) by 10–20 mm Hg. Hypoxemia starts when the bronchoscope is inserted into the trachea, and worsens after the instillation of local anesthetics and saline into the lower airways. Arterial oxygen saturation (SaO_2) can be reduced further by bronchoalveolar lavage (BAL). Additionally, suction during bronchoscopy causes alveolar closure by reducing end-expiratory volume and positive end-expiratory pressure [1, 11, 12].

Cardiac arrhythmias can be caused by hypoxemia during flexible bronchoscopies in 11–40% of cases; however, in most cases, they are not clinically significant. According to the international guidelines, bronchoscopy and BAL should be avoided if PaO_2 cannot be raised to ≥75 mmHg or SaO_2 to >90% while receiving oxygen treatment [1, 13]. Avoiding bronchoscopy and giving empirical treatment, or intubating and applying mechanical ventilation during bronchoscopy, are the alternative approaches in such high-risk patients with hypoxemia. Severe complications can be caused by endotracheal intubation and mechanical ventilation, whereas NIV can be an acceptable alternative in many cases, particularly those with immunosuppression or severe pneumonia [14–16]. However, in cases of respiratory distress within 48 h of extubation, NIV does not lower the reintubation rate, in-hospital mortality, and length of stay in the intensive care unit or hospital, and it can increase mortality due to cardiac ischemia, fatigue of respiratory muscles, pneumonia due to aspiration, and complications of reintubation [17, 18].

In comparison to high-flow oxygen alone, NIV can improve oxygenation during bronchoscopy in high-risk patients with severe hypoxemia. In these high-risk patients, NIV or intubation should be applied instead of oxygen therapy alone in any case, even if bronchoscopy is not required [1, 19, 20]. Currently, there are no published studies directly comparing NIV with intubation during bronchoscopy in large patient populations with hypoxemia. NIV has been suggested as a safe and effective alternative during bronchoscopy in hypoxemic patients with immunosuppression by only small and underpowered studies showing no clear outcome benefit regarding the clinical relevance of oxygenation improvement [21].

31.1.2 Sleep-Related Respiratory Disorders

Bronchoscopy leads to hypoxemia by causing ventilation-perfusion mismatch as a result of obstruction by the bronchoscope, suction, instillation of lavage fluid into the alveoli, and provocation of latent obstructive sleep apnea by sedation [22]. Furthermore, in cases with obesity-hypoventilation syndrome, the risk of hypoxemia is higher as they also have high partial arterial carbon dioxide pressures ($PaCO_2$) [23].

In obstructive sleep apnea, mechanical ventilation improves hypoxemia by reversing the negative inspiratory forces. The pressure applied to the oropharynx via NIV compensates for the hypotonicity of the muscles in the upper airway. CPAP during bronchoscopy has been shown to be effective in expanding the collapsed pharyngeal airway [24, 25].

During the intubation of obese patients, nasal CPAP applied with a nasal pillow through one nostril has been shown to be beneficial in ventilation in some cases by keeping the airway open and thus, improving the visualization of anatomic landmarks and passage of the bronchoscope through the larynx. Airway protection with endotracheal intubation is usually necessary during fiberoptic intubation for the most difficult airways. However, in some cases, CPAP may provide sufficient ventilation and may be better than a laryngeal mask airway, but it may cause gastric insufflation [26].

31.1.3 Pediatric Patients

As the airways of young children are narrower and more collapsible, during bronchoscopy, they have a higher risk for hypoxemia and hypercapnia. Furthermore, flexible bronchoscopy increases airway resistance and reduces tidal volume and peak tidal inspiratory and expiratory flows in this group of pediatric patients. CPAP, when used during bronchoscopy, reverses these effects by widening the laryngeal opening and preventing collapse of the lateral pharyngeal walls. Consequently, tidal volumes and flows are maintained within normal limits in young children [27–29].

31.1.4 Postoperative Respiratory Distress

After a thoracic or abdominal surgery, intubation and mechanical ventilation may be required for the respiratory distress caused by mucus plugging. However, complications such as lung injury, poor surgical outcome, and prolonged hospital stay can result from invasive mechanical ventilation. In hypoxemia despite maximum supplemental oxygen on spontaneous breathing, flexible bronchoscopy on NIV improves ventilation and oxygen exchange by providing safe and successful removal of the mucus plugs from the airways without the need for intubation [1, 30].

31.1.5 Chronic Obstructive Pulmonary Disease

In severe emphysema, bronchoscopy causes air trapping and thus increases functional residual capacity (FRC) by 17% when the scope is inserted transnasally. Intrinsic positive end-expiratory pressure in these cases can be reversed by positive-pressure ventilation. NIV can also be useful during bronchoscopy in COPD cases with hypercapnia and pneumonia [1, 31].

31.1.6 Expiratory Collapse of Central Airways

In expiratory collapse of central airways, NIV can be used as an alternative for conservative treatment. NIV can be beneficial in maintaining airway patency, facilitating drainage of secretions, and improving expiratory flow. Improvements in spirometric values, sputum production, atelectasis, and exercise tolerance by nasal CPAP have been shown in small studies [32–35]. Increased transmural pressure in the central airways (pneumatic stenting) as a result of the increased intraluminal pressure by NIV and consequent increase in the luminal area of the airway is the most probable therapeutic mechanism although alternative mechanisms have been proposed [33, 36].

As NIV is shown to reverse central airway collapse regardless of the mechanism of action, it can be utilized in these cases during bronchoscopy to maintain patency of the airways by titrating the pressure to limit airway collapse to a level < 50% during exhalation. However, prospective studies are required to confirm the improvements by NIV objectively regarding dyspnea, functional status, and severity of airway collapse, as the pertinent data is still limited currently [1].

31.2 NIV During Bronchoscopy—Contraindications

The contraindications of NIV during bronchoscopy are the same as in other applications of NIV: high aspiration risk, inability to protect the airway (e.g., indications for emergency intubation), psychomotor agitation, respiratory failure due to status asthmaticus or neurologic disease, facial deformities, and recent surgery in the mouth, esophagus, or stomach. Refractory hypoxemia with $SaO_2 \leq 85\%$ despite optimal oxygen therapy with a high fraction of inspired oxygen (FiO_2), secretions difficult to clear, acidosis, or mental changes are other significant contraindications to bronchoscopy on NIV. In all cases having contraindications to NIV, endotracheal intubation should be considered [1, 18, 37].

31.3 NIV During Bronchoscopy—Technique

Usually, a full-face mask connected to the ventilator is secured to the patient's face with straps. The bronchoscope is advanced through the dual-axis swivel adaptor on the mask and then inserted through the mouth or nares (Figs. 31.1, and 31.2). For facilitating advancement of the bronchoscope through the swivel adaptor, silicone or jelly lubricant is used. The tight disposable cap on the adaptor prevents air leaks. Bronchoscopy is performed in a standard fashion by continuously monitoring with electrocardiography and pulse oximetry. Lidocaine 1% is used at a dose of ≤300 mg for topical anesthesia of the larynx. Complete airway examination is performed by advancing the bronchoscope through the trachea and more distal airways. For the decision of using NIV-facilitated bronchoscopy, $PaO_2/FiO_2 < 300$ mmHg or oxygen saturation of ≤92% despite FiO_2 of 1.0 on spontaneous breathing has been used as a definition of severe hypoxemia, provided that oxygen saturation can be improved by NIV before bronchoscopy. BAL is performed by wedging the tip of the bronchoscope in the pertinent bronchial segment and then instilling and retrieving 3–5 30-mL aliquots of physiologic saline [1, 16, 20, 21].

Clinical indications determine the settings for NIV. For refractory hypoxemia or hypercarbia in COPD, a 5-cm H_2O setting for CPAP and a 15–17-cm H_2O setting for pressure-support ventilation are suitable. FiO_2 maintained at 1.0 during bronchoscopy is reduced to the pre-bronchoscopy level if the SaO_2 can be kept at a level > 92%. In a severely hypoxemic patient, positive-pressure ventilation should be maintained for ≥30 min after a bronchoscopy performed on NIV. NIV can be discontinued after this watchful period, provided that SaO_2 remains >92% and there is no evidence of respiratory distress [1].

When required, bronchoscopy can be performed in the upright or supine position and on or off NIV to check the response of airway narrowing to CPAP. Generally, CPAP at a level of 7–10 cm H_2O can provide sufficient airway patency in excessive dynamic airway collapse or tracheobronchomalacia although this has not been confirmed yet by large studies [32, 35]. During exhalation, to reach an airway caliber that is ≥50% of that during inspiration, the pressure can be increased by 3-cm H_2O increments in patients with various degrees of expiratory central airway collapse. The optimal CPAP setting that will maintain airway patency has not been studied

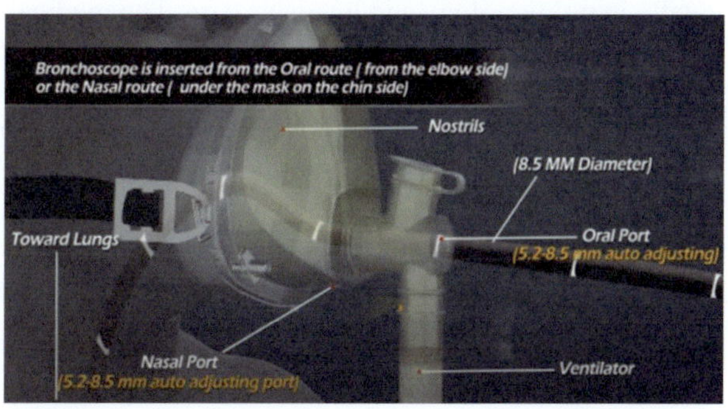

Fig. 31.1 The flexible bronchoscope is inserted through the oral port of an oronasal noninvasive ventilation mask. The nasal port is under the mask on the chin side

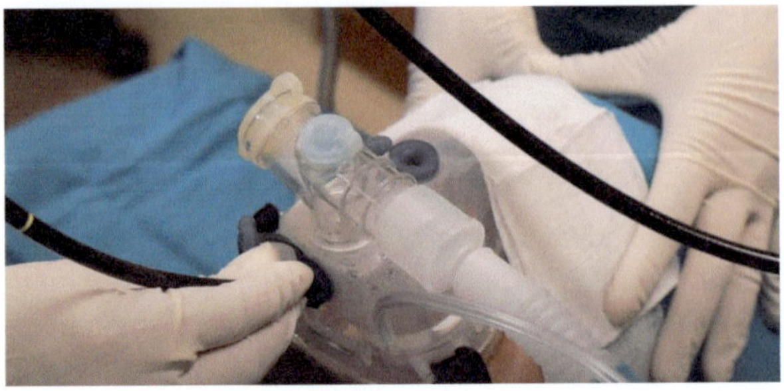

Fig. 31.2 The flexible bronchoscope is inserted through the nasal port under the mask on the chin side in a patient on noninvasive ventilation

systematically. When the collapse of central airways occurs, it should be documented with a photograph and/or video in the upright and supine position and on and off CPAP to assess the airway narrowing and its response to CPAP [1].

NIV-facilitated bronchoscopy can be performed through a NIV helmet by applying 10–20 cm H_2O pressure support, 8–15 cm H_2O positive end-expiratory pressure, and lowest FiO_2 for $SaO_2 \geq 92\%$, or through an oronasal, full-face or modified total full-face mask with a synthetic plastic cylinder in it allowing insertion of bronchoscope through the mouth or nose but not interfering with the ventilator circuit. The disposable cap from a swivel adaptor seals the cylinder and prevents air leak [16, 37]. If a nasal mask is used, the bronchoscope is inserted orally through a bite block while the patient is ventilated nasally.

31.4 NIV During Bronchoscopy—Complications, Risk Factors, and Predictors of Failure

NIV can be continued during bronchoscopy in patients already requiring NIV prior to bronchoscopy [2, 7], but it can also be initiated primarily to facilitate bronchoscopy [16, 19–21, 31].

In a critically ill patient, the challenge is not the bronchoscopic procedure per se but the complexity of the case. The critically ill patient on NIV has an increased risk of hemodynamic instability, bleeding, air trapping, and pneumothorax. It is not simply inserting the bronchoscope and performing the diagnostic or therapeutic procedure. Thus, a bronchoscopic study should be supervised in person by an expert, ideally in pulmonology and intensive care. The medical team should be fully knowledgeable about the potential pathophysiological changes due to bronchoscopy in a critically ill patient on NIV: increase in airway resistance, functional residual capacity, peak inspiratory pressure, positive end-expiratory pressure (PEEP) and alveolar collapse, decrease in tidal volume, dynamic/static lung compliance, and gas exchange besides the accompanying cardiovascular effects [38–40].

Having a robust indication and no contraindications, preparing everything necessary before bronchoscopy with a definite idea of what should be done, trained personnel, appropriate lighting conditions, and good wall suction are ideal [38]. The risk factors and predictors of failure and complications during NIV-assisted flexible bronchoscopy are poor nutritional status, lower Glasgow Coma Scale <11–13, more severe physiologic derangement, high severity-of-illness scores (APACHE II score $\geq$ 29, SAPS II $\geq$35), lower PaO_2, SaO_2 and/or pH (<7.25), higher $PaCO_2$ or white blood cell count, higher respiratory rate ($\geq$35), $PaO_2/FiO_2 \leq 146$ (175 for adult respiratory distress syndrome-ARDS) after 1 h of NIV, excessive secretions, deterioration during bronchoscopy, poor patient-ventilator interaction, excessive mask leak, left heart disease (ischemic heart disease or heart failure), pneumonia, and ARDS (Table 31.1) [38, 41–43].

It may be required to stop the bronchoscopy for several minutes as clinically significant hypoxemia may occur with some frequency. Close monitoring and making adjustments as needed on the noninvasive mechanical ventilator is critical during these periods when the scope is out of the airway. The period of risk for the patient can extend beyond the procedure, mainly owing to gas exchange and compliance alterations. Thus, close monitoring should continue post-bronchoscopy and should be long enough to ensure the stability of the patient, without overlooking recovery to preprocedure PEEP level [38, 42].

Table 31.1 The risk factors and predictors of failure and complications during and after NIV-assisted flexible bronchoscopy [41–43]

Lower PaO_2 ($\leq$49 mmHg)
Lower SaO_2 ($\leq$83%)
$PaO_2/FiO_2 \leq 146$ (175 for ARDS) after 1 h of NIV
Higher $PaCO_2$ ($\geq$55 mmHg)
Lower pH ($\leq$7.25)
Higher WBC ($\geq$14,400/mm^3)
Lower Glasgow coma scale ($\leq$11–13)
Higher APACHE II score ($\geq$29)
Higher SAPS II score ($\geq$35)
Higher respiratory rate ($\geq$35/min)
Excessive secretions
Excessive mask leak
Poor patient-ventilator interaction
Poor nutritional status
Pneumonia
ARDS
Left heart disease (ischemic heart disease, heart failure, condition post MI)

PaO_2, partial arterial oxygen pressure, *SaO_2* arterial oxygen saturation; *PaO_2/FiO_2* partial arterial oxygen pressure/fraction of inspired oxygen, *ARDS* adult respiratory distress syndrome, *NIV* noninvasive ventilation, *$PaCO_2$* partial arterial carbondioxide pressure, *pH* acidity or basicity, *WBC* white blood cell count, *APACHE* Acute Physiology and Chronic Health Evaluation, *SAPS* Simplified Acute Physiology Score, *MI* myocardial infarction

31.5 NIV During Conventional Bronchoscopy

The articles on NIV-assisted diagnostic and therapeutic procedures performed mostly by flexible bronchoscopy have increased in the last two decades; however, the number of high-quality and large studies with prospective, controlled, randomized, and/or multicentric design is still limited in this field.

Although bronchial washing and BAL were the only procedures performed during NIV-assisted flexible bronchoscopy in most of the previous case reports, case series, and studies [16, 19, 37, 44–46], over the last decade, there has been an increasing number of articles on NIV-assisted bronchoscopic procedures such as endobronchial biopsy (EBB), brushing and/or transbronchial biopsy (TBB), and bronchial washing and/or BAL (Table 31.2) [47–49].

Nasal [44, 47], oronasal [44, 48, 49], full-face [19, 44, 46, 49] or modified full face mask [37], or helmet [16] have been used to perform diagnostic or therapeutic procedures during conventional bronchoscopy.

The duration of NIV-assisted bronchoscopy should be kept as short as possible: 8–14 min [2, 16, 19, 44]. Intubation may be required in 8–10% of the patients within the 24 h after NIV-assisted bronchoscopy [2, 16, 37, 44–47].

Table 31.2 Diagnostic and therapeutic procedures performed by conventional and interventional bronchoscopy assisted by noninvasive ventilation

Diagnostic bronchoscopic procedures
Bronchial washing/aspiration
Bronchoalveolar lavage
Brushing
Endobronchial biopsy
Transbronchial biopsy
Endobronchial ultrasound-guided transbronchial needle aspiration
Therapeutic bronchoscopic procedures
Bronchial washing/aspiration
Bronchoalveolar lavage
Foreign body removal
Baloon dilatation
Stenting
Percutaneous tracheostomy and tracheostomy tube placement
Flexible bronchoscopy-guided nasotracheal intubation
Argon plasma coagulation
Electrocautery
Laser therapy
Cryotherapy

31.5.1 Diagnostic Conventional Bronchoscopy

Bronchial washing/aspiration performed together with BAL, brushing, endobronchial biopsy, and/or transbronchial biopsy under NIV has been reported in some articles. This procedure is mainly used to determine the etiology of pulmonary infections [45, 47–49].

BAL under NIV has been shown to be feasible, safe, and efficient in determining the definitive etiologic diagnosis in community-acquired, nosocomial, or ventilator-associated pneumonias and in pneumonias in immunocompromised patients [16, 19, 37, 44–49]. Four to five 25-ml aliquots or three 50-ml aliquots of saline solution can be instilled, and about 45% (33–55%) can be retrieved as a BAL specimen. BAL has a diagnostic yield of 67–72% in patients with pneumonia and can lead to treatment changes in 34–80% of these patients [2, 19, 44, 47].

Brushing has also been performed under NIV, mainly for the diagnosis of pulmonary infections [6, 9, 44, 47, 49]. Particularly protected-specimen brush is used to obtain specimens for microbiologic examination in pulmonary infections [4, 47].

EBB under NIV support is reported to be safe and with diagnostic results [9, 44, 45, 47–49]. It has been used together with BAL, bronchial washing, brushing, and/or TBB in the diagnosis of mainly pulmonary infections [9, 45] and malignancy [47, 48].

TBB has been more frequently utilized in recent years. It has a higher risk of complications (pneumothorax, bleeding) than bronchial washing, BAL, brushing, and EBB in patients undergoing bronchoscopy with NIV support [6, 8, 9, 44]. TBB has been performed mainly for diffuse lung infiltrates due to infection, malignancy, and interstitial lung disease [8, 9, 44]. It should be emphasized that NIV-assisted TBB has to be performed in centers with extensive experience in NIV and TBB. More research is required to clearly define the utility and safety of this approach.

31.5.2 Therapeutic Conventional Bronchoscopy

Bronchial washing/aspiration and/or BAL under NIV can also be used for therapeutic purposes to remove the secretions from the airways, most commonly for pneumonia and atelectasis in patients with ineffective cough [4, 6, 9, 42, 44–47, 49]. In spontaneously breathing Coronavirus Disease 2019 (COVID-19) patients with $SaO_2 < 92\%$ despite a FiO_2 of 100%, bronchial washing/aspiration or BAL has been performed effectively and safely under NIV for therapeutic purposes, mainly for clearing secretions and mucous plugs [50].

31.6 NIV during Interventional Bronchoscopy

Interventional diagnostic [5, 6, 51, 52] and therapeutic procedures [5, 7, 53–59] under NIV have been reported in a quite limited number of articles. These interventional bronchoscopic procedures facilitated by NIV include endobronchial ultrasound-guided transbronchial needle aspiration (EBUS-TBNA), foreign body removal, balloon dilatation, airway stenting, percutaneous tracheostomy and tracheostomy tube placement, fiberoptic bronchoscopy-guided nasotracheal intubation, argon plasma coagulation, electrocautery, laser therapy, and cryotherapy (Table 31.2).

31.6.1 Diagnostic Interventional Bronchoscopy

EBUS-TBNA is the only diagnostic interventional procedure reported to be performed under NIV support. Only case reports or case series constitute the pertinent literature [6, 51, 52].

Although the EBUS bronchoscope with a wider diameter than a conventional bronchoscope would be expected to have a more pronounced effect on lung mechanics and gas exchanges, NIV-assisted EBUS-TBNA has been successfully and safely performed under conscious or deep sedation in acute respiratory failure with $PaO_2/FiO_2 < 200$ mmHg [6].

Two reported cases of small cell lung cancer with wide mediastinal involvement and in acute respiratory failure [51] and one case of renal cell carcinoma with a 2-cm metastasis adjacent to the right upper lobe apical and anterior segmental bronchi and in chronic respiratory failure [52] have been safely diagnosed by EBUS-TBNA owing to the stable tidal volume and reduced work of breathing provided by NIV.

31.6.2 Therapeutic Interventional Bronchoscopy

Therapeutic interventional bronchoscopy performed with NIV support has been reported in a limited number of patients [6, 7, 46, 53–59].

Foreign body removal has been described in four pediatric cases of aspirated pen cap by using laser, guidewire, and balloon catheter guided by short-working-length flexible bronchoscopy with the support of a novel NIV technique (*nasopharyngeal oxygen with intermittent nose close and abdomen compression*) that was routinely applied for oxygenation, airway, and ventilation in the intensive care unit setting. After confirmation of the diagnosis and location of the aspirated pen cap, a balloon catheter, while being kept parallel to the bronchoscope, was passed through the hole of the aspirated pen cap. Pretreatment with a laser was also required before removal of the pen caps in two cases: for debulking the granulation tissue in one and for enlarging the size of the cap hole in the other. Guide wires were utilized in three cases to facilitate the procedure of passing the balloon catheter through the cap hole. Aspirated pen caps were successfully retrieved in the first attempts with no significant complications in all four cases [53].

In another case, a patient on home oxygen and NIV due to chronic obstructive pulmonary disease-related chronic respiratory failure had accidentally aspirated a pea into the left lower lobe bronchus. Removal of the pea by NIV-assisted flexible bronchoscopy under sedation with fentanyl and midazolam resulted in significant attenuation of dyspnea. During the foreign body removal, the same ventilator he used at home was used with a flexible bronchoscopy-dedicated mask. PEEP and pressure support were periodically adjusted during the procedure to prevent bronchoscopy-induced hypoxia and to maintain an adequate level of minute ventilation. There were no complications related to the procedure [7].

Balloon dilatation is another method performed during therapeutic interventional bronchoscopy assisted with NIV; however, balloon dilatation under NIV has been reported in retrospective studies in only a limited number of patients [6, 55, 57].

In a retrospective study evaluating the feasibility of therapeutic flexible bronchoscopy under moderate sedation and NIV in hypoxemic patients with central airway obstruction, balloon dilatation was performed with electrocautery, argon plasma coagulation, and/or cryotherapy in 5 out of 15 patients on NIV. The type of procedures, procedure time, success rate, the lowest SaO_2 during procedure, and improvement of PaO_2 were similar in the NIV and control (artificial airway-general anesthesia) groups. However, there was less reduction in systolic blood pressure and heart rate during the procedure, shorter admission time (35 h vs 55 h) before procedures, and lower procedural fees ($540 vs $975) in the NIV group than those in the 14-patient control group [55].

In another retrospective study in infants undergoing flexible endoscopy supported with a novel NIV technique (*pharyngeal oxygen with nose closure and abdominal compression without any mask or laryngeal mask airway*), 129 aero-esophageal tract lesions were determined in 38 infants. They were airway lesions in 83.3% (bronchial granulations, bronchomalacia, tracheomalacia) and esophageal lesions in 35.7%. There were no significant complications, but bradycardia or desaturation was reversible within 60 sec in 19%. The endoscopy findings led to changes in the management of all 38 infants. Of these, 18 received 37 therapeutic interventional procedures: balloon dilatations (14), laser treatment (13), and stenting (10). In 9 infants, 14 balloon dilatations were performed for stenosis in the larynx, trachea, and bronchi. Only 7 (16.7%) underwent surgeries [57].

Stenting is performed for significant central airway stenosis due to distortion, scar stricture, extrinsic compression, malacia, or excessive dynamic collapse of the airway wall [7, 57].

By using flexible bronchoscopy supported with a novel NIV technique (*pharyngeal oxygen with nose closure and abdominal compression without any mask or laryngeal mask airway*), stenting of central airways was performed for the management of severe tracheomalacia, carina malacia, and bronchomalacia in 6 of 38 infants with severe bronchopulmonary dysplasia [57]. In these infants, 10 stenting procedures (17%) were safely and successfully accomplished. In most of the studies on interventional therapeutic flexible bronchoscopy under NIV, stenting is excluded as it is much harder and riskier than the other therapeutic interventional procedures during NIV-assisted flexible bronchoscopy [55].

Percutaneous tracheostomy and tracheostomy tube placement can be performed by NIV-assisted flexible bronchoscopy [7, 42]. In a retrospective study on the risk and complications of NIV-assisted flexible bronchoscopy, percutaneous tracheostomy and tracheostomy tube placement were performed in 12 (24%) out of 50 patients, and complications occurred in 2 (16%) of 12 patients [42].

Fiberoptic bronchoscopy-guided nasotracheal intubation under continuous NIV support with 100% oxygen and by using a specially designed face mask has been reported in a single-center randomized study that compared NIV to bag-valve-mask ventilation for preoxygenation prior to intubation. The pulse SaO_2 after preoxygenation and minimum SaO_2 during intubation were significantly higher, and the severe hypoxemic events were less frequent in the NIV group [58].

Argon plasma coagulation is a heat treatment used to ablate small endobronchial tumors and granulation tissues, to make cuts in the web-like simple airway stenosis, and to stop visible endoluminal bleeding [6]. In a retrospective study on flexible bronchoscopy in conjunction with NIV in hypoxemic patients with central airway obstruction, argon plasma coagulation was utilized in 12 out of 15 patients in the NIV group and in 10 out of 14 patients in the artificial airway-general anesthesia group. The NIV group had less complications, shorter admission time, and lower procedure fee than the control group [55].

Electrocautery is another heat treatment used in the ablation of endobronchial tumors and granulation tissues, to make cuts in web-like simple airway stenosis and to stop endoluminal visible bleeding [6]. Electrocautery was performed in the palliation of central airway obstruction in 2 of 15 in the NIV group and in 3 of 14 in the artificial airway-general anesthesia group in the retrospective study mentioned in the previous paragraph. NIV support during flexible bronchoscopy guaranteed stable oxygenation, good patient tolerance, and minor complications in line with most of the studies on flexible bronchoscopy under NIV [55].

Laser therapy is applied for similar indications as electrocautery mentioned above [53, 54, 57]. In a retrospective study, infants with vallecular cyst coexisting with laryngomalacia were diagnosed and treated by laser therapy through flexible endoscopy with novel NIV of sustained pharyngeal inflation support. All infants (14 supported with bi-nasal prongs NIV and 4 with tracheal intubation before procedure) were supported with only a nasopharyngeal NIV during diagnostic and therapeutic bronchoscopy. A laser was used to treat 13 lesions in the same bronchoscopy session. The mean laser therapy time was 18.1 min (15.5–21.6 min), and the total bronchoscopy time lasted 24.6 min (19.7–28.6 min). Revision laser therapy was needed in three infants, 4 days later. No desaturation, bradycardia, or pneumothorax occurred. After flexible bronchoscopy with laser therapy, all infants were supported only with bi-nasal prongs NIV with considerably lower pressure and weaned off before discharge 8.4 days later. Six-month follow-up showed many clinical improvements [54].

In another retrospective study in infants undergoing flexible endoscopy supported with NIV of pharyngeal oxygen with nose closure and abdominal compression without any mask or laryngeal mask airway, 13 laser-plasty procedures were safely and effectively performed for subglottic narrowing, and granulations in trachea or bronchi in 7 infants out of a total of 38 infants with 129 aerotract lesions [57].

Cryotherapy is a cold bronchoscopic procedure used for ablating or extracting endobronchial tumors or granulation tissue, removing a foreign body or clot, and reducing mucous overproduction in chronic bronchitis.

In a retrospective study on flexible bronchoscopy under NIV in hypoxemic patients with central airway obstruction, cryotherapy was utilized in 13 out of 15 patients in the NIV group and in 10 out of 14 patients in the artificial airway-general anesthesia group. No significant complications occurred in all 29 patients, but the NIV group had less complications, shorter admission time, and lower procedure fee than the control group [55].

31.7 Conclusion

NIV is a safe and effective alternative to endotracheal intubation and mechanical ventilation for facilitating bronchoscopy in high-risk patients with severe hypoxemia. Most of the diagnostic and therapeutic procedures have been performed effectively and safely during NIV-assisted conventional or interventional bronchoscopy. However, the appropriate indications and contraindications of NIV during bronchoscopy should be meticulously considered for each case before the procedure.

NIV-assisted bronchoscopic study should be supervised in person by an expert, ideally in pulmonology and intensive care. The medical team, as well as being fully knowledgeable about the risk factors, predictors of failure, pathophysiological changes due to bronchoscopy and potential complications, should also be ready to cope with the complications in a critically ill patient on NIV.

The most frequently performed and reported diagnostic and therapeutic procedures during NIV-assisted bronchoscopy have been bronchial washing/aspiration and BAL. The rest of the NIV-assisted conventional or interventional procedures have been performed less frequently and reported in a limited number of patients. Thus, to fill the gap in this field, there is a need for high-quality research and publications on NIV-assisted conventional and interventional bronchoscopy for diagnostic and therapeutic purposes.

References

1. Murgu SD, Pecson J, Colt HG. Bronchoscopy during noninvasive ventilation: indications and technique. Respir Care. 2010;55(5):595–600.
2. Baumann HJ, Klose H, Simon M, Ghadban BSA, Hennigs JK, Kluge S. Fiber optic bronchoscopy in patients with acute hypoxemic respiratory failure requiring noninvasive ventilation – a feasibility study. Crit Care. 2011;15:R179. http://ccforum.com/content/15/4/R179
3. Ambrosino N, Guarracino F. Unusual applications of noninvasive ventilation. Eur Respir J. 2011;38:440–9.
4. Esquinas A, Zuil M, Scala R, Chiner E. Bronchoscopy during non-invasive mechanical ventilation: a review of techniques and procedures. Arch Bronconeumol. 2013;49(3):105–12.
5. Cabrini L, Nobile L, Cama E, Borghi G, Pieri M, Bocchino S, Zangrillo A. Non-invasive ventilation during upper endoscopies in adult patients: a systematic review. Minerva Anestesiol. 2013;79:683–94.
6. Pelaia C, Bruni A, Garofalo E, Rovida S, Arrighi E, Cammarota G, Navalesi P, Pelaia G, Longhini F. Oxygenation strategies during flexible bronchoscopy: a review of the literature. Respir Res. 2021;22:253. https://doi.org/10.1186/s12931-021-01846-1.
7. Skoczyński S, Minarowski Ł, Tobiczyk E, Oraczewska A, Glinka K, Ficek K, Mróz R, Barczyk A. Noninvasive ventilation-facilitated bronchofiberoscopy in patients with respiratory failure. In: Pokorski M, editor. Advances in pulmonary medicine: research and innovations. Advances in experimental medicine and biology, vol. 1160. Cham: Springer; 2019. p. 53–64. https://doi.org/10.1007/5584_2019_375.
8. Agarwal R, Khan A, Aggarwal AN, Gupta D. Bronchoscopic lung biopsy using noninvasive ventilatory support: case series and review of literature of NIV-assisted bronchoscopy. Respir Care. 2012;57(11):1927–36.
9. Sircar M, Jha OK, Chabbra GS, Bhattacharya S. Noninvasive ventilation-assisted bronchoscopy in high-risk hypoxemic patients. Indian J Crit Care Med. 2019; https://doi.org/10.5005/jp-journals-10071-23219.
10. Scala R. Flexible bronchoscopy during non-invasive positive pressure mechanical ventilation: are two better than one? Panminerva Med. 2016;58(3):211–21.
11. Payne CB Jr, Goyal PC, Gupta SC. Effects of transoral and transnasal fiberoptic bronchoscopy on oxygenation and cardiac rhythm. Endoscopy. 1986;18(1):1–3.
12. Katz AS, Michelson EL, Stawicki J, Holford FD. Cardiac arrhythmias, frequency during fiberoptic bronchoscopy and correlation with hypoxemia. Arch Intern Med. 1981;141(5):603–6.
13. Goldstein RA, Rohatgi PK, Bergofsky EH, Block ER, Daniele RP, Dantzker DR, et al. Clinical role of bronchoalveolar lavage in adults with pulmonary disease. Am Rev Respir Dis. 1990;142(2):481–6.
14. Hilbert G, Gruson D, Vargas F, Valentino R, Gbikpi-Benissan G, Dupon M, et al. Noninvasive ventilation in immunosuppressed patients with pulmonary infiltrates, fever, and acute respiratory failure. N Engl J Med. 2001;344(7):481–7.
15. Mutlu GM, Factor P. Complications of mechanical ventilation. Respir Care Clin N Am. 2000;6(2):213–52.
16. Antonelli M, Pennisi M, Conti G, Bello G, Maggiore SM, Michetti V, et al. Fiberoptic bronchoscopy during noninvasive positive pressure ventilation delivered by helmet. Intensive Care Med. 2003;29(1):126–9.
17. Keenan SP, Powers C, McCormack DG, Block G. Noninvasive positive-pressure ventilation for postextubation respiratory distress: a randomized controlled trial. JAMA. 2002;287(24):3238–44.
18. Esteban A, Frutos-Vivar F, Ferguson ND, Arabi Y, Apezteguía C, Gonzalez M, et al. Noninvasive positive-pressure ventilation for respiratory failure after extubation. N Engl J Med. 2004;350(24):2452–60.

19. Antonelli M, Conti G, Rocco M, Arcangeli A, Cavaliere F, Proietti R, Meduri GU. Noninvasive positive-pressure ventilation versus conventional oxygen supplementation in hypoxemic patients undergoing diagnostic bronchoscopy. Chest. 2002;121(4):1149–54.
20. Maitre B, Jaber S, Maggiore SM, Bergot E, Richard JC, Bakthiari H, et al. Continuous positive airway pressure during fiberoptic bronchoscopy in hypoxemic patients: a randomized double-blind study using a new device. Am J Respir Crit Care Med. 2000;162(3 Pt 1):1063–7.
21. Antonelli M, Conti G, Riccioni L, Meduri GU. Noninvasive positive-pressure ventilation via face mask during bronchoscopy with BAL in high-risk hypoxemic patients. Chest. 1996;110(3):724–8.
22. Chhajed PN, Aboyoun C, Malouf MA, Hopkins PM, Plit M, Grunstein RR, Glanville AR. Management of acute hypoxemia during flexible bronchoscopy with insertion of a nasopharyngeal tube in lung transplant recipients. Chest. 2002;121(4):1350–4.
23. Mokhlesi B, Tulaimat A. Recent advances in obesity hypoventilation syndrome. Chest. 2007;132(4):1322–36.
24. Popper RA, Leidinger MJ, Williams AJ. Endoscopic observations of the pharyngeal airway during treatment of obstructive sleep apnea with nasal continuous positive airway pressure-A pneumatic splint. West J Med. 1986;144(1):83–5.
25. Borowiecki B, Pollak CP, Weitzman ED, Rakoff S, Imperato J. Fibro-optic study of pharyngeal airway during sleep in patients with hypersomnia obstructive sleep-apnea syndrome. Laryngoscope. 1978;88(8 Pt 1):1310–3.
26. Aoyama K, Yasunaga E, Takenaka I, Kadoya T, Sata T, Shigematsu A. Positive pressure ventilation during fibreoptic intubation: comparison of the laryngeal mask airway, intubating laryngeal mask and endoscopy mask techniques. Br J Anaesth. 2002;88(2):246–54.
27. Schnapf BM. Oxygen desaturation during fiberoptic bronchoscopy in pediatric patients. Chest. 1991;99(3):591–4.
28. Kuna ST, Bedi DG, Ryckman C. Effect of nasal airway positive pressure on upper airway size and configuration. Am Rev Respir Dis. 1988;138(4):969–75.
29. Trachsel D, Erb TO, Frei FJ, Hammer J. Swiss Paediatric respiratory research group. Use of continuous positive airway pressure during flexible bronchoscopy in young children. Eur Respir J. 2005;26(5):773–7.
30. Dellinger RP. Fiberoptic bronchoscopy in adult airway management. Crit Care Med. 1990;18(8):882–7.
31. Da Conceicao M, Genco G, Favier JC, Bidallier I, Pitti R. Fiberoptic bronchoscopy during non-invasive positive-pressure ventilation in patients with chronic obstructive lung disease with hypoxemia and hypercapnea. Ann Fr Anesth Reanim. 2000;19(4):231–6.
32. Wiseman NE, Duncan PG, Cameron CB. Management of tracheobronchomalacia with continuous positive airway pressure. J Pediatr Surg. 1985;20(5):489–93.
33. Rozycki HJ, Van Houten ML, Elliott GR. Quantitative assessment of intrathoracic airway collapse in infants and children with tracheobronchomalacia. Pediatr Pulmonol. 1996;21(4):241–5.
34. Ferguson GT, Benoist J. Nasal continuous positive airway pressure in the treatment of tracheobronchomalacia. Am Rev Respir Dis. 1993;147(2):457–61.
35. Adliff M, Ngato D, Keshavjee S, Brenaman S, Granton JT. Treatment of diffuse tracheomalacia secondary to relapsing polychondritis with continuous positive airway pressure. Chest. 1997;112(6):1701–4.
36. Davis S, Jones M, Kisling J, Angelicchio C, Tepper RS. Effect of continuous positive airway pressure on forced expiratory flows in infants with tracheomalacia. Am J Respir Crit Care Med. 1998;158(1):148–52.
37. Heunks LM, de Bruin CJ, van der Hoeven JG, van der Heijden HF. Non-invasive mechanical ventilation for diagnostic bronchoscopy using a new face mask: an observational feasibility study. Intensive Care Med. 2010;36(1):143–7.

38. Elizalde-González JJ. Bronchoscopy in the ICU. Simple procedures in difficult cases. Med Crit. 2023;37(2):66–8.
39. Hyzy RC, McSparron JI. Noninvasive ventilation in adults with acute respiratory failure: benefits and contraindications. In: Parsons PE, Finlay G, editors. UpToDate. Wolters Kluwer. Last updated: May 08, 2023. https://www.uptodate.com/contents/noninvasive-ventilation-in-adults-with-acute-respiratory-failure-benefits-and-contraindications.
40. Gong Y, Sankari A. Noninvasive ventilation. In: StatPearls [Internet]. NCBI Bookshelf. A service of the National Library of Medicine, National Institutes of Health. Treasure Island: StatPearls Publishing; 2023. Last Update: December 11, 2022. https://www.ncbi.nlm.nih.gov/books/NBK578188/.
41. Murphy PB, Zoumot Z, Polkey MI. Noninvasive ventilation and lung volume reduction. Clin Chest Med. 2014;35:251–69.
42. Skoczyński S, Ogonowski M, Tobiczyk E, Krzyzak D, Brozek G, Wierzbicka A, et al. Risk factors of complications during noninvasive mechanical ventilation-assisted flexible bronchoscopy. Adv Med Sci. 2021;66:246–53.
43. Saillard C, Mokart D, Lemiale V, Azoulay E. Mechanical ventilation in cancer patients. Minerva Anestesiol. 2014;80:712–25.
44. Scala R. Noninvasive mechanical ventilation during bronchoscopy: key technical and clinical evidence. In: Esquinas AM, editor. Noninvasive mechanical ventilation: theory, equipment, and clinical applications. 2nd ed. Cham: Springer; 2016. p. 607–20. https://doi.org/10.1007/978-3-319-21653-9_71.
45. Lucena CM, Martínez-Olondris P, Badia JR, Xaubet A, Ferrer M, Torres A, et al. Fiberoptic bronchoscopy in a respiratory intensive care unit. Med Intensiva. 2012;36:389–95.
46. Giugliano CC, Cerpa FA, Keymer JE, Perez RA, Romero CP, Budini HR, et al. Clinical and breathing behavior in subjects undergoing bronchoscopy supported with noninvasive mechanical ventilation. Respir Med. 2018;2:106.
47. Chiner E, Sancho-Chust JN, Llombart M, Senent C, Camarasa A, Signes-Costa J. Fiberoptic bronchoscopy during nasal non-invasive ventilation in acute respiratory failure. Respiration. 2010;80:321–6.
48. Guziejko K, Minarowski Ł, Mróz R. Case report: case report: non-invasive mechanical ventilation in combination with bronchoscopy in the treatment of respiratory failure of lung cancer patient. F1000Res. 2022;11:1130. https://doi.org/10.12688/f1000research.124457.1.
49. Korkmaz Ekren P, Basarik Aydogan B, Gurgun A, Tasbakan MS, Bacakoglu F, Nava S. Can fiberoptic bronchoscopy be applied to critically ill patients treated with noninvasive ventilation for acute respiratory distress syndrome? Prospective observational study. BMC Pulm Med. 2016;16:89.
50. Patrucco F, Failla G, Ferrari G, Galasso T, Candoli P, Mondoni M, et al. Bronchoscopy during COVID-19 pandemic, ventilatory strategies and procedure measures. Panminerva Med. 2021;63:529–38.
51. Jha OK, Yadav S, Sircar M, Gupta N. Endobronchial ultrasound bronchoscopy in patients with acute respiratory failure on noninvasive ventilation: report of two cases. Indian J Chest Dis Allied Sci. 2022;64:292–6.
52. Ito T, Okachi S, Ikenouchi T, Ushijima F, Ohashi T, Ogawa M, et al. Endobronchial ultrasound-guided transbronchial needle aspiration under non-invasive positive pressure for the diagnosis of lung metastasis due to renal cell carcinoma in a patient with respiratory failure. Respir Med Case Rep. 2020;29:101028. https://doi.org/10.1016/j.rmcr.2020.101028.
53. Soong W-J, Tsao P-C, Lee Y-S, Yang C-F, Liao J, Jeng M-J. Retrieving difficult aspirated pen caps by balloon catheter with short working-length flexible endoscopy and noninvasive ventilation support in intensive care unit. Int J Pediatr Otorhinolaryngol. 2015;79:484–1489.

54. Soong W-J, Yang C-F, Lee Y-S, Tsao P-J, Lin C-H, Chen C-H. Vallecular cyst with coexisting laryngomalacia: successful diagnosis and laser therapy by flexible endoscopy with a novel noninvasive ventilation support in infants. Pediatr Pulmonol. 2020;55:1–7. https://doi.org/10.1002/ppul.24796.
55. Chen X, Zhou Y, Yu H, Peng Y, Xia L, Liu N, et al. Feasibility analysis of flexible bronchoscopy in conjunction with noninvasive ventilation for therapy of hypoxemic patients with central airway obstruction: a retrospective study. PeerJ. 2020;8:e8687. https://doi.org/10.7717/peerj.8687.
56. Tale S, Meitei SP, Prakash V, Negi A, Mishra M, Sindhwani G. Bronchoscopic cryotherapy for acute hypoxemic respiratory failure in three mechanically ventilated patients: a case series. Indian J Crit Care Med. 2021;25:94–6.
57. Soong W-J, Tsao P-C, Yang C-F, Lee Y-S, Lin C-H, Chen C-H. Flexible endoscopy with non-invasive ventilation enables clinicians to assess and manage infants with severe bronchopulmonary dysplasia. Front Pediatr. 2022;10:837329. https://doi.org/10.3389/fped.2022.837329.
58. Nong L, Liang W, Yu Y, Xi Y, Liu D, Zhang J, et al. Noninvasive ventilation support during fiberoptic bronchoscopy-guided nasotracheal intubation effectively prevents severe hypoxemia. J Crit Care. 2020;56:12–7.
59. Guarracino F, Cabrini L, Baldassarri R, Cariello C, Covello RD, Landoni G, et al. Non-invasive ventilation-aided transoesophageal echocardiography in high-risk patients: a pilot study. Eur J Echocardiogr. 2010;11:554–6.

32 Noninvasive Mechanical Ventilation (NIV) During Transesophageal Echocardiography

Michael Hannon, Emily Seif, Mark A. Marinescu, and Kunal Panda

32.1 Introduction

Transesophageal echocardiography (TEE) is a commonly performed procedure among multiple disciplines, including cardiologists, anesthesiologists, and intensivists. It is performed on a wide spectrum of patients from the outpatient clinic to the intubated ICU patient. It is commonly utilized to assess valvular disease and heart function when transthoracic echocardiography proves inadequate. Another common indication is for intraoperative monitoring of the cardiac status and for procedural guidance. Noninvasive ventilation can be used to help support the cardiac and respiratory status in higher-risk patients undergoing TEE while avoiding the need for intubation.

32.2 Physiology of Positive Airway Pressure in Patients with Heart Failure and Valvular Disease

Cardiac function is impacted in several ways by the application of positive pressure ventilation (PPV). It can have beneficial or deleterious effects depending on the underlying pathophysiology and patient volume status. An increase in intrathoracic pressure is well described in the literature with the use of PPV. This increased

M. Hannon · E. Seif · M. A. Marinescu
Department of Cardiology, University of Rochester School of Medicine & Dentistry, Rochester, NY, USA
e-mail: Michael_Hannon@urmc.rochester.edu; Emily_Seif@urmc.rochester.edu; Mark_Marinescu@urmc.rochester.edu

K. Panda (✉)
Department of Anesthesiology and Perioperative Medicine, University of Rochester School of Medicine & Dentistry, Rochester, NY, USA
e-mail: kunal_panda@urmc.rochester.edu

© The Author(s), under exclusive license to Springer Nature Switzerland AG 2025

K. Panda et al. (eds.), *Noninvasive Ventilatory Approaches in Interventional Procedures*, Noninvasive Ventilation. The Essentials,
https://doi.org/10.1007/978-3-032-05328-2_32

intrathoracic pressure typically decreases right ventricle (RV) and left ventricle (LV) preload, while increasing RV afterload and decreasing LV afterload. Positive end expiratory pressure (PEEP) is typically set greater than zero and has beneficial or deleterious consequences depending on the underlying physiology. In patients with incomplete exhalation, air trapping may occur, further reducing preload. Also, by preventing the lungs from returning to functional residual capacity, pulmonary vascular resistance may be increased. Alternatively, PEEP can aid in alveolar recruitment and displace alveolar edema. Another beneficial effect of PEEP is the reduction of left ventricular afterload, which can be useful in patients with numerous left ventricular pathologies. At low levels (~5–8 cm H_20), PEEP can even lower PVR via helping to recruit additional alveolar units and mitigate hypoxia-mediated vasoconstriction. This recruitment increases the overall pulmonary arteriolar cross-sectional area, thereby reducing intrapulmonary shunting and improving oxygenation. However, high levels of PEEP (~ > 15 cm H_20) can lead to vascular compression, which leads to an increase in PVR that can negatively impact RV function. PEEP decreases venous return to the RV, which reduces preload to the RV and also ultimately the LV. At moderate to high PEEP (8–15 cm H_2O), the RV cardiac output may be decreased in those with RV failure or significant dependence on preload [1]. These effects on the RV can be particularly deleterious in patients with severe RV dysfunction, such as those with massive pulmonary emboli or significant pulmonary arterial hypertension. These patients require close monitoring of hemodynamics and titration of PEEP.

32.3 NIV in Contrast to Other Modes of Oxygen Delivery

NIV allows the patient to reach an increased level of sedation that allows the TEE exam to be performed in a more comprehensive manner while avoiding general anesthesia (and its deleterious hemodynamic changes) and endotracheal intubation.

Oxygen can be delivered in a number of ways, including nasal cannula, venti masks, non-rebreather mask, high flow nasal cannula, continuous positive airway pressure (CPAP), or bilevel positive airway pressure (BiPAP). Only BiPAP assists with ventilation. CPAP aids oxygen by providing PEEP, thereby mitigating hypoxia by avoiding atelectasis, but it will not be helpful with ventilation in the patient that has significant respiratory depression as a result of sedation.

32.4 NIV—Technical Considerations for TEE

There are two main methods commonly used to deliver NIV during TEE. Nasal mask (Fig. 32.1) or nasal prongs allow the oropharynx to be readily accessible and permit easy manipulation of the TEE probe. The other approach is the use of specialized face masks for NIV, which have a port that allows for passage of the TEE probe. Endoscopy Mask (VBM Medizintechnik), Endoscopy Mask (DEAS), and Janus (Biomedical) are three such masks that allow TEE to be performed while maintaining a full-face seal.

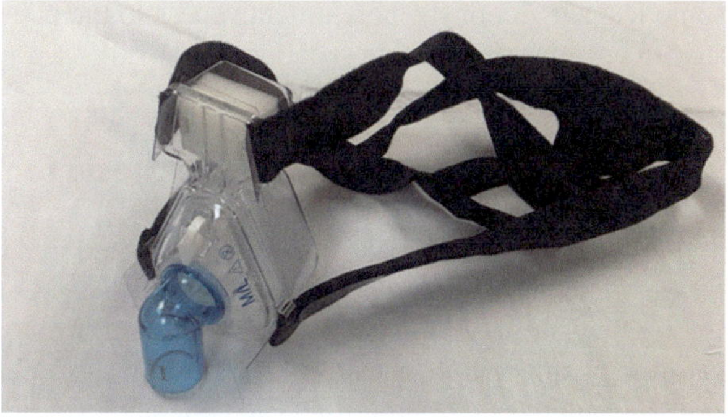

Fig. 32.1 Nasal Mask that is routinely used for all TEE cases done by cardiology at our institution

Gastro-laryngeal tube (GLT) is a supraglottic airway device that has a dedicated channel for endoscopy, which has also been described for facilitating TEE. A recently performed randomized prospective trial looked at this device in two groups receiving sedation and analgesia (propofol and fentanyl) for TEE. One group had a nasal cannula for oxygen delivery (22 patients), and the other had GLT (22 patients). All patients in the GLT group had the TEE probe passed on the first attempt, while only 11 patients in the sedation and analgesia group had first-attempt success. There was increased proceduralist satisfaction reported in this study with the use of GLT, while similar patient satisfaction was reported in both groups. On the other hand, higher propofol dose, procedural duration, and length of stay in the recovery area were noted in the GLT group [2].

Typically, the patient is started on CPAP with a pressure of 5 cm of H_20 (or patient's home CPAP level) and FiO_2 of 40% to allow for patient acclimation to the mask before sedation is administered. Once the patient is sedated and if their respiratory drive appears significantly depressed, then the transition to BiPAP can be made. Typically, we start with an inspiratory pressure (IPAP) of 10 cm H_2O and an expiratory pressure (EPAP) of 5 cm H_2O and titrate as needed to achieve adequate minute ventilation, chest rise, and adequate pulse oximetry. The delta pressure on BiPAP can be increased as needed to ensure adequate ventilation. The insertion of the TEE probe can be quite stimulating, and the patient's respiratory rate often increases on probe passage. If desaturation occurs during the procedure, EPAP and FiO_2 can be increased as needed.

The use of end-tidal CO_2 ($ETCO_2$) monitoring can be performed while using NIV and can help identify respiratory depression earlier than pulse oximetry. This technique was studied in a population of 200 patients undergoing TEE. There were 90 patients identified as having respiratory depression via capnography obtained from a nasal cannula monitor. The criteria used to determine respiratory depression were the loss of the $ETCO_2$ waveform for greater than or equal to 15 seconds, $ETCO_2$ change from baseline of greater than 10 mmHg, or $ETCO_2$ of greater than or equal to 50 mmHg. However, the only interventions used in this study were jaw repositioning, verbal and tactile stimulation, and increased nasal cannula oxygen [3]. Capnography monitoring may be aided by full-face mask use; however, there can be issues with obtaining a good seal and accurate monitoring, as there will be some leakage out of the port. Attentiveness to the patient's clinical status is necessary to ensure safety during sedation.

32.5 Sedation and Topical Anesthesia for TEE

To perform a TEE, the probe needs to be inserted into the esophagus. This requires a level of sedation that typically leads to some depression of the respiratory drive. Intermittent doses of fentanyl and midazolam are commonly used agents in the cardiology suite, while anesthesiologists may use bolus dosing or continuous infusions of sedatives like propofol. The patient's level of consciousness and alertness is evaluated continuously to achieve a level of sedation of 2–3 on the modified Wilson sedation scale. Typically, additional doses are needed incrementally over time to maintain an adequate level of sedation. Lidocaine spray or topical lidocaine is also commonly used as an adjunct to aid in numbing the oropharynx before TEE probe passage. While the concentration of lidocaine may vary depending on the type available, the maximal dose is typically 4.5 mg/kg (max total 300 mg) of lidocaine. One percent lidocaine solution contains 10 mg of lidocaine per 1 ml. Reversal agents such as naloxone (if using fentanyl) or flumazenil (if using midazolam) should be readily available but are rarely needed in our experience with judicious use of sedation and close patient monitoring.

32.6 Contraindications to NIV in TEE

There are several contraindications to the use of NIV during TEE. If the patient is not able to protect their own airway or is in extremis and needs to be intubated for another reason, then NIV is not appropriate. Patients must also be able to manage their own secretions prior to sedation. Those with facial trauma or in whom the mask cannot maintain an adequate seal are also not appropriate candidates. Significant recent upper gastrointestinal bleeding is also another contraindication. The patient must also be on an empty stomach. There must also be appropriate and experienced staff available to monitor the patient during the procedure, with resuscitation equipment readily available.

Those with a known history of a difficult airway or severe upper airway obstruction should also not undergo NIV for TEE, and consideration should be given to endotracheal tube placement before TEE imaging rather than face the possibility of requiring emergent intubation.

Substance use (heavy alcohol) or opioid replacement therapy (buprenorphine/naloxone or methadone) is not an absolute contraindication to the use of NIV. At our institution, we have safely used moderate sedation and NIV in this patient population. However, those performing the procedure should be familiar with the pharmacology of these agents and adjust sedation medications accordingly.

32.7 TEE and Associated Procedures

TEE is used for many different clinical scenarios in cardiology. It is used for diagnostic purposes when transthoracic imaging is not adequate, such as to better evaluate prosthetic valves or to evaluate for endocarditis. In addition, it is also used for a wide variety of procedures. Electrical cardioversion for cases of atrial flutter or fibrillation is a very commonly performed procedure. TEE allows for definitive evaluation of thrombus in the left atrial appendage, and NIV can help to improve the comfort of the patient undergoing cardioversion by allowing deeper sedation. There are many additional structural heart procedures where TEE can be used in combination with NIV to safely accomplish the procedure. These procedures are discussed in a separate chapter on structural heart procedures (Chap. 36).

32.8 TEE Complications

There are several serious complications that can occur during TEE. The most feared and concerning complication is significant trauma or perforation of the esophagus. This is rare but can be life-threatening. The incidence of this ranges from 0.01 to 0.03% [4]. Perforation may not be readily apparent during the procedure, but there can be significant blood or clots noted after probe removal. The patient may also have a significant cough, voice changes, pain, and subcutaneous emphysema. NIV can help to minimize the incidence of several complications associated with TEE, such as hypoxia, and avoid the need for endotracheal intubation.

Oropharyngeal, dental, or gastric trauma may also occur after TEE; however, these are also uncommon. After the procedure, the patient should be monitored and observed until the effects of sedation have worn off as some complications may not be as apparent while the patient is sedated.

32.9 Conclusion

1. Noninvasive ventilation (NIV) is a rational approach in heart failure patients during TEE procedures.
2. The hemodynamic effect of NIV can be mixed depending on the underlying pathophysiology, but NIV can often be titrated to have an overall positive effect.
3. Use of NIV can allow better TEE images to be obtained and also increase patient comfort during the procedure by safely allowing increased depth of sedation.

References

1. Alviar CL, Miller PE, McAreavey D, et al. Positive pressure ventilation in the cardiac intensive care unit. J Am Coll Cardiol. 2018;72(13):1532–53. https://doi.org/10.1016/j.jacc.2018.06.074.

2. Calim M, Uysal H, Kahraman Ay N, Karaaslan K, Daskaya H. Utility of the gastro-laryngeal tube during transesophageal echocardiography: a prospective randomized clinical trial. Medicine (Baltimore). 2022;101(50):e32269. https://doi.org/10.1097/MD.0000000000032269.
3. Adams L, Butas S, Spurlock D Jr. Capnography (ETCO2), respiratory depression, and nursing interventions in moderately sedated adults undergoing transesophageal echocardiography (TEE). J Perianesth Nurs. 2015;30(1):14–22. https://doi.org/10.1016/j.jopan.2013.07.009.
4. Côté G, Denault A. Transesophageal echocardiography-related complications. Can J Anaesth. 2008;55(9):622–47. https://doi.org/10.1007/BF03021437.

NIV Procedures: Endovascular Procedures, Pacemaker, Jugular Catheters

33

Laurent Asiama, Christopher Galton, and Joseph W. Dooley

Abbreviations

BIPAP	Bi-level positive airway pressure
CPAP	Continuous positive airway pressure
CMV	Controlled mechanical ventilation
EPAP	Expiratory positive airway pressure
IPAP	Inspiratory positive airway pressure
LMA	laryngeal mask airway
LAAO	Left atrial appendage occlusion
NIV	Noninvasive ventilation
PAVI	Percutaneous aortic valve implantation

L. Asiama
University of Rochester School of Medicine and Dentistry, Rochester, NY, USA
e-mail: Laurent_Asiama@URMC.Rochester.edu

C. Galton
Departments of Anesthesiology and Perioperative Medicine, Emergency Medicine, University of Rochester Medical Center, Rochester, NY, USA
e-mail: Christopher_Galton@URMC.Rochester.edu

J. W. Dooley (✉)
Departments of Anesthesiology and Perioperative, Medicine, Neurosurgery, University of Rochester Medical Center, Rochester, NY, USA
e-mail: joseph_dooley@urmc.rochester.edu

© The Author(s), under exclusive license to Springer Nature Switzerland AG 2025

K. Panda et al. (eds.), *Noninvasive Ventilatory Approaches in Interventional Procedures*, Noninvasive Ventilation. The Essentials,
https://doi.org/10.1007/978-3-032-05328-2_33

33.1 Introduction

Noninvasive ventilation (NIV) is a method of positive pressure ventilatory support without the use of adjuncts for invasive mechanical ventilation, such as an endotracheal tube, tracheostomy appliance, or laryngeal mask airway (LMA). In NIV, airway pressure is delivered via external interfaces such as face masks, nasal masks, or helmets. Noninvasive ventilation works physiologically by exerting its effects on the pulmonary and cardiovascular systems through the application of positive airway pressure [1]. NIV improves oxygenation and reduces the work of breathing. It improves oxygenation by opening atelectatic areas of the lung, which reduces shunt (ventilation/perfusion mismatch). It reduces the work of breathing by offloading some or all of the work of breathing to the ventilator. For patients with congestive heart failure, positive pressure ventilation reduces the risk of heart failure exacerbation and pulmonary edema by decreasing the pressure gradient across the left ventricular wall. This decreases the left ventricular wall tension (afterload), which decreases myocardial oxygen demand.

Due to its minimal intrusive nature, NIV reduces the need for and the risks associated with general anesthesia and invasive mechanical ventilation. These risks include nosocomial lung infections, barotrauma, and hemodynamic instability [1, 2]. Furthermore, some NIV modes, such as continuous positive airway pressure (CPAP), applied to anesthetized patients provide more efficient ventilation with a significantly lower peak airway pressure compared with controlled mechanical ventilation (CMV) [3].

Modern NIV modes are classified into (1) continuous positive airway pressure (CPAP), which applies a constant positive pressure during both inspiration and expiration, and (2) bi-level positive airway pressure (BiPAP), which provides separate positive pressure settings during inspiration (IPAP) and expiration (EPAP). Noninvasive ventilation modes such as CPAP and BiPAP have been used to manage several respiratory conditions in the clinical setting. Since the advent of NIV technologies, they have been employed primarily in the intensive care unit to treat both acute and chronic respiratory failure resulting from various pathologies, including cardiogenic pulmonary edema, pneumonia, and COPD exacerbation. With the increasing understanding and research of NIV, clinicians have been exploiting the application of NIV to treat and manage a large number of conditions in other clinical settings. One such way is the use of NIV by anesthesiologists to manage patients undergoing minimally invasive surgeries. In this chapter, after a brief discussion of patient selection for NIV and limitations of NIV, we discuss how noninvasive ventilation has been applied by anesthesiologists for endovascular procedures, pacemaker insertion, and internal jugular vein catheter placement.

33.2 Patient Populations for NIV Procedures

The indication of NIV requires careful patient analysis. While NIV can be used for most patients, certain features have been used to select patients for NIV. In general, NIV has been used for patients with significant comorbidities that increase their risk of complications from general anesthesia and mechanical ventilation. Such populations include elderly patients, obese patients, and patients with preexisting lung diseases. NIV has also been recommended postoperatively for those patients undergoing thoracic, cardiac, or upper abdominal surgeries who are at increased risk for postoperative respiratory complications.

While some indications are related to the risk for systemic complications under general anesthesia, others are specific to the patient's characteristics, irrespective of the general anesthesia risk. Some of these include the severity of the patient's upper airway obstruction, mask interference with the surgical field, the level of required hyperventilation, and the severity of orthopnea. To this effect, NIV has been safely used in patients requiring low levels of hyperventilation, mild obstructive sleep apnea, and patients who need to avoid hypoventilation.

33.3 Limitations of NIV

NIV is contraindicated in patients in respiratory arrest, those unable to fit the mask, those unable to manage the secretions, uncooperative patients, patients with hemodynamic shock, and patients at significant risk for aspiration. The majority of complications related to the use of NIV are related to the use of the mask; the most common of which is the discomfort that comes with the mask and its associated pressure on the face. Other complications include skin rash related to hypersensitivity to the mask material and nasal bridge ulcers, which are very rare. Physically, the strap that fixes the nasal mask can interfere with the surgical field in some cases. NIV is also not advised for patients who have severe obstruction of the upper airway. NIV may not be adequate for patients who need aggressive hyperventilation because of increased intracranial pressure [4].

Further, Schwartz et al. [5] have reported the interaction between magnets embedded in CPAP masks and cardiac-implanted electronic devices (CEIDs) such as pacemakers. In this report, patients with dual-chamber pacemakers experienced episodes of asynchronous pacing with the use of magnet-embedded CPAP masks. Hence, CPAP masks secured with magnetic clips should be avoided in patients with CIEDs.

33.4 NIV for Endovascular Procedures

Cardiovascular disease remains the leading cause of mortality in the Western world. Patients undergoing cardiac and peripheral vascular procedures often present with significant comorbidities. For example, patients presenting for coronary and valvular interventions may have ventricular dysfunction and arrhythmias. Invasive cardiac and endovascular surgeries requiring general anesthesia may be particularly challenging since the anesthesiologist has to consider the patient's comorbidities when determining the anesthetic plan. These procedures often have stringent anesthetic requirements to provide acceptable surgical conditions while ensuring patient comfort. While general anesthesia with endotracheal ventilation has been proven adequate for patients undergoing invasive cardiac procedures, this technique could have unintended consequences, especially in patients with significant comorbidities.

In general, patients who undergo general anesthesia for cardiac procedures are more likely to develop pulmonary hypertension, right ventricular failure, and hyperactive airways [2, 6, 7]. In a study by Taggart et al. [8], 66% of patients who underwent cardiopulmonary bypass experienced significant hypoxemia and respiratory dysfunction as measured by alveolar-arterial oxygen gradients in the immediate days following surgery. In daily practice, when the risks of surgical complications and prolonged post-procedure respiratory failure are high, the decision to undergo surgery poses a significant dilemma for both physicians and patients. Therefore, patients may choose not to undergo an otherwise recommended surgical procedure. Given these concerns, alternatives to endotracheal intubation, such as noninvasive ventilation (NIV), are being considered for patients presenting for minimally invasive cardiac and endovascular procedures. Since NIV provides ventilatory support without endotracheal intubation, the risk of postoperative complications may be lessened. Thus, NIV is postulated to minimize the adverse effects of invasive mechanical ventilation while offering a similar degree of efficacy.

NIV has been employed with deep sedation for catheter ablation of atrial fibrillation [9]. For this procedure, deep sedation or general anesthesia is preferred over local anesthesia alone since patients are required to lie motionless for several hours. In addition, the repeated stimuli from ablation are often painful. In specific patients where general anesthesia is relatively contraindicated, deep sedation is recommended. Deep sedation, however, presents with the challenge of requiring frequent manipulation of the patient's airway and titration of the administered oxygen flow rate to ensure adequate oxygenation and ventilation. Relative to endotracheal intubation, NIV was shown to mitigate these challenges while decreasing the risk of hemodynamic, respiratory, and neurological problems secondary to inadequate ventilation [10]. NIV, therefore, can be used as a viable ventilatory management strategy in procedures requiring deep sedation since it can be used to treat respiratory depression and hypoxia induced by deep sedation.

Endovascular procedures for aortic aneurysm repair (EVAR or TEVAR) require the patient to breathe hold multiple times during the procedure. This requires either a relatively alert and cooperative patient or a completely anesthetized patient whose ventilation can be held at frequent points during the procedure. There is little or no role for NIV in these procedures at this time.

33.5 NIV for Permanent Pacemaker Placement

There is little or no literature on the use of NIV for pacemaker placement. At our institution, for placement of transvenous, percutaneous pacemaker leads, light to moderate sedation is almost always adequate. For patients who are unable to lie flat or who require deep sedation due to claustrophobia when under a full-body drape, NIV would be an acceptable option. For patients having permanent pacemaker placement, deep sedation or general anesthesia is usually required due to the need to create a relatively large subcutaneous pocket for the pacemaker generator. In most cases, the airway and oxygenation can be maintained with nasal cannula oxygen and gentle manipulation of the airway. These manipulations include oropharyngeal airway placement, nasopharyngeal airway placement, and jaw thrust. When the above measures are inadequate to provide adequate oxygen and ventilation, either a laryngeal mask airway (LMA) or an endotracheal tube is placed, and the patient is mechanically ventilated. NIV has been used occasionally in this setting. Barriers to more frequent use of NIV include access to and familiarity with NIV equipment, as well as the straps used to secure the CPAP or BiPAP mask encroaching upon the surgical field.

33.6 NIV for Internal Jugular Vein Catheter Placement

Internal jugular vein catheters can usually be placed using local anesthesia with no sedation or light to moderate sedation. These catheters include traditional double and triple-lumen central venous catheters and dialysis catheters. Patients who are unable to lie flat due to orthopnea or who are claustrophobic may require deeper sedation. Similarly, patients requiring tunneled catheter placement may require deeper sedation. If these patients are unable to oxygenate and ventilate adequately with supplemental oxygen delivered either via nasal cannula or a conventional face mask, NIV is a reasonable alternative.

33.7 Conclusions

Noninvasive ventilation has been used for select patients with acute respiratory failure and acute on chronic respiratory failure managed in the intensive care unit for decades. More recently, NIV has been used in the operating room and procedural suites when sedation issues, patient positioning issues, and/or patient comorbidities have resulted in the patient having inadequate oxygenation and/or ventilation. Using NIV can improve these parameters when invasive mechanical ventilation with an endotracheal tube is determined to be either too risky to the patient due to comorbidities or when endotracheal intubation is determined to be more than is needed to perform the procedure. Barriers to NIV include poor cooperation, poor secretion management, and risk for aspiration. There is a role for NIV use for patients undergoing endovascular procedures, pacemaker placement, and internal jugular vein line placement.

References

1. Cabrini L, Nobile L, Plumari VP, Landoni G, Borghi G, Mucchetti M, Zangrillo A. Intraoperative prophylactic and therapeutic non-invasive ventilation: a systematic review. Br J Anaesth. 2014 Apr;112(4):638–47.
2. Cabrini L, Plumari VP, Nobile L, Olper L, Pasin L, Bocchino S, Landoni G, Beretta L, Zangrillo A. Non-invasive ventilation in cardiac surgery: a concise review. Heart Lung Vessel. 2013;5(3):137–41.
3. Bratzke E, Downs J, Smith R. Intermittent CPAP: a new mode of ventilation during general anesthesia. Anesthesiology. 1998;89:334–40.
4. Yamamoto F, Kato R, Sato J, Nishino T. Anaesthesia for awake craniotomy with non-invasive positive pressure ventilation. Br J Anaesth. 2003 Mar;90(3):382–5.
5. Schwartz Y, Wasserlauf J, Sahakian AV, Knight B. Inappropriate activation of pacemaker magnet response mode by CPAP masks. Pacing Clin Electrophysiol. 2019;42(8):1158–61. https://doi.org/10.1111/pace.13693. Epub 2019 Apr 29
6. Wynne R, Botti M. Postoperative pulmonary dysfunction in adults after cardiac surgery with cardiopulmonary bypass: clinical significance and implications for practice. Am J Crit Care. 2004;13:384–93.
7. Guarracino F, Cabrini L, Baldassarri R, Petronio S, De Carlo M, Covello RD, Landoni G, Gabbrielli L, Ambrosino N. Noninvasive ventilation for awake percutaneous aortic valve implantation in high-risk respiratory patients: a case series. J Cardiothorac Vasc Anesth. 2011 Dec;25(6):1109–12.
8. Taggart DP, el-Fiky M, Carter R, Bowman A, Wheatley DJ. Respiratory dysfunction after uncomplicated cardiopulmonary bypass. Ann Thorac Surg. 1993 Nov;56(5):1123–8.
9. Zangrillo A, Mazzone P, Oriani A, Pieri M, Frau G, D'Angelo G, Sartini C, Capucci R, Belletti A, Bella PD, Monaco F. Noninvasive ventilation during left atrial appendage closure under sedation: preliminary experience with the Janus mask. Ann Card Anaesth. 2019;22(4):400–6.
10. Sbrana F, Ripoli A, Formichi B. Anesthetic management in atrial fibrillation ablation procedure: adding non-invasive ventilation to deep sedation. Indian Pacing Electrophysiol J. 2015;15(2):96–102.

Applications of NIV in Patients Undergoing Coronary Angiography

34

Michal Kozlowski and Marek Jędrzejek

34.1 Introduction and Terminology

The most widespread method of mechanical ventilation is intermittent positive pressure ventilation (IPPV). This method utilizes repeated application of pressures higher than the alveolar pressure to generate flow. Noninvasive ventilation represents a type of mechanical ventilation in which the connection between the ventilator and patient airways does not require endotracheal intubation. In most cases, special face masks are used, which cover both the nose and the mouth and provide a proper seal to prevent excessive leakage.

The role of mechanical ventilation is to deliver mechanical breaths. There are several types of mechanical breaths which can be defined based on five variables: type of trigger, mode of phase shift, mode of gas delivery control, breath size target, and baseline pressure. It is beyond the scope of this chapter to extensively discuss these variables. Therefore, many types of breaths may be distinguished based on combinations of the abovementioned variables.

Mode of ventilation can be defined as a specific behavior of the ventilation system which utilizes one or more predefined types of mechanical breaths. There are many ventilator modes with no universal nomenclature. As far as the application of NIV in coronary angiography is considered, two modes should be mentioned:

1. CPAP (continuous positive airway pressure)—In this setting, the ventilator maintains a positive (higher than atmospheric) pressure in the airways throughout the respiratory cycle, which is commonly referred to as PEEP (positive end-

M. Kozlowski (✉) · M. Jędrzejek
Department of Cardiology and Structural Heart Diseases, Medical University of Silesia, Katowice, Poland

© The Author(s), under exclusive license to Springer Nature Switzerland AG 2025

K. Panda et al. (eds.), *Noninvasive Ventilatory Approaches in Interventional Procedures*, Noninvasive Ventilation. The Essentials,
https://doi.org/10.1007/978-3-032-05328-2_34

expiratory pressure). This keeps alveoli open, reduces atelectasis, decreases ventilation/perfusion mismatch, and therefore improves oxygenation.
2. NIPSV (noninvasive pressure support ventilation)—In this mode, additional pressure is applied on top of PEEP during inspiration, which decreases the work of breathing.

Both modes should only be used in conscious, cooperative patients with adequate respiratory drive.

34.2 Coronary Angiography Procedures—Overview

Coronary angiography is an invasive procedure during which radiopaque contrast is selectively administered to the right and left coronary arteries with a diagnostic catheter that is introduced through radial or femoral arteries. The purpose of the study is to visualize epicardial coronary arteries in search of atherosclerotic plaques that obstruct coronary flow, leading to ischemia. The procedure is performed with local anesthesia, in a catheterization lab, under fluoroscopic guidance. The patient has to stay in a supine position for the whole duration of the procedure.

According to the guidelines of the European Society of Cardiology, indications to perform coronary angiography include [1–3] the following:

1. Mild or no symptoms of coronary artery disease in patients on medical treatment in whom noninvasive tests indicate high annual event risk (3% and over).
2. Symptoms of coronary artery disease (angina) in subjects with a high-risk clinical profile, especially if symptoms are refractory to pharmacotherapy. This category typically includes subjects with multiple cardiovascular risk factors and typical angina at a low level of exercise.
3. Inconclusive of conflicting results on noninvasive tests performed to diagnose coronary artery disease.
4. Qualification for elective cardiac surgery procedures.
5. ST-elevation myocardial infarction (STEMI).
6. Non-ST-segment elevation myocardial infarction (NSTEMI).

Based on the results of coronary angiography, the physician who performs the procedure may immediately proceed with coronary angioplasty. This is usually the case in acute coronary syndromes.

In case of stable patients, coronary angiography can always be deferred. Therefore, there is no role for an upfront use of noninvasive ventilation in patients undergoing elective procedures. When a patient presents with myocardial infarctions (both STEMI and NSTEMI), coronary angiography should be performed within a specific timeframe to improve flow in narrowed/occluded coronary arteries. In the case of STEMI, when considering treatment approaches (fibrinolysis vs primary PCI), the maximum expected delay from diagnosis to primary PCI is 120 min. However, if primary PCI is chosen as the treatment strategy, even shorter time targets are recommended: $\leqslant$ 60 min when the patient is admitted to a hospital in which primary PCI can be performed and $\leqslant$ 90 min when the patient has to be transferred to another hospital. In the case of NSTEMI, coronary angiography has to be performed within 24 hours from hospital admission, unless the patient is considered to have a very high risk of in-hospital mortality—in such cases, a time target below 120 min is recommended.

Patients with acute coronary syndromes can present with various symptoms. These include chest pain that is often described as squeezing, heaviness, pressure, or tightness. The pain can radiate to the jaw or left upper extremity. Instead of pain, patients can report dyspnea or nausea. The general patient condition is related to several factors: amount of ischemic myocardium, presence of complications (acute valvular dysfunction, septal rupture, free wall rupture), and presence of significant arrhythmias. Therefore, the overall condition of subjects with acute myocardial infarction can range from "stable patients" with no respiratory failure and adequate cardiac output to "critical patients" with overt signs of cardiopulmonary failure. NIV is especially helpful in patients with acute respiratory failure caused by acute left ventricular systolic dysfunction, a condition commonly leading to cardiac pulmonary edema [4].

34.3 Pathophysiology and Symptoms of Cardiac Pulmonary Edema

Pulmonary edema is a condition in which there is abnormal extravascular accumulation of fluid in the lung parenchyma. This diminishes gas exchange, reduces respiratory system compliance, and elevates airway resistance, ultimately leading to acute respiratory failure. This condition may be caused by an abrupt increase in hydrostatic pressure in pulmonary capillaries due to acute left ventricular systolic and/or diastolic dysfunction (acute coronary syndromes, myocarditis), valvular heart diseases (acute mitral or aortic regurgitation, critical aortic stenosis), and arrhythmias (ventricular tachycardia, atrial fibrillation with rapid ventricular response, severe bradycardia due to a second- or third-degree heart block).

Symptoms of cardiac pulmonary edema include dyspnea that is exacerbated in a supine position (orthopnea), tachypnea, increased work of breathing, and respiratory failure with hypoxemia and hypercapnia. Clinical examination reveals fine or coarse crackles during inspiration. Lung ultrasound typically shows diffuse B-lines that can be detected in all examined areas [5]. Pulse oximetry reveals SaO_2 below 90% which usually corresponds to PaO_2 less than 60 mmHg in arterial blood gases with normal $PaCO_2$ levels (type 1 respiratory failure).

34.4 Treatment of Cardiac Pulmonary Edema

In most cases, cardiac pulmonary edema is not accompanied by low cardiac output. Such cases have a better prognosis and do not require inotropic support. Treatment of cardiac pulmonary edema involves several aspects [6]:

1. Oxygen therapy—preferred options include continuous positive airway pressure (CPAP), pressure support ventilation (PSV), or high-flow nasal cannula.
2. Intravenous diuretics.
3. Intravenous vasodilators to reduce afterload (if blood pressure is high).
4. Specific treatment for the underlying condition that is the cause of acute heart failure, e.g., revascularization in case of acute coronary syndrome, cardioversion in case of atrial fibrillation with fast ventricular rhythm, pacing in case of severe bradycardia, etc.

In case of acute coronary syndromes, cardiac pulmonary edema may be caused by systolic dysfunction of the left ventricle, bradycardia due to advanced heart block, or acute mitral regurgitation. The best-established treatment in these scenarios is coronary angiography with treatment of occluded/severely narrowed coronary arteries as soon as possible. As mentioned earlier, one of the key symptoms of acute pulmonary edema is orthopnea, which practically excludes the possibility of performing coronary angiography, because the patient has to stay in a supine position for the whole duration of the procedure. Therefore, rapid treatment of respiratory failure that accompanies pulmonary edema expedites interventional treatment and improves prognosis in acute coronary syndromes.

34.5 Scientific Rationale Behind Noninvasive Ventilation

A large meta-analysis of 15 clinical trials that compared CPAP or NIPSV with standard oxygen therapy in subjects with acute cardiogenic pulmonary edema showed a substantial mortality benefit that favored noninvasive ventilation (mortality rate reduced by 45%, statistically significant results for CPAP but not for NIPSV). Both techniques also reduced the need for intubation [7]. Another randomized study compared the effects of pre-hospital CPAP initiation in subjects with acute pulmonary edema and investigated if immediate CPAP would be better than delayed CPAP in this population [8]. The time delay between the "early" and "late" CPAP groups was only 15 minutes. Study showed that patients in the "early" group had significantly lower dyspnea clinical score, better arterial blood gases, lower intubation rate, and lower in-hospital mortality than the "late" CPAP group.

To sum up, in case of cardiac pulmonary edema that is caused by acute myocardial infarction, we can expect two major benefits of noninvasive ventilation: (1) a lower mortality due to proven effectiveness of these therapies in treatment of respiratory failure and (2) improved short- and long-term outcomes of acute coronary syndromes treatment due to faster revascularization.

34.6 Noninvasive Ventilation during Coronarography—Step-by-Step Approach

1. Patient selection

   All patients with respiratory failure due to pulmonary edema in the setting of acute myocardial infarction represent the population that would benefit from noninvasive ventilation. Therapy should be started as soon as possible if no contraindications exist (see special considerations section below).

2. Preparation

   Preparation can be divided into patient preparation and equipment preparation.

   - Patient preparation requires the removal of dentures that are not fixed permanently. Male subjects with excessive facial hair have to be shaved. Contraindications to NIV should be considered at this point.
   - Equipment preparation entails the selection of a properly sized mask (usually 3 sizes are available: small, medium, and large) and ventilator assembly. All equipment should be stored in one place. Ideally, the ventilator should be readily available with tubes and a filter already attached.

3. Mode selection

   As mentioned earlier, CPAP has the most robust clinical evidence and is easy to set up. Therefore, we recommend CPAP to be the first choice in the treatment of cardiac pulmonary edema. Settings should be set before the mask is placed on the subject's face. Providing PEEP, which is the cornerstone of CPAP mode, keeps the alveoli open during the whole breathing cycle and improves gas exchange.

4. Settings

   Initial CPAP settings include a PEEP value of at least 5 cm of water and FiO_2 of 1,0 (Picture 34.1). PEEP values can be uptitrated to 10 cm of water or more based on the effects of intervention. FiO_2 should be decreased as soon as improvement in oxygen saturation is achieved, since there is evidence that hyperoxia may increase infarct size and in-hospital mortality [9]. PEEP values

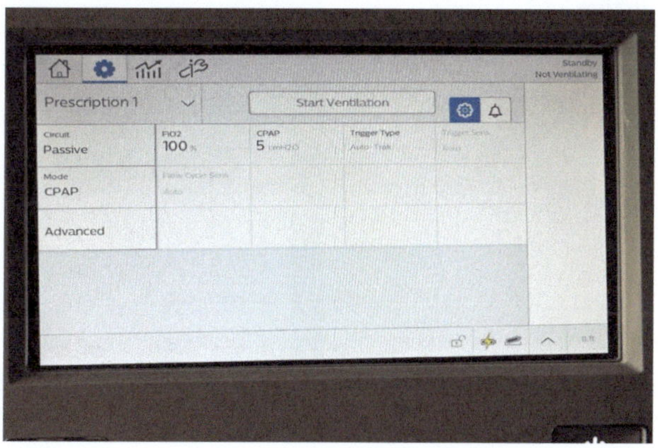

Picture 34.1 Basic CPAP settings

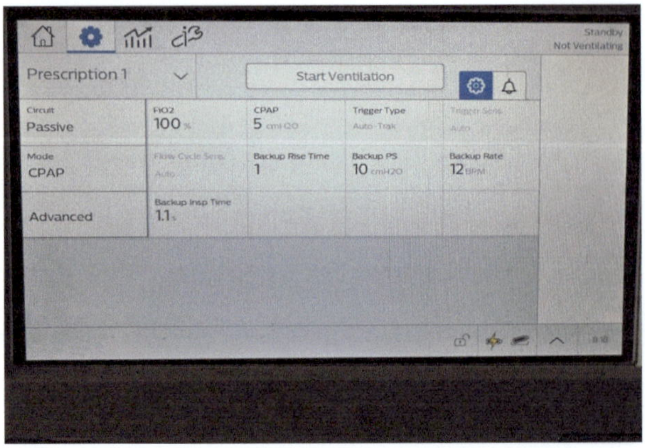

Picture 34.2 Initial CPAP settings with apnea backup

greater than 10 cm of water and SaO_2 values above 92% are not recommended in subjects with COPD.

Basic CPAP settings do not protect patients from apnea. Subjects with acute pulmonary edema usually present with tachypnea, but this can change rapidly. In addition, adequate supervision of subjects' ventilation may not occur during coronary angiography. Therefore, we recommend always setting a backup respiratory rate (e.g., 12 breaths per minute) with some level of pressure support (e.g., 10 cm of water). This is presented in Picture 34.2.

5. Supervision

Patients undergoing NIV require vital signs monitoring during the whole duration of the procedure. A transient drop in blood pressure can be expected. Since CPAP and NIPSV modes don't allow for specifying tidal volumes, attention should be paid to avoid hypoventilation and CO_2 accumulation. This can be accomplished by setting an appropriate minute ventilation alarm (Picture 34.3). It should be stressed that if noninvasive ventilation fails to provide clinical improvement, intubation should not be delayed.

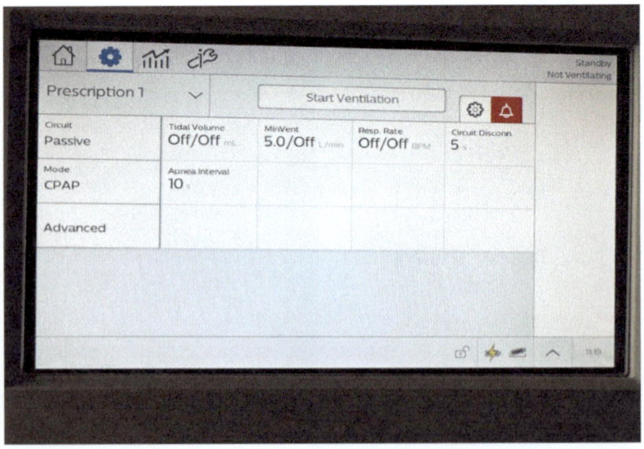

Picture 34.3 Minute ventilation alarm setup

34.7 Special Considerations

Patients with acute coronary syndromes may feel nauseated or experience vomiting. This may be a result of ischemia (most common in the case of inferior myocardial infarction) or due to the administration of opioid analgesics. It should be stressed that an inability to adequately protect the airways from aspiration is a contraindication to NIV. Antiemetic drugs, such as metoclopramide or ondansetron, represent an option, but an individual decision has to be made in each case.

CPAP is a simple and very effective procedure provided that patients are properly selected for this intervention. Subjects have to be conscious, understand the indications and potential benefits, because this would increase compliance. Noninvasive ventilation may not be well tolerated by patients with dementia and other conditions with an impaired state of consciousness, since they may try to remove the facial mask during coronary intervention. Intravenous sedatives may be administered judiciously to improve compliance.

34.8 Role of NIV in Elective Procedures

As mentioned earlier, elective coronary procedures are performed in stable patients without respiratory failure. Unfortunately, all invasive procedures can have complications that are sometimes life-threatening and require immediate action. One of such cases includes acute vessel closure, which occurs when there is loss of flow in a previously patent coronary artery during the procedure. This requires immediate action to restore flow, but at the same time, deterioration of the patient's medical condition can be expected due to myocardial ischemia. If the area of ischemia is high, acute pulmonary edema can occur, and NIV can be used in such cases to improve ventilation and provide the operator time to finish the procedure.

34.9 Conclusions

NIV in the CPAP mode is the preferred ventilation mode for treatment of respiratory failure due to pulmonary edema. Application of NIV may expedite coronary angiography procedures in cases of myocardial infarction complicated by acute left ventricular dysfunction. Basic initial settings include FiO_2 of 100% and PEEP of 5 cm of water. Apnea support and minute ventilation alarms should always be programmed.

References

1. Knuuti J, Wijns W, Saraste A, Capodanno D, Barbato E, Funck-Brentano C, Prescott E, Storey RF, Deaton C, Cuisset T, Agewall S, Dickstein K, Edvardsen T, Escaned J, Gersh BJ, Svitil P, Gilard M, Hasdai D, Hatala R, Mahfoud F, Masip J, Muneretto C, Valgimigli M, Achenbach S, Bax JJ, ESC Scientific Document Group. 2019 ESC Guidelines for the diagnosis and man-

agement of chronic coronary syndromes: the task force for the diagnosis and management of chronic coronary syndromes of the European Society of Cardiology (ESC). Eur Heart J. 2020;41(3):407–77.

2. Ibanez B, James S, Agewall S, Antunes MJ, Bucciarelli-Ducci C, Bueno H, Caforio ALP, Crea F, Goudevenos JA, Halvorsen S, Hindricks G, Kastrati A, Lenzen MJ, Prescott E, Roffi M, Valgimigli M, Varenhorst C, Vranckx P, Widimský P, ESC Scientific Document Group. 2017 ESC Guidelines for the management of acute myocardial infarction in patients presenting with ST-segment elevation: the Task Force for the management of acute myocardial infarction in patients presenting with ST-segment elevation of the European Society of Cardiology (ESC). Eur Heart J. 2018;39(2):119–77. https://doi.org/10.1093/eurheartj/ehx393.
3. Byrne RA, Rossello X, Coughlan JJ, Barbato E, Berry C, Chieffo A, Claeys MJ, Dan G-A, Dweck MR, Galbraith M, Gilard M, Hinterbuchner L, Jankowska EA, Jüni P, Kimura T, Kunadian V, Leosdottir M, Lorusso R, Pedretti RFE, Rigopoulos AG, Gimenez MR, Thiele H, Vranckx P, Wassmann S, Wenger NK, Ibanez B, ESC Scientific Document Group. 2023 ESC Guidelines for the management of acute coronary syndromes: developed by the task force on the management of acute coronary syndromes of the European Society of Cardiology (ESC). Eur Heart J. 2023;44(38):3720–826. https://doi.org/10.1093/eurheartj/ehad191.
4. Bello G, De Santis P, Antonelli M. Non-invasive ventilation in cardiogenic pulmonary edema. Ann Transl Med. 2018;6(18):355. https://doi.org/10.21037/atm.2018.04.39. PMID: 30370282; PMCID: PMC6186545
5. McDonagh TA, Metra M, Adamo M, Gardner RS, Baumbach A, Böhm M, Burri H, Butler J, Čelutkienė J, Chioncel O, Cleland JGF, Coats AJS, Crespo-Leiro MG, Farmakis D, Gilard M, Heymans S, Hoes AW, Jaarsma T, Jankowska EA, Lainscak M, Lam CSP, Lyon AR, McMurray JJV, Mebazaa A, Mindham R, Muneretto C, Piepoli MF, Price S, Rosano GMC, Ruschitzka F, Skibelund AK, ESC Scientific Document Group. 2021 ESC Guidelines for the diagnosis and treatment of acute and chronic heart failure: developed by the Task Force for the diagnosis and treatment of acute and chronic heart failure of the European Society of Cardiology (ESC) With the special contribution of the Heart Failure Association (HFA) of the ESC. Eur Heart J. 2021;42(36):3599–726. https://doi.org/10.1093/eurheartj/ehab368.
6. Soldati G, Demi M, Demi L. Ultrasound patterns of pulmonary edema. Ann Transl Med. 2019;7(Suppl 1):S16. https://doi.org/10.21037/atm.2019.01.49. PMID: 31032297; PMCID: PMC6462619
7. Masip J, Roque M, Sánchez B, Fernández R, Subirana M, Expósito JA. Noninvasive ventilation in acute cardiogenic pulmonary edema: systematic review and meta-analysis. JAMA. 2005;294(24):3124–30. https://doi.org/10.1001/jama.294.24.3124. PMID: 16380593
8. Plaisance P, Pirracchio R, Berton C, Vicaut E, Payen D. A randomized study of out-of-hospital continuous positive airway pressure for acute cardiogenic pulmonary oedema: physiological and clinical effects. Eur Heart J. 2007;28(23):2895–901. https://doi.org/10.1093/eurheartj/ehm502. Epub 2007 Oct 29. PMID: 17967821
9. Stub D, Smith K, Bernard S, et al. Air versus oxygen in ST-segment-elevation myocardial infarction. Circulation. 2015;131:2143–50.

NIV Procedures in Right Heart Catheterization

35

Marek Grabka

35.1 Right Heart Catheterization in Patients Treated with NIV

In the majority of cases of noninvasive ventilation and right heart catheterization, we are dealing with a situation where the RHC procedure is performed in a patient already treated with NIV. There is a quite large group of patients with chronic lung disease requiring diagnosis of pulmonary hypertension. The most common indications for right heart catheterization in a patient ventilated with NIV are suspicion of pulmonary hypertension in the course of lung diseases (group 3 of PH), suspicion of chronic thromboembolic pulmonary hypertension (CTEPH; group 4 PH), qualification for lung transplantation (LTx) or heart transplantation (HTx) with concomitant severe heart failure, and rare cases of suspected other types of concomitant pulmonary arterial hypertension (PAH, group I). In general, pulmonary hypertension in a patient with lung disease is suspected on the basis of echocardiography. It should be remembered that usually clinical symptoms in a patient with lung disease, with and without pulmonary hypertension, cannot be distinguished. Due to the nature of the underlying disease, clinical symptoms do not determine the coexistence of pulmonary hypertension.

35.1.1 RHC in Patients with Suspicion of Type 3 Pulmonary Hypertension

Patients with lung disease and suspicion of severe pulmonary hypertension based on echocardiography, including patients with diagnosed PH where there is a lack of clarity about the appropriateness of the PH-targeted medication, should be referred

M. Grabka (✉)
Ist Department of Cardiology, Upper Silesian Medical Centre, Katowice, Ochojec, Poland

© The Author(s), under exclusive license to Springer Nature Switzerland AG 2025

K. Panda et al. (eds.), *Noninvasive Ventilatory Approaches in Interventional Procedures*, Noninvasive Ventilation. The Essentials,
https://doi.org/10.1007/978-3-032-05328-2_35

to a pulmonary hypertension referral center. It should be remembered that pulmonary hypertension cannot be diagnosed or ruled out on the basis of echocardiography. For this purpose, the only valid diagnostic test to confirm or exclude PH is invasive right heart catheterization. Typically, RHC is performed using a Swan–Ganz catheter. It is a special, usually two-lumen catheter consisting of a proximal and distal canal and an air-filled balloon at the end of the catheter (Fig. 35.1). The catheter makes it possible to measure the pressure in specific heart chambers and cardiac output using thermodilution, as well as calculate pulmonary resistance and obtain the pulmonary capillary wedge pressure. The examination is usually performed via the jugular vein and alternatively via the femoral vein. The examination is safe in the hands of an experienced operator and has a small percentage of possible complications, usually mild. Serious complications such as pulmonary artery damage are very rare (0.03–0.7%). The measurement of the pressure in the inferior or superior vena cava (depending on the vascular access), right atrium, right ventricle, pulmonary artery, and the wedge pressure is the standard (RHC pressure curves are illustrated in Fig. 35.2a–e). The measurements made enable the diagnosis or exclusion of pulmonary hypertension and specify its type.

Despite the limited possibilities of pulmonary hypertension treatment in patients with chronic lung disease, the current ESC guidelines recommend right heart catheterization if there is a high probability that the diagnosis of pulmonary hypertension confirmation in a particular patient will influence treatment decisions (recommendation class IC) [1]. Because the majority of patients with advanced lung disease develop pulmonary hypertension, a discussion about the assessment of pulmonary hypertension severity in these patients is important. The purpose is to select the patients who would obtain the benefits from the administration of PAH treatment drugs. According to the current recommendations from 2022, we categorize pulmonary hypertension related to underlying lung diseases into severe and moderate categories based on the result of pulmonary resistance measured during catheterization. Based on the results of two studies [2, 3], it was established that PVR > 5 is associated with a worse prognosis and suggests consideration of treatment with pulmonary artery-targeted drugs.

The majority of chronic obstructive pulmonary disease (COPD) and interstitial lung disease (ILD) cases, patients developing pulmonary hypertension, fortunately, have a mild form of PH. Only 1–5% of patients have a severe form of the disease

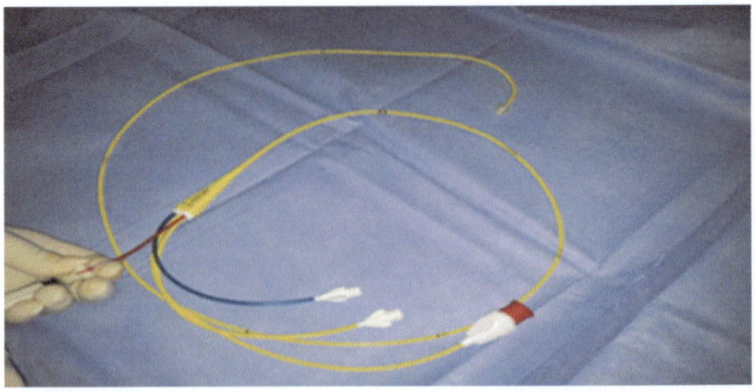

Fig. 35.1 Swan–Ganz catheter

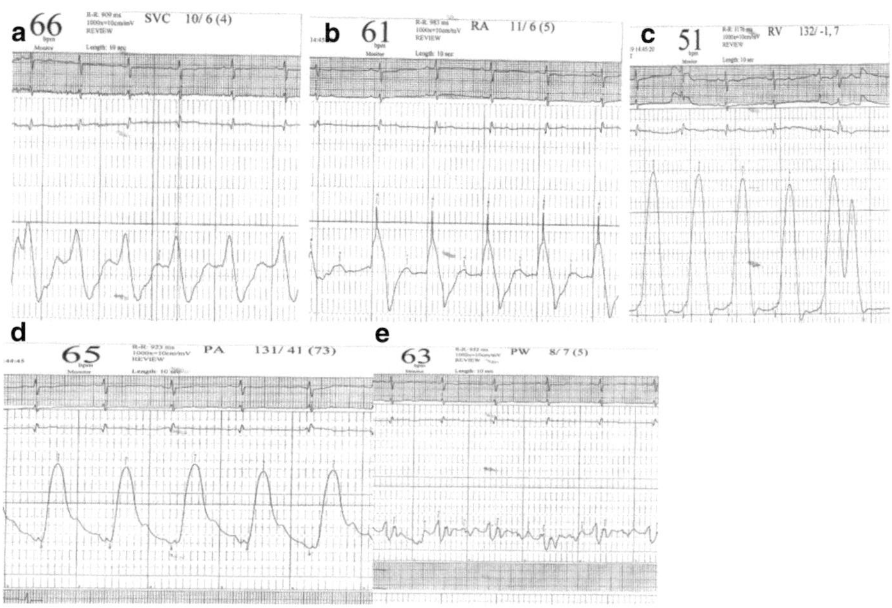

Fig. 35.2 (**a–e**) Pressure curves obtained during RHC : a SVC, b RA, c RV, d PA, e wedge

and may require targeted treatment. While the recommendations from 2015 stated that there were no indications for RHC in the course of lung diseases, apart from exceptional cases, the current recommendations even suggest performing RHC if there are noninvasive features to suspect the effectiveness of pulmonary artery-targeted drugs. Therefore, noninvasive tests assessing the prognosis of a patient with PH and lung disease play a very important role at present, in order to avoid a situation in which we perform an invasive pulmonary circulation test only to confirm the diagnosis in a patient with no chance of targeted PH therapy success. Performing an invasive procedure associated with potential complications without any benefits for the patient's treatment should be avoided. It is important to realize that all targeted drugs for pulmonary hypertension have an ultimate primary mechanism of action of pulmonary arteriolar vasodilation. Therefore, in the case of very advanced interstitial lesions or a significant degree of fibrosis as well as severe airway obstruction, PH targeted treatment probably will not be effective, and also, no benefit from undergoing a diagnostic RHC will be obtained. Moreover, in some cases, progression of hypoxia could be caused by ventilation and perfusion mismatch associated with the intensification of perfusion of fibrotic parts of the lung by vasodilating drugs [4]. Studies of PH-targeted drugs, as well as long-term oxygen therapy in pulmonary hypertension connected with lung diseases, have until now shown variable results and only partial improvement of pulmonary parameters (reduction of mPAP and PVR). Moreover, only partial improvement of some clinical parameters without lasting clinical benefits and without evidence of life prolongation was obtained in clinical trials [5]. In the current guidelines [1], apart from the fact that the inclusion of targeted drugs in these patients is left to the individual decision, the only drug suggested for consideration (recommendation IIb) in the treatment of pulmonary hypertension in the course of lung diseases is the inhaled form of treprostinil. In conclusion, the indications for right heart catheterization in suspected pulmonary hypertension in the course of lung disease are limited to cases where there is a large probability that PH-targeted drugs may bring clinical benefit. Apart from echocardiography, qualification for RHC in patients with lung disease should be based on the assessment of the severity of lung disease in imaging tests and functional assessment (FEV1, FEV1/VC, DLCO). In the case of advanced obstruction or a significantly reduced DLCO, the benefits of RHC will probably be limited. Usually, in a patient treated with NIV, the lung disease is rather advanced, and probably the benefit of RHC performance is so small that it may not outweigh the risks associated with the procedure, despite the quite low procedural risk in general.

35.1.2 RHC in a Patient with Suspected CTEPH (Chronic Thromboembolic Pulmonary Hypertension)

Patients with chronic lung disease and chronic right ventricular failure with abdominal organs, pelvic veins, and lower limbs venous stasis have an increased risk of venous thromboembolism (DVT and PE) [6]. Among patients who have had a pulmonary embolism, 1–5% develop chronic thromboembolic pulmonary hypertension (CTEPH). Surprisingly, approximately 20% of patients with diagnosed CTEPH have no history of symptomatic pulmonary embolism. Type 4 pulmonary hypertension (CTEPH) should always be suspected in a patient with echocardiographic and clinical features of pulmonary hypertension and coexisting post-thrombotic syndrome or a history of deep vein thrombosis. In such patients, before qualifying for RHC, it is worth performing ventilation and perfusion scintigraphy in order to look for a ventilation and perfusion "mismatch." The test has high specificity (90–100%) and similarly high sensitivity in detecting CTEPH (94–100%) [7]. If the mismatch disorders and the presence of echocardiographic and clinical features of pulmonary hypertension are documented, in addition to right heart catheterization, pulmonary arteriography should be performed at the same time, in order to qualify for specific CTEPH treatment. Of course, the decision to perform arteriography should take into consideration the current kidney function. It should be remembered that during this diagnostic procedure, the patient receives a large (usually 200 ml) dose of nephrotoxic contrast agent. Moreover, we should remember that in general patients with CTEPH and chronic right ventricular failure have an increased probability of chronic kidney disease.

35.1.3 RHC in a Patient Qualified for Lung (LTx) or Heart (HTx) Transplantation

Another specific group of patients undergoing RHC is patients with advanced lung/heart disease qualified for transplantation. Right heart catheterization should always be performed in qualifying for transplantation and in order to determine the urgency of transplantation. This examination should be performed on a patient on the LTx/HTx waiting list at least every 12 months to assess the severity of the disease. The criteria for qualifying a patient for an urgent transplant list include: right atrial pressure >15 mm Hg and low cardiac index (<1.8–2 l/min/m^2) [8].

35.1.4 Other Indications for RHC in a Patient with Lung Disease

The rarest group of patients undergoing right-sided catheterization is patients with a coincidence of chronic lung disease requiring NIV treatment and pulmonary arterial hypertension with underlying systemic connective tissue disease, idiopathic pulmonary hypertension (IPAH), or congenital heart disease. Of course, each time, we may deal with patients suspected of any form of pulmonary hypertension listed in the ESC guidelines (Fig. 35.3), initially not suffering from lung disease, but treated with NIV due to secondary changes in the lungs.

35.2 Substantive and Technical Aspects of NIV in a Patient Undergoing Right Heart Catheterization (RHC)

Noninvasive ventilation by generating high pressure in the airways and thus in the chest reduces venous return and preload of the right ventricle but also contributes to increasing pulmonary resistance. It also reduces left ventricular afterload and thus can increase cardiac output in left ventricular failure, while the reduction in preload can reduce output in a normally functioning ventricle. From the respiratory point of view, NIV increases alveolar recruitment and residual tidal volume by reducing respiratory effort and increasing oxygenation. These mechanisms collectively lead to the anti-edematous effect of this form of oxygen therapy, which, avoiding endotracheal intubation, is used in the treatment of acute left ventricular failure [9] and may also be used in the treatment of post-reperfusion pulmonary oedema, which can rarely be a complication of pulmonary artery angioplasty [10]. It is important to remember the existing contraindications to NIV. These include cardiac arrest, anatomical obstructions within the craniofacial and oral cavity, some mental disorders, poor treatment tolerance, bleeding from the upper gastrointestinal tract, vomiting, or recent surgery of the upper gastrointestinal or upper respiratory tract.

From the physiology of NIV point of view, this method is relatively contraindicated in isolated acute right ventricular failure. In such a case, NIV-induced decrease in right ventricular preload and increase in pulmonary resistance may exacerbate RV failure. The same properties of NIV can be used in chronic right ventricular

Fig. 35.3 Clinical classification of pulmonary hypertension

GROUP 1 Pulmonary arterial hypertension (PAH)
- 1.1 Idiopathic
  - 1.1.1 Non-responders at vasoreactivity testing
  - 1.1.2 Acute responders at vasoreactivity testing
- 1.2 Heritable[a]
- 1.3 Associated with drugs and toxins[a]
- 1.4 Associated with:
  - 1.4.1 Connective tissue disease
  - 1.4.2 HIV infection
  - 1.4.3 Portal hypertension
  - 1.4.4 Congenital heart disease
  - 1.4.5 Schistosomiasis
- 1.5 PAH with features of venous/capillary (PVOD/PCH) involvement
- 1.6 Persistent PH of the newborn

GROUP 2 PH associated with left heart disease
- 2.1 Heart failure:
  - 2.1.1 with preserved ejection fraction
  - 2.1.2 with reduced or mildly reduced ejection fraction[b]
- 2.2 Valvular heart disease
- 2.3 Congenital/acquired cardiovascular conditions leading to post-capillary PH

GROUP 3 PH associated with lung diseases and/or hypoxia
- 3.1 Obstructive lung disease or emphysema
- 3.2 Restrictive lung disease
- 3.3 Lung disease with mixed restrictive/obstructive pattern
- 3.4 Hypoventilation syndromes
- 3.5 Hypoxia without lung disease (e.g. high altitude)
- 3.6 Developmental lung disorders

GROUP 4 PH associated with pulmonary artery obstructions
- 4.1 Chronic thrombo-embolic PH
- 4.2 Other pulmonary artery obstructions[c]

GROUP 5 PH with unclear and/or multifactorial mechanisms
- 5.1 Haematological disorders[d]
- 5.2 Systemic disorders[e]
- 5.3 Metabolic disorders[f]
- 5.4 Chronic renal failure with or without haemodialysis
- 5.5 Pulmonary tumour thrombotic microangiopathy
- 5.6 Fibrosing mediastinitis

failure, where careful application of positive airway pressure leads to decompression of the overloaded right ventricle by lowering the preload. Device settings should be determined by the patient's condition and not by the fact of performing an invasive test. The effect of positive pressure in the chest generated by NIV on pulmonary parameters (decreased cardiac output, increased pulmonary resistance) should be taken into consideration during the RHC procedure. However, these changes have not been quantitatively validated so far, and it should be remembered that changes in the pulmonary circulation parameters due to NIV can be variable among individuals.

35.3 Summary

In conclusion to this chapter, it should be noted that among patients who are qualified for RHC, NIV patients are rather rare. Each case of a NIV patient qualified for RHC should be considered in terms of the benefits of the procedure and the impact of its results on the patient's treatment. In my opinion, patients with end-stage respiratory failure will not benefit from RHC, and the main beneficiaries of RHC may be patients with mild or moderate lung disease.

References

1. Humbert M, et al. 2022 ESC/ERS Guidelines for the diagnosis and treatment of pulmonary hypertension. Eur Heart J. 2022;43(38):3618–731.
2. Zeder K, Avian A, Bachmaier G, Douschan P, Foris V, Sassmann T, et al. Elevated pulmonary vascular resistance predicts mortality in COPD patients. Eur Respir J. 2021;58:2100944.
3. Olsson KM, Hoeper MM, Pausch C, Grunig E, Huscher D, Pittrow D, et al. Pulmonary vascular resistance predicts mortality in patients with pulmonary hyper-tension associated with interstitial lung disease: results from the COMPERA registry. Eur Respir J. 2021;58:2101483.
4. Andersen CU, et al. Pulmonary hypertension in chronic obstructive and interstitial lung diseases. Int J Cardiol. 2013;168(3):1795–804.
5. Arif R, et al. Treatment of pulmonary hypertension associated with COPD:a systematic review. ERJ Open Res. 2022;8:00348–2021.
6. Xiaofang F, et al. The prevalence and clinical features of pulmonary embolism in patients with AE- COPD: a meta-analysis and systematic review. PLoS One. 2021; https://doi.org/10.1371/journal.pone.0256480.
7. Florczyk M, et al. Pulmonary hypertension in contemporary imaging. Expert consensus statement of the polish clinical forum for cardiovascular imaging. Kardiol Pol. 2014;72(1):89–106.
8. Mularek-Kubzdela T, et al. Lung transplantation in patients with pulmonary arterial hypertension: the opinion of the Polish Cardiac Society Working Group on Pulmonary Circulation. Polish Cardiac Society J. 2022;
9. Masip J, et al. Indications and practical approach to non-invasive ventilation in acute heart failure. Eur Heart J. 2018;39:17–25.
10. Moriyama K, et al. Noninvasive positive pressure ventilation against reperfusion pulmonary edema following percutaneous transluminal pulmonary angioplasty. Case Rep Anesthesiol. 2011;2011:204538.

Noninvasive Mechanical Ventilation (NIV) in Valvular Heart Disease and Left Atrial Occlusion Procedures

36

Fallon France, Daniel Rubinger, Ravie Abozaid, and Kunal Panda

36.1 Introduction

Patients with heart failure due to valvular heart disease undergoing cardiac procedures represent a medically challenging patient population with special considerations. Often, these are patients who require an essential procedure but are deemed high-risk candidates for anesthesia. Some patients may even appear to have normal functional status preoperatively, but they can decompensate quickly with sedation. Noninvasive ventilation (NIV) can be used in these cases to support both the cardiac and respiratory status of the patient. This chapter will discuss the physiology of positive airway pressure as it relates to heart failure patients, the advantages and disadvantages of NIV, and the evidence behind the use of NIV during some common transcatheter cardiology procedures.

36.2 Physiology of Positive Airway Pressure in Patients with Valvular Heart Disease

The cardiovascular and pulmonary systems are highly integrated; therefore, it is important to consider the effects of ventilation on the underlying cardiovascular physiology. When positive airway pressure is applied by way of NIV, multiple physiologic changes occur. Both the right ventricle (RV) and pulmonary capillaries are compressed, leading to increases in RV afterload and pulmonary vascular resistance (PVR), while the increased intrathoracic pressure will also result in decreased

F. France · D. Rubinger · R. Abozaid · K. Panda (✉)
Department of Anesthesiology & Perioperative Medicine, University of Rochester School of Medicine & Dentistry, Rochester, NY, USA
e-mail: fallon_france@urmc.rochester.edu; daniel_rubinger@urmc.rochester.edu; Ravie_abozaid@urmc.rochester.edu; kunal_panda@urmc.rochester.edu

© The Author(s), under exclusive license to Springer Nature Switzerland AG 2025

K. Panda et al. (eds.), *Noninvasive Ventilatory Approaches in Interventional Procedures*, Noninvasive Ventilation. The Essentials,
https://doi.org/10.1007/978-3-032-05328-2_36

venous return and preload. On the other hand, in the setting of pulmonary edema or atelectasis, NIV can increase lung recruitment and thereby reduce PVR. In addition, the positive pleural pressure also causes compression of the left ventricle (LV). This increase in transmural pressure can increase cardiac output. Unlike the increase in RV afterload, LV afterload is decreased by activation of the baroreceptor reflex in response to increased aortic pressure [1]. Therefore, the overall hemodynamic effects of NIV are dependent on whether the type of heart failure is preload or afterload-dependent. NIV can reduce cardiac output in preload-dependent states, while increasing it in afterload-dependent states [2].

The left ventricle is particularly susceptible to ischemia in patients with aortic stenosis (AS), which can reduce cardiac output. The bottleneck effect of the stenotic valve, causing increased pressure in the left ventricle with decreased pressure in the aortic root, leads to low coronary perfusion pressure [3]. General anesthesia or procedural sedation can lead to hypotension and compensatory tachycardia. Hypotension further reduces coronary perfusion pressure while tachycardia increases myocardial oxygen demand. Critical aortic stenosis is dependent on the atrial kick for diastolic filling of the stiff, hypertrophied left ventricle; therefore, it is important to maintain sinus rhythm and avoid hypovolemia in such patients to optimize preload [4]. NIV can allow procedural sedation in patients with AS while reducing the untoward effects of hypoventilation. However, NIV can reduce preload in these preload-dependent patients, which has to be balanced against the potential respiratory benefits in individual patients.

The LV diastolic volume is increased in aortic regurgitation (AR), leading to LV dilation over time, which compromises LV ejection. Significant AR also leads to an increase in left atrial pressure and pulmonary edema. Faster heart rates are ideal to limit the time in diastole, which allows for forward flow and reduces backflow through the aortic valve. Reductions in SVR also encourage forward flow. NIV support is therefore well-suited in these patients due to the decrease in preload and afterload it provides [5].

In mitral regurgitation (MR), the left atrium receives increased volume and pressure. Over time, the pulmonary artery pressures can increase, causing eventual right heart failure. The LV has chronic increased work due to larger volumes, which can eventually lead to LV failure. The most important hemodynamic goal for patients with MR is to maintain forward flow. Additionally, the regurgitant volume can be decreased with higher heart rates to shorten back flow during systole, and decreased systemic vascular resistance due to anesthetic agents will promote forward flow [5]. Patients with severe mitral regurgitation (MR) have high preload and are typically afterload dependent. Similarly to patients with AR, NIV can provide respiratory support in these patients with pulmonary edema and can reduce preload and afterload, thereby improving cardiac output [6].

36.3 Transcatheter Aortic Valve Replacement—TAVR

An alternative for patients who are considered high risk for surgical valve replacement is a transcatheter aortic valve replacement (TAVR). Approved for use by the US FDA in 2012, the number of TAVR procedures performed annually has exceeded surgical aortic valve replacement since 2017. While initially established for native valve aortic stenosis, TAVR procedures are now increasingly being used in aortic regurgitation, as well as valve-in-valve reoperation procedures for prior bioprosthetic surgical or previous TAVR valves. Interestingly, while the first TAVR procedure in 2002 was performed with mild sedation and noninvasive ventilation, subsequent TAVR procedures were primarily performed under general anesthesia. Advantages of general anesthesia include allowing for TEE placement, prevention of patient movement, and improved device deployment, thereby decreasing complication risks of paravalvular leak and valve malpositioning [7]. However, as operators obtained more experience with the procedure and sheath delivery systems became smaller, TAVR procedures have shifted to being performed under local anesthesia with sedation. In the STS-ACC TVT TAVR Registry [8], the amount of TAVRs performed under sedation has increased from 5.1% in 2014 to 33% in 2016 and 64% in 2019.

The STS-ACC TVT TAVR registry found that conscious sedation was associated with lower 30-day mortality, decreased length of stay, and fewer inotropic drugs compared to general anesthesia. Similarly, a recent meta-analysis of 14,388 patients demonstrated an improvement in mortality, stroke, or major vascular complication without any difference in paravalvular leak in patients with conscious sedation compared to general anesthesia [9]. One of the landmark randomized trials called the SOLVE-TAVI (Comparison of Second-Generation Self-Expandable Versus Balloon-Expandable Valves and General Versus Local Anesthesia in TAVI) trial demonstrated no difference in composite endpoint of mortality, stroke, myocardial infarction, infection requiring antibiotic treatment, and acute kidney injury at 30 days but showed a reduction in the use of inotropes and vasopressors in the conscious sedation group [10].

A cohort of patients that may benefit from NIV during sedation for TAVR procedures includes those with underlying pulmonary disease such as COPD or interstitial lung disease and those with orthopnea or pulmonary edema from aortic valve disease. A case series demonstrated the safety of performing TAVR with patients undergoing sedation assisted with NIV in four patients with pulmonary fibrosis and one patient with silicosis [11]. When TEE guidance is deemed necessary for TAVR procedures, NIV has been used successfully to avoid endotracheal intubation [12].

36.4 Percutaneous Left Atrial Appendage Closure

A percutaneous left atrial appendage occlusion (LAAO) device acts to close off the LAA to decrease clot formation and subsequently reduce a patient's stroke risk. Stroke is a very common cardiovascular event, and it is estimated that atrial fibrillation increases the stroke risk fivefold [13]. Patients with atrial fibrillation can decrease thromboembolic complications with vitamin K antagonists or other anticoagulants. In those intolerant of anticoagulation due to bleeding risk, LAAO offers an alternative to decrease stroke risk. These can be placed percutaneously via transseptal puncture. One such device, the WATCHMAN™ Implant (Boston Scientific, USA), was approved for use in Europe in 2005 and by the FDA in 2015.

For WATCHMAN™ placement, general anesthesia has typically been utilized to ensure the patient remains still during deployment into the LAA. Additionally, TEE is often utilized throughout the procedure to guide placement. Chan et al. [14] demonstrated the safety and efficacy of placing the WATCHMAN™ as well as another LAA occlusion device under conscious sedation with midazolam and fentanyl. Zangrillo et al. [15] published a preliminary case series of three patients where the WATCHMAN™ was placed under deep sedation. This group utilized a Janus mask for noninvasive ventilation, which is a specialized full-face mask with a dedicated endoscope port that enables TEE placement in non-intubated patients [16]. The authors maintained conscious sedation with a combination of midazolam, propofol, and remifentanil. The LAA occlusion procedures were all successful and had no complications. However, in one of the cases, the echocardiographer noted that the initial placement of the TEE probe was difficult. In a follow-up retrospective case-controlled study in 2019, Zangrillo et al. [17] compared deep sedation with a Janus mask against general anesthesia. There was a high degree of surgeon and anesthesiologist satisfaction in both cohorts. The authors conclude that sedation with NIV is a viable alternative to general anesthesia for the WATCHMAN™ procedure.

More recently, Kleinecke et al. [18] published a cohort study that compared 196 patients undergoing conscious sedation with midazolam and propofol with 115 patients undergoing general anesthesia for WATCHMAN™ placement. The conscious sedation group had a lower number of implantation attempts, less use of contrast media, and shorter procedure and fluoroscopy times. Five cases undergoing conscious sedation had to be converted to general anesthesia, due to either LAA perforation (one), aspiration (one), or acute respiratory failure (three). The authors conclude that both techniques are safe and effective, with the sedation group requiring shorter postoperative monitoring and fewer resources.

36.5 Percutaneous Mitral Valve Repair—MitraClip

Transcatheter edge-to-edge repair (TEER) with MitraClip™ (Abbot, Wetzlar, Germany) is a recently introduced technique for the treatment of severe MR. It is especially attractive in high-risk patients, as cardiopulmonary bypass, sternotomy, bleeding, and tissue trauma may be avoided [19, 20]. A major concern after mitral valve surgery is increased left ventricular afterload following elimination of the low-impedance regurgitant pathway into the left atrium; this may result in impaired left ventricular systolic performance and low cardiac output. Patients with MR also have varying degrees of pulmonary hypertension and increased pulmonary vascular resistance, a major risk factor for mortality and worse outcomes after both cardiac and noncardiac surgery [21].

The MitraClip™ procedure is most often conducted under general anesthesia with mechanical ventilation of the lungs. However, data on the acute hemodynamic consequences of the MitraClip™ procedure during anesthesia are scarce [22, 23] and, to our knowledge, have not been reported to date. A recent retrospective study compared conscious sedation using remifentanil and dexmedetomidine with general anesthesia and found that the conscious sedation group utilized less vasopressors and had higher mean arterial pressures [24].

36.6 Percutaneous Mitral Valve Replacement

Transcatheter mitral valve replacement (TMVR) is a new approach that avoids surgical mitral valve replacement and avoids risks of cardiopulmonary bypass, sternotomy, and bleeding, as the other minimally invasive approaches to valve repairs and replacements. Much of the data regarding TMVR procedures is case studies as this procedure is not yet part of common clinical practice. For example, in 2019, 1120 TMVRs were done at 301 centers across the United States compared with 10,460 transcatheter mitral valve repairs during that same year [25]. In a case series published by Cubeddu et al. [26], TMVRs were done under sedation using intracardiac echocardiography, which they referred to as a "minimalist approach" since one of their objectives was to avoid TEE. There have been reports of using sedation for MVR, but data are limited regarding NIV for these procedures, as this is a novel procedure.

36.7 Conclusion

1. Patients with heart failure due to valvular heart disease are particularly sensitive to the effects of general anesthesia; therefore, it is appropriate to find alternative methods of sedation to facilitate transcatheter cardiac procedures.
2. Procedures including TAVR, percutaneous LAA closures, percutaneous TEER, and MVR are becoming increasingly common as an alternative to surgical replacement in high-risk patients.
3. NIV can allow these procedures to be performed safely under sedation in high-risk patients with poor cardiopulmonary reserve.
4. Reduction in preload and afterload associated with NIV is particularly beneficial in patients with significant mitral or aortic regurgitation and can improve cardiac output in these patients.

References

1. Alviar CL, Miller PE, McAreavey D, Katz JN, Lee B, Moriyama B, Soble J, van Diepen S, Solomon MA, Morrow DA. Positive pressure ventilation in the cardiac intensive care unit. J Am Coll Cardiol. 2018;72(13):1532–53.
2. Hieda M. Noninvasive positive pressure ventilation for acute decompensated heart failure. Heart Fail Clin. 2020;16(3):271–82.
3. Hensley FA, Martin DE, Gravlee GP. A practical approach to cardiac anesthesia. Lippincott Williams & Wilkins; 2012.
4. Horak JWS. Emergent management of the airway. New pharmacology and the control of comorbidities in cardiac disease, ischemia, and valvular heart disease. Crit Care Clin. 2000;16(3):411–27.
5. Abhijit Paul SD. Valvular heart disease and anaesthesia. Indian J Anaesth. 2017;61(9):721–7.
6. Bellone A, Barbieri A, Ricci C, Iori E, Donateo M, Massobrio M, et al. Acute effects of non-invasive ventilatory support on functional mitral regurgitation in patients with exacerbation of congestive heart failure. Intensive Care Med. 2002;28(9):1348–50.
7. Guarracino F, Covello RD, Landoni G, Baldassarri R, Stefani M, Cariello C, et al. Anesthetic management of transcatheter aortic valve implantation with transaxillary approach. J Cardiothorac Vasc Anesth. 2011;25(3):437–43.
8. Carroll JD, Mack MJ, Vemulapalli S, Herrmann HC, Gleason TG, Hanzel G, et al. STS-ACC TVT registry of Transcatheter aortic valve replacement. J Am Coll Cardiol. 2020;76(21):2492–516.
9. Ahmed A, Mathew DM, Mathew SM, Awad AK, Varghese KS, Khaja S, et al. General anesthesia versus local anesthesia in patients undergoing Transcatheter aortic valve replacement: an updated meta-analysis and systematic review. J Cardiothorac Vasc Anesth. 2023;37(8):1358–67.
10. Thiele H, Kurz T, Feistritzer HJ, Stachel G, Hartung P, Lurz P, et al. General versus local anesthesia with conscious sedation in Transcatheter aortic valve implantation: the randomized SOLVE-TAVI trial. Circulation. 2020;142(15):1437–47.
11. Guarracino F, Cabrini L, Baldassarri R, Petronio S, De Carlo M, Covello RD, et al. Noninvasive ventilation for awake percutaneous aortic valve implantation in high-risk respiratory patients: a case series. J Cardiothorac Vasc Anesth. 2011;25(6):1109–12.
12. Pieri M, Landoni G, Cabrini L. Noninvasive ventilation during endoscopic procedures: rationale, clinical use, and devices. J Cardiothorac Vasc Anesth. 2018;32(2):928–34.
13. Vahanian A, Beyersdorf F, Praz F, Milojevic M, Baldus S, Bauersachs J, et al. 2021 ESC/EACTS guidelines for the management of valvular heart disease: developed by the task force for the management of valvular heart disease of the European Society of Cardiology (ESC) and the European Association for Cardio-Thoracic Surgery (EACTS). Eur Heart J. 2021;43(7):561–632.
14. Chan NY, Lau CL, Tsui PT, Lo YK, Mok NS. Experience of left atrial appendage closure performed under conscious sedation. Asian Cardiovasc Thorac Ann. 2015;23(4):394–8.
15. Zangrillo A, Mazzone P, Votta CD, Villari N, Della Bella P, Monaco F. Prolonged transesophageal echocardiography during percutaneous closure of the left atrial appendage without general anesthesia: the utility of the Janus mask. Can J Anaesth. 2016;63(8):962–5.
16. Cabrini L, Landoni G. A novel non-invasive ventilation mask to prevent and manage respiratory failure during fiberoptic bronchoscopy, gastroscopy and transesophageal echocardiography. Heart Lung Vessel. 2015;7(4):297–303.
17. Zangrillo A, Mazzone P, Oriani A, Pieri M, Frau G, D'Angelo G, et al. Noninvasive ventilation during left atrial appendage closure under sedation: preliminary experience with the Janus mask. Ann Card Anaesth. 2019;22(4):400–6.
18. Kleinecke C, Allakkis W, Buffle E, Liu X-X, Mohrez Y, Gloekler S, et al. Impact of conscious sedation and general anesthesia on periprocedural outcomes in Watchman left atrial appendage closure. Cardiol J. 2021;28(4):519–27.

19. Franzen O, van der Heyden J, Baldus S, Schlüter M, Schillinger W, Butter C, et al. MitraClip® therapy in patients with end-stage systolic heart failure. Eur J Heart Fail. 2011;13(5):569–76.
20. Feldman T, Foster E, Glower DD, Kar S, Rinaldi MJ, Fail PS, et al. Percutaneous repair or surgery for mitral regurgitation. N Engl J Med. 2011;364(15):1395–406.
21. Kottenberg E, Dumont M, Frey UH, Heine T, Plicht B, Kahlert P, et al. The minimally invasive MitraClip™ procedure for mitral regurgitation under general anaesthesia: immediate effects on the pulmonary circulation and right ventricular function. Anaesthesia. 2014;69(8):860–7.
22. Siegel RJ, Biner S, Rafique AM, Rinaldi M, Lim S, Fail P, et al. The acute hemodynamic effects of MitraClip therapy. J Am Coll Cardiol. 2011;57(16):1658–65.
23. Biner S, Siegel RJ, Feldman T, Rafique AM, Trento A, Whitlow P, et al. Acute effect of percutaneous MitraClip therapy in patients with haemodynamic decompensation. Eur J Heart Fail. 2012;14(8):939–45.
24. Berger C, Said E, Haller K, Nordine M, Reinthaler M, Landmesser U, et al. Dexmedetomidine sedation combined with remifentanil in MitraClip procedures is feasible and improves hemodynamics. J Cardiothorac Vasc Anesth. 2023;37(1):50–7.
25. Mack M, Carroll JD, Thourani V, Vemulapalli S, Squiers J, Manandhar P, Deeb GM, Batchelor W, Herrmann HC, Cohen DJ, Hanzel G, Gleason T, Kirtane A, Desai N, Guibone K, Hardy K, Michaels J, DiMaio JM, Christensen B, Fitzgerald S, Krohn C, Brindis RG, Masoudi F, Bavaria J. Transcatheter mitral valve therapy in the United States: a report from the STS/ACC TVT registry. Ann Thorac Surg. 2022;113(1):337–65.
26. Cubeddu RJ, Sarkar A, Navas V, Navia JL. 'Minimalist approach' for transcatheter mitral valve replacement using intracardiac echocardiography and conscious sedation: a case series. Eur Heart J Case Rep. 2020;4(3):1–5.

NIV Tube Adaptor for Nasogastric Enteral Nutrition

37

María Paula Garcia-Garcia, Oscar Ivan Quintero, and Antonio M. Esquinas

37.1 Nutrition in Noninvasive Ventilation Nutrition

37.1.1 Overview

Treating respiratory distress is a priority in acute respiratory failure patients, making nutrition a challenging aspect of critically ill patients' treatment. Noninvasive ventilation (NIV) is increasingly used as a tool to prevent endotracheal intubation. However, patients are frequently denied or delayed adequate nutritional support, given that providing either oral or enteral nutrition has been perceived as unsafe during NIV due to the increased risk of aspiration [1].

Current international nutrition guidelines include recommendations for the nutrition management of critically ill patients with invasive mechanical ventilation, including nutrition risk screening, initiation and mode of nutrition delivery, energy and protein targets, and formula composition. Nevertheless, guidelines on nutrition management in noninvasive ventilation (NIV) are nonexistent [2–5], and applicability of existing nutrition guidelines in invasive mechanical ventilation is debatable in this scenario.

Only one literature review has been published on the nutrition management of critically ill adult patients requiring NIV. Sixteen studies were identified, with no consensus on the route of nutrition and none addressing the barriers to adequate nutrition provision [6]. However, identified challenges in nutrition management in NIV patients included NIV interruption while providing oral nutrition, high costs and risk of infection in parenteral nutrition (PN), and air leakages due to physical

M. P. Garcia-Garcia (✉) · O. I. Quintero
Centro de Investigaciones Clínicas, Fundación Valle del Lili, Cali, Colombia

A. M. Esquinas
Unidad de Cuidado Intensivo, Hospital Morales Meseguer, Murcia, Spain

© The Author(s), under exclusive license to Springer Nature Switzerland AG 2025

K. Panda et al. (eds.), *Noninvasive Ventilatory Approaches in Interventional Procedures*, Noninvasive Ventilation. The Essentials,
https://doi.org/10.1007/978-3-032-05328-2_37

interference of a nasogastric tube (NGT) with the use of NIV mask. Ultimately, all types of nutrition compromise patients' respiratory function [6].

Similarly, NIV is increasingly used in the support of acute respiratory failure in critically ill pediatric patients admitted to the intensive care unit (ICU). One of the major challenges in pediatric NIV is finding an optimal fitting mask that limits air leakage, patient discomfort, and patient-ventilator asynchrony, in particular for younger children and those with facial anomalies [3]. Such complications contribute to NIV treatment failure in up to 30% of pediatric cases [4, 5]. Commercially available masks limit their usage given that they do not appropriately take into account the large variation in face shapes and sizes throughout childhood development or those with specific facial features due to genetic syndromes [3, 6].

Personalizing a mask by 3D scanning and printing techniques, based on age-related 3D anthropometric data, holds a promising future to reduce air leakage and hence improve pediatric NIV effectiveness [7–9]. Recently, it was described the successful use of a simple anesthetic (nose–mouth) mask for NIV in a 4-year-old child with specific facial features admitted to the pediatric ICU for acute hypoxic respiratory failure [10]. This anesthetic mask is connected to a 5-point headgear using an in-house developed, 3D-printed reusable quick-release adaptor. As it comes in several sizes and has demonstrated lower air leakage at various positive pressure levels when compared with a commercially available pediatric NIV mask, this innovative mask may serve as an effective and less costly alternative to commercially available NIV pediatric masks.

It is well known that NIV and enteral nutrition prevent starvation, malnutrition, dehydration, pneumonia, and hypoxia and in turn increase survival and patients' quality of life and alleviate symptoms of respiratory insufficiency. Nevertheless, it has been described that the majority of ICU patients do not receive nutritional support upon admission. A French observational study estimated that approximately 60% of NIV patients are starved during the first 2 days of treatment [11].

Moreover, pulmonary diseases are selectively treated by inhaled drugs. Interruption of NIV to administer aerosol therapy is associated with adverse effects for the patient. Technically, NIV impairs aerosol therapy and oral and enteral feeding.

Whether early enteral nutrition should be provided in these patients or not remains controversial, due to its association with airway complications, longer duration of NIV, and hospitalization stay. This chapter will focus on enteral nutrition and NIV.

37.1.2 Strategies for Providing Nutrition in Noninvasive Ventilation

Over the years, clinicians have used different strategies to overcome the increased risk of air leaks when using feeding tubes and NIV concomitantly; some of these strategies include the following:

1. Strapping the mask tighter. But this can deform and block the feeding tube and could lead to skin lesions.
2. Passing the feeding tube (or tubes) through an existing port in the mask. However, tubes must be withdrawn each time the interface is required to be removed, which is not ideal for the patient [12].
3. During the COVID-19 pandemic, Renato Favero created the "Charlotte valve," a 3D printed piece of bioplastic. The valve enables the transformation of a cheap snorkeling mask into a new total face mask, allowing the provision of continuous NIV to a greater number of patients. The new 3D printed valve allows the connection of a simple-branch circuit on one side and the passage of NGT on the other side. Thus, NIV could be carried on for long periods of time concomitantly with continuous enteral feeding, without any additional air leaks. The new snorkeling mask, specially equipped with a 3D printed valve, enables the connection of the simple-branch circuit of the ventilator on the right side and the air-proof passage of a nasogastric feeding tube on the other side [13].

Development of special NIV masks with a port for NGT is often complex to set up, costly, and consequently unavailable in all clinical scenarios [1, 14].

A new tube and inhaler adaptor for NIV (TIA-NIV) was developed from the need for a NIV mask design that acted as one system, aiming to allow simultaneously enteral tube placement while on NIV, by improving the adjustment of the mask, while preventing one of NIV's major complications, interface leakage [15, 16]. Its design creates an interface between the ventilator circuit and the NIV mask. The proximal part corresponds to the oro-nasal mask end, while the distal end contains two openings that allow the passage of up to two enteric tubes at the same time with different diameters.

In addition, given that patients with acute respiratory distress and NIV often require aerosol therapy, a metered-dose inhaler port (MDIP) for medication delivery was incorporated on top of the main body of the adaptor, in order to allow adequate aerosol delivery (Fig. 37.1).

The initial TIA-NIV prototype has proven in studies to improve NIV support effectiveness by significantly reducing air leaks, in addition to ameliorating patients' subjective comfort (19). Furthermore, this adapter has shown potential use in difficult airway in post-extubation failure by creating an adequate mask seal while maintaining an airway exchange catheter in place, providing practicality in the intensive care unit [15].

Moreover, the TIA-NIV could potentially reduce skin lesions associated with the use of enteric tubes and oro-nasal masks and be used as part of the 3D anthropometric masks in pediatrics, reducing air leaks, ensuring successful ventilation, and feeding.

This TIA-NIV is a low-cost, easy-to-use device that has been shown to solve therapeutic problems in the clinical setting. However, more studies are needed to further evaluate the clinical impact of TIA-NIV in acute respiratory failure patient's management.

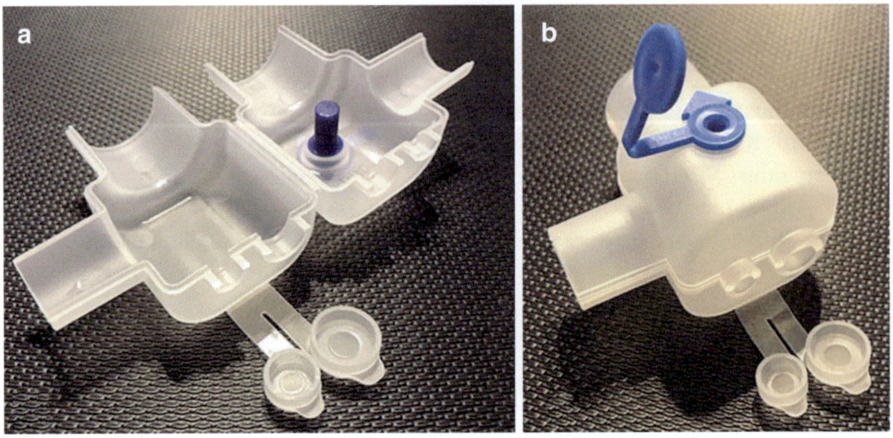

Fig. 37.1 (**a**) TIA-NIV opened. (**b**) Closed TIA-NIV with opened MDIP and enteral feeding ports

37.2 Summary

The integration of nutritional support in patients undergoing noninvasive ventilation (NIV) remains a significant clinical challenge, largely due to the perceived risk of aspiration and technical difficulties associated with delivering enteral nutrition concurrently with respiratory support. While comprehensive guidelines exist for nutrition in invasively ventilated patients, there is a striking absence of equivalent recommendations for those on NIV. Current evidence, drawn from limited studies, highlights inconsistent practices, with no consensus on the safest or most effective route of nutritional delivery.

Critically ill adults and pediatric patients treated with NIV frequently experience delayed or inadequate nutritional intake, often leading to malnutrition, prolonged hospital stays, and increased morbidity. Pediatric NIV poses unique challenges due to the variability in facial anatomy and the limitations of commercially available masks, which contribute to significant air leakage, poor mask fit, and patient-ventilator asynchrony. Emerging 3D printing technologies and personalized masks show promise in overcoming these limitations by enhancing mask fit and comfort.

In both adult and pediatric populations, multiple innovative strategies have been explored to mitigate the interaction between feeding systems and NIV interfaces. These include modifying existing NIV masks with ports for nasogastric tubes, utilizing 3D-printed adapters like the Charlotte valve for integrated feeding and ventilation, and the development of specialized multi-functional interfaces such as the Tube and Inhaler Adapter for NIV (TIA-NIV). The TIA-NIV device enables simultaneous enteral feeding and aerosol medication delivery without compromising ventilatory support, significantly reducing air leakage and improving patient comfort.

Despite these technological advances, most ICU patients on NIV remain undernourished, with observational data suggesting that up to 60% receive no nutritional support in the first 48 hours. Therefore, further research is required to evaluate the safety, efficacy, and clinical outcomes of innovative NIV-nutrition integration tools. Personalized interface designs, especially for pediatric populations, and low-cost adaptable systems like the TIA-NIV adapter, represent a promising direction toward optimizing both ventilation and nutritional support in this vulnerable patient population.

References

1. Singer P, Rattanachaiwong S. To eat or to breathe? The answer is both! Nutritional management during noninvasive ventilation. Crit Care. 2018;22(1):27. https://doi.org/10.1186/s13054-018-1947-7.
2. Viner Smith E, Ridley EJ, Rayner CK, Chapple LS. Nutrition management for critically ill adult patients requiring non-invasive ventilation: a scoping review. Nutrients. 2022;14(7):1446. https://doi.org/10.3390/nu14071446.
3. Hovenier R, Goto L, Huysmans T, van Gestel M, Klein-Blommert R, Markhorst D, Dijkman C, Bem RA. Reduced air leakage during non-invasive ventilation using a simple anesthetic mask with 3D-printed adaptor in an anthropometric based pediatric head-lung model. Front Pediatr. 2022;10:873426. https://doi.org/10.3389/fped.2022.873426.
4. Lopez J, Pons-Odena M, Medina A, Molinos-Norniella C, Palanca-Arias D, Demirkol D, et al. Early factors related to mortality in children treated with bi-level noninvasive ventilation and CPAP. Pediatr Pulmonol. 2021;56:1237–44. https://doi.org/10.1002/ppul.25246.
5. Mayordomo-Colunga J, Medina A, Rey C, Diaz JJ, Concha A, Los Arcos M, et al. Predictive factors of non-invasive ventilation failure in critically ill children: a prospective epidemiological study. Intensive Care Med. 2009;35:527–36. https://doi.org/10.1007/s00134-008-1346-7.
6. Barker N, Willox M, Elphick HE. A review of the benefits, challenges, and the future for interfaces for long term non-invasive ventilation in children. Int J Resp Pulm Med. 2018;5:23937. https://doi.org/10.23937/2378-3516/1410077.
7. Wu YY, Acharya D, Xu C, Cheng B, Rana S, Shimada K. Custom-fit three- dimensional-printed BiPAP mask to improve compliance in patients requiring long-term noninvasive ventilatory support. J Med Device. 2018;12:0310031–8. https://doi.org/10.1115/1.4040187.
8. Amirav I, Luder AS, Halamish A, Raviv D, Kimmel R, Waisman D, et al. Design of aerosol face masks for children using computerized 3D face analysis. J Aerosol Med Pulm Drug Deliv. 2013;26:1–7. https://doi.org/10.1089/jamp.2013.1069.
9. Shikama M, Nakagami G, Noguchi H, Mori T, Sanada H. Development of personalized fitting device with 3-dimensional solution for prevention of NIV oronasal mask-related pressure ulcers. Respir Care. 2018;63:1024–32. https://doi.org/10.4187/respcare.05691.
10. Muller GJ, Hovenier R, Spijker J, van Gestel M, Klein-Blommert R, Markhorst D, et al. Non-invasive ventilation for pediatric hypoxic acute respiratory failure using a simple anesthetic mask with 3D printed adaptor: a case report. Front Pediatr. 2021;9:710829. https://doi.org/10.3389/fped.2021.710829.
11. Terzi N, Darmon M, Reignier J, Ruckly S, Garrouste-Orgeas M, Lautrette A, et al. Initial nutritional management during noninvasive ventilation and outcomes: a retrospective cohort study. Crit Care. 2017.; Epub ahead of publication;21:293.
12. Otero DP, Domínguez DV, Fernández LH, Magariño AS, González VJ, Klepzing JV, Montesinos JV. Preventing facial pressure ulcers in patients under non-invasive mechanical ventilation: a randomised control trial. J Wound Care. 2017;26(3):128–36. https://doi.org/10.12968/jowc.2017.26.3.128. PMID: 28277990
13. Lemyze M, Mascot M, Orfi A. Enteral feeding and non-invasive ventilation during the COVID-19 crisis: a new snorkeling mask specially fit to provide both concomitantly. Clin Nutrit (Edinburgh, Scotland). 2020;39(12):3852–3. https://doi.org/10.1016/j.clnu.2020.09.048.

14. Minev I, Stefanov C. Is the gastric tube a burden for the noninvasive ventilation? Crit Care. 2015;19(Suppl 1):P220. https://doi.org/10.1186/cc14300.
15. Quintero Osorio OI, Arenas JV, Cuervo JA, Ospina Tascón GA. Non-invasive ventilation and airway exchange catheter using a novel adapter in a difficult airway patient with post-extubation respiratory failure. Respirol Case Rep. 2020;8(5):e00558. Published 2020 Apr 18. https://doi.org/10.1002/rcr2.558.
16. Quintero OI, Sanchez AI, Chavarro PA, Casas IC, Ospina Tascón GA. Impact of using a novel gastric feeding tube adaptor on patient's comfort and air leaks during non-invasive mechanical ventilation. Arch Bronconeumol. 2020;56(6):353–9. English, Spanish. https://doi.org/10.1016/j.arbres.2019.10.002. Epub 2019 Nov 13. PMID: 31732357

38 NIV Procedures: Upper Gastrointestinal Endoscopy

Robert Pieczyrak and Aleksandra Oraczewska

Upper tract endoscopy is considered to be the best technique to visualize the mucosa of the upper gastrointestinal (GI) tract. Introduced to the medical practice over one hundred years ago, first as rigid and semirigid gastroscopy and finally, after the optic fiber's breakthrough of optical developed in the 1950s, as gastroscopy with the use of flexible endoscopes.

Upper tract endoscopy may be ordered due to diagnostic or therapeutic purposes and may be elective or urgent.

One of the main contraindications to performing endoscopic procedures is acute respiratory insufficiency, so the first patient with such a condition must be stabilized, and later we can proceed with the endoscopy. An unconscious patient requires intubation to perform the endoscopic procedures.

During the endoscopy with the use of intravenous sedatives or anesthetics, the proper continuous vital signs surveillance is recommended, ECG and blood pressure monitoring, respiratory rate monitoring, saturation monitoring, and a nasal canula with oxygen supply.

During the upper tract endoscopy, sedatives are administered to patients who do not meet the requirement for general anesthesia to improve patients' comfort and endoscopist accuracy. Sedation as well as general anesthesia increases the risk of respiratory insufficiency and increases the risk of life-threatening conditions (respiratory, cardiovascular, neurological) as a consequence of desaturation, hypoxemia, and tissue hypoxia which is relatively rare in case of healthy individuals but rises in patients referred to the endoscopy with a heavy burden of overlapped comorbidities. Therefore, high-risk patients may expect complications during the endoscopy [1–5].

R. Pieczyrak (✉)
Department of Internal Medicine, Rheumatology and Clinical Immunology, Medical University of Silesia, Katowice, Poland

A. Oraczewska
Department of Lung Diseases and Tuberculosis, Faculty of Medical Sciences in Zabrze, Medical University of Silesia in Katowice, Katowice, Poland

© The Author(s), under exclusive license to Springer Nature Switzerland AG 2025

K. Panda et al. (eds.), *Noninvasive Ventilatory Approaches in Interventional Procedures*, Noninvasive Ventilation. The Essentials,
https://doi.org/10.1007/978-3-032-05328-2_38

NIV could be dedicated to prevent respiratory insufficiency in high-risk patients, including obese patients with the risk of hypoventilation while sedated, patients with a medical history of respiratory diseases as chronic obstructive pulmonary disease (COPD), interstitial lung disease, pneumonia, cardio-vascular diseases like coronary heart disease, and chronic heart failure, and patients with neurological disorders.

NIV can allow safer sedation in uncooperative patients with such risk factors. NIV may also be used for pre-oxygenation before intubation.

Insufficient respiration due to primary respiratory disorders of different mechanisms (obstruction, restriction, abnormal gas exchange) or as a consequence of endoscopy (laryngospasm, aspiration, increased intra-abdominal pressure with impact on diaphragm function, vagal nerve reaction) may lead to hypoxemia and further to cardiovascular complications, eventually with cardiac arrest, brain ischemia, and fatal outcome.

Worldwide use of intravenous sedation with pharmacoanesthetics (i.e., propofol) in endoscopy to improve patients' comfort and assure the high-quality endoscopic procedures may be the next risk factor that triggers respiratory insufficiency [6, 7].

Patients under NIV sometimes need diagnostic procedures in the area of the upper GI tract, like endoscopic inspection, biopsy in the area of suspected mucosal lesions, polypectomy, etc., or require the therapeutic endoscopy due to urgent disorders like bleeding management, stricture dilatation, or foreign body removal, etc. [8]

NIV mask has a special shape to cover firmly the face, nose, and mouth area, providing smooth and unlimited flow of oxygen during inspiration and the exhalation of the air from the airways through the one-directional valve.

Noninvasive ventilation is much less harmful to patients, so the invention of the mask adapted to the endoscopy procedures, allowing to introduction of the flexible endoscope shaft to the mouth with an acceptable air leak, was much needed.

The next problem is the inability to provide positive pressure in the airways during ventilation with the mask.

Finally, such a mask was introduced to clinical practice first as a prototype, later as a commercial product, and now may be widely used if needed. To overcome this problem, dedicated endoscopic NIV helmets have been designed to facilitate the performance of upper GI endoscopic procedures.

38.1 Techniques

The high-flow nasal canula (HFNC), which provides oxygen, is one of the possible techniques used in GI endoscopy.

HFNC providing oxygen, reducing the dead space, is one of the possible techniques used in GI endoscopy [5]. It allows for to provision of 100% oxygen, and it can increase CPAP depending on oxygen flow. The mechanism depends on the prolongation of apnea time. The oxygen administered by the canula has to be heated and humidified; otherwise, it may lead to severe mucosal damage in the upper airways and to lung injury. HFNC may facilitate safe upper GI endoscopy procedures; however, it has to be acknowledged that an open mouth will decrease the positive airway pressure, which is generated by increasing flow. This may be partially minimized by the introduction of an asymmetric nasal cannula, which has a greater ability to increase upper airway pressure. Moreover, an asymmetric cannula was found to better facilitate CO_2 washout; therefore, this method should be safer in terms of type 2 respiratory failure risk.

That technique may be applied to patients with chronic obstructive pulmonary disease (COPD), essential obesity, obstructive sleep apnea, and pulmonary fibrosis who require advanced endoscopic procedures of a longer duration. HFNC can help avoid intubation [8].

During the endoscopy with the use of intravenous anesthetics, the proper continuous surveillance is recommended, including ECG and blood pressure monitoring, respiratory rate, and saturation.

The regular nasal canula with oxygen supply is used separately or combined with the bite-blocking device used in GI endoscopy, which protects the endoscope shaft from mechanical damage by the teeth. When combined with the nasal canula, this will provide 100% oxygen flow to the nose and decrease the risk of desaturation [9, 10].

Another way to improve ventilation comfort is the face mask, which provides a 100% oxygen flow through the mouth and nose, leading to an increase in oxygen concentration in low pharynx and larynx. The face mask is easy to use and common in hospitals with an improvised aperture to introduce the endoscope through the bite block and perform the upper tract endoscopy. It supplies 100% oxygen but does not provide CPAP (continuous positive airway pressure). The dedicated face mask may be used, with two different ports: one to adjust the ventilation system and the second to intubate the upper GI tract. An endoscopic face mask may provide both CPAP and IPPV (intermittent positive pressure ventilation), reducing the risk of desaturation.

The idea of providing effective ventilation by covering the nose area separately is another approach to maintain ventilation during the endoscopy procedures, while still having open access to the mouth. That is the nasal endoscopic mask that supplies oxygen, decreases the risk of desaturation, and, due to the closed attachment to the nostrils by the inflatable seal or self-sealing cushion, allows to ventilate effectively, keeping IPPV (intermittent positive pressure ventilation). The port allows attachment of the respiratory system [11].

The NIV mask placed during the upper GI tract endoscopy when the endoscope shaft is already introduced that does not require endoscope withdrawal is the Janus mask (consisting of two halves) which is applied to the patient's face during the ongoing procedure [12].

The introduction of noninvasive methods of respiratory support and dedicated interfaces for endoscopy enables procedures to be performed safely even in patients with respiratory failure, without the need to intubate patients and minimizing the risk of respiratory complications.

References

1. McQuaid KR, Laine L. A systematic review and meta-analysis of randomized, controlled trials of moderate sedation for routine endoscopic procedures. Gastrointest Endosc. 2008;67:910–23.
2. Metzner J, Domino KB. Risks of anesthesia or sedation outside the operating room: the role of the anesthesia care provider. Curr Opin Anaesthesiol. 2010;23:523–31.
3. Cabrini L, Nobile L, Cama E, Borghi G, Pieri M, Bocchino S, et al. Non-invasive ventilation during upper endoscopies in adult patients. A systematic review. Minerva Anestesiol. 2013;79:683–94.
4. Gregory S, Siderowf A, Golaszewski AL, McCluskey L. Gastrostomy insertion in ALS patients with low vital capacity: respiratory support and survival. Neurology. 2002;58:485–7.
5. Nay MA, Fromont L, Eugene A, Marcueyz JL, Mfam WS, Baert O, et al. High-flow nasal oxygenation or standard oxygenation for gastrointestinal endoscopy with sedation in patients at risk of hypoxaemia: a multicentre randomised controlled trial (ODEPHI trial). Br J Anaesth. 2021;127(1):133–42.
6. Nishimura M. High-flow nasal cannula oxygen therapy devices. Respir Care. 2019;64:735–42.
7. Shao LJZ, et al. Trials Comparison of two supplement oxygen methods during gastroscopy with intravenous propofol anesthesia in obese patients: study protocol for a randomized controlled trial. Trials. 2018;19:602. https://doi.org/10.1186/s13063-018-2994-8.
8. Basavana G, Gowri G, Preet MS. Recent developments in devices used for gastrointestinal endoscopy sedation. Clin Endosc. 2021;54:182–92.
9. Respa O2 delivery bite block (internet). Mentor (OH): STERIS; c2019 (cited 2019 Sep 14). https://www.steris.com/healthcare/products/endoscopy-devices/gi-procedure-products/bite-blocks/respao2-bite-block
10. Using OxyshieldTM (internet). Achenmühle: OxyshieldTM; c2019 (cited 2019 Sep 14). http://www.oxy-shield.com/UsingOxyshield
11. Dimou F, Huynh S, Dakin G, et al. Nasal positive pressure with the SuperNO2 VATM device decreases sedation-related hypoxemia during pre-bariatric surgery EGD. Surg Endosc. 2019;33:3828–32.
12. Cabrini L, Landoni G. A novel non-invasive ventilation mask to prevent and manage respiratory failure during fiberoptic bronchoscopy, gastroscopy and transesophageal echocardiography. Heart Lung Vessel. 2015;7(4):297–303.

39 Noninvasive Positive Pressure Ventilation During Feeding Tube Placement

Claudia De Petro, Agata Lax, Antonello Nicolini, Eleonora Volpato, and Paolo Banfi

39.1 Introduction

Patients who have difficulty swallowing, problems with their appetite, or an inability to take adequate nutrition through the mouth can benefit from feeding tube placement (FTP) to avoid weight loss, correct significant nutritional deficiencies, and retard the general deterioration related to inadequate nutritional intake [1]. FTP is indicated in neuromuscular diseases (NMD), as dysphagia and muscular weakness are common causes of malnutrition, and weight loss is a poor prognostic factor.

As NMD progresses, patients' respiratory muscles cannot sustain autonomous respiration; the use of mechanical ventilation is the cornerstone of pulmonary medicine and critical care to improve symptomatology and gas exchange [2].

C. De Petro
Department of Pathophysiology and Transplantation, University of Milan, Milan, Italy

Respiratory Unit and Cystic Fibrosis Adult Center, Fondazione IRCCS Ca' Granda Ospedale Maggiore Policlinico, Milan, Italy
e-mail: claudia.depetro@unimi.it

A. Lax · A. Nicolini · P. Banfi (✉)
IRCCS Fondazione Don Carlo Gnocchi ONLUS, Milan, Italy
e-mail: alax@dongnocchi.it; pabanfi@dongnocchi.it

E. Volpato
IRCCS Fondazione Don Carlo Gnocchi ONLUS, Milan, Italy

Department of Psychology, Università Cattolica del Sacro Cuore, Milan, Italy
e-mail: evolpato@dongnocchi.it

© The Author(s), under exclusive license to Springer Nature Switzerland AG 2025

K. Panda et al. (eds.), *Noninvasive Ventilatory Approaches in Interventional Procedures*, Noninvasive Ventilation. The Essentials,
https://doi.org/10.1007/978-3-032-05328-2_39

39.2 FTP Disease Spectrum

Since the crucial aim of FTP is to guarantee adequate nutritional intake, the disease spectrum for its use is wide, and it can be divided into the following:

1. Oncological diseases: (i.e., stenotic neoplasms of the maxillofacial region or the upper gastrointestinal tract): FTP can be used palliatively or before surgery, radiotherapy, or chemotherapy, and removed when the patient recovers.
2. Gastroenteric diseases (i.e., Crohn's disease): FTP is the most useful nutritional measure in malnourished patients with gastroenteric diseases, when supplementary nutritional drinks are not effective.
3. Pulmonary disorders (i.e., cystic fibrosis, tracheal tract fistulas): Especially in cystic fibrosis, FTP improves nutritional status and stabilizes lung function. It is superior to the use of nasogastric tubes and it is associated with less side effects.
4. Neurological disorders causing dysphagia (i.e., neuromuscular diseases, dementia, cerebral palsy, stroke): FTP is helpful and highly effective, and in stroke-affected patients, it allows, in parallel, adequate training to reenable swallowing. Neuromuscular diseases are the most common field of FTP application.

39.3 NMD as Progressive Muscular Dysfunction

NMD encompasses a wide range of rare diseases which mainly manifest with motor and/or respiratory dysfunction. In amyotrophic lateral sclerosis (ALS), the hallmark is a progressive asymmetric weakness with both upper and lower motoneuron signs. It is broadly classified into limbic onset (80% cases) and bulbar onset (20%), while a small percentage presents with respiratory symptoms only [3].

In the natural history of neuromuscular pathology, bulbar dysfunction is the end-stage point of the disease, and it can manifest as impairment of the following:

- Upper airway muscles, leading to collapsibility and hypotonia that increase airflow resistance
- Inspiratory and expiratory muscles, leading to chronic global lung failure as the respiratory pump fails to support an increased respiratory workload and, likewise, the thoracic muscles fail to generate enough force
- Cough reflex, leading to decreased airway protection
- Dysphagia may lead to weight loss, malnutrition, dehydration, sialorrhea, frequent hospitalization and reduced quality of life, and increased risk of aspiration pneumonia

In the end, dysphagia and muscular weakness are the major causes of morbidity and mortality in ALS and NMD, so FTP is often performed to manage and improve the patient's nutritional status.

Video-fluoroscopic swallowing evaluation (VFSE) or fiberoptic evaluation of swallowing (FEES) remains the main investigative technique for the assessment of dysphagia in neuromuscular conditions, allowing the direct visualization of swallowing safety and efficiency, i.e., aspiration and the presence of residue, respectively. This is very important given the high incidence of "silent" aspiration in this patient population. There always remains the question of when to start and how often to do the examination.

39.4 Methods of Feeding Tube Insertion

- *Percutaneous endoscopic gastrostomy (PEG)*: It is performed under local anesthesia as an endoscope is inserted down the esophagus into the stomach. The light on the tip of the probe shines through the stomach and skin, marking the spot where the PEG tube should be inserted by the surgeon through a small incision.
- *Radiologically inserted G-tube (RIG)*: It is performed under local anesthesia as a nasogastric tube is inserted into the stomach to insufflate air into it. A radiologist uses ultrasounds to find the correct spot to insert the tube, then a RIG tube is inserted with the aid of fluoroscopy. A gastropexy is held in place with sutures called T-tacs that are removed about 14 days after the procedure.
- *Percutaneous radiological gastrostomy (PRG)*: It is performed under local anesthesia as a nasogastric tube is placed into the stomach to insufflate air into it. Fluoroscopy of the abdomen is undertaken, and the position of the nasogastric tube is identified (This is the main difference from the RIG). Then, the spot for the gastric puncture is chosen, and it must be equidistant from the greater and lesser curves of the stomach.

39.5 General Indications and Initial Management

Before proceeding with FTP, it is necessary to perform a proper swallowing assessment (see above) and make sure that diet modification is not sufficient to ensure normal nutritional intake. It is still possible to perform FTP and maintain partial oral nutrition by taking advantage of the patient's remaining resources.

Generally, FTP should be considered when nutritional intake has been qualitatively and quantitatively inadequate for a 2–3-week period of time. It should not be considered a terminal measure for patients with short life expectancy, and the ethical aspect must be considered while decision-making should always be individualized [2, 3].

Eventually, we have to maximize the following:

- Dietary prescription of high-protein and high-calorie supplements
- Food and fluids consistency (i.e., blending food, thickeners, agents)
- Swallowing hygiene (i.e., chin-tuck maneuver, supraglottic swallowing, and postural changes)

When the above measures do not improve the patient's nutritional status, FTP is indicated. Contraindications to FTP are as follows:

- Serious coagulation disorders
- Abdominal abnormalities (i.e., interposed organs, marked peritoneal carcinomatosis, severe ascites, peritonitis)
- Psychiatric disorders (i.e., anorexia nervosa, severe psychosis) [1]

39.6 FTP in MND and NPPV Support

The main challenge of FTP in NMD is to establish the correct timing of intervention. The patient should attend multiple outpatient visits annually according to the clinical status of the disease. When the vital capacity (VC) starts reducing and mealtime increases, follow-up visits should be anticipated, and each time, nutritional status (i.e., body weight or BMI) and respiratory function (i.e., Blood Gas analysis (BGA), forced vital capacity-FVC, maximal inspiratory pressure-MIP, maximal expiratory pressure-MEP, or Sniff nasal inspiratory pressure-SNIP) must be assessed, as well as early signs of dysphagia or dysarthria [4].

FTP is indicated when.

- Symptoms of bulbar progression occur (i.e., prolonged mealtime; ending meal prematurely because of fatigue; family concerns).
- Weight loss exceeds 10% during the follow-up period.

As for the current guidelines, FTP should be performed before VC or forced vital capacity (FVC) falls below 50% of prediction, since the lower it is, the higher the risk of respiratory impairment. However, different studies have demonstrated that the outcomes in subjects with FVC >50% and FVC <50% did not differ with respect to long-term survival. Furthermore, it is known that FVC is not the best indicator of phrenic insufficiency, which has been identified as the main cause of pulmonary symptoms in NMD patients.

To overcome these difficulties, NPPV has been proposed to optimize lung function during FTP [5].

39.7 Procedure

In our experience, all subjects are admitted into the pneumology ward the day before the procedure, and biochemistry, hematic, and coagulation samples are withdrawn while BGA and EKG are performed.

A specially trained respiratory physiotherapist fits the patient with a nasal mask or through the tracheostomy cannula, depending on the patient's features, and NPPV is initiated. NPPV ventilation modality is patient-based and depends on their needs, in order to maintain oxygen saturation > 92%. According to different case reports and clinical reviews, the most common modalities are CPAP, low-span bi-level, spontaneous/timed (S/T), and assist-control ventilation (ACP). It i's important to consider mask leaks, respiratory rate, estimated minute ventilation, and signs of hypoventilation [2].

It's necessary to suspend anticoagulant therapy and maintain fasting for at least 12 h before the procedure. It's recommended to start antibiotic prophylaxis 1 h before FTP [6].

In the endoscopy unit, conscious sedation with midazolam is administered, and clinical and biological variables are monitored so that the pulmonologist or the respiratory physiotherapist can adjust NPPV parameters to maintain $SPO_2 > 95\%$ during the positioning. Note that oxygen can compensate for mouth air leaks to obtain a $SpO_2 \geq 92\%$. NPPV is continued via an oronasal mask when the procedure finishes, while secretions are managed.

39.8 Sedation and Secretions

Conscious sedation is nowadays the most widely used and safe approach for FTP, mainly because of the adverse events linked to the administration of general anesthesia in NMD patients.

In fact, although anesthesia with propofol has proved safe for different procedures, there is evidence that cardiorespiratory side effects may occur more frequently and that assisted ventilation may be necessary. Assisted ventilation and oro-tracheal intubation (OTI) during a procedure in NMD is a poor prognostic factor, and it can commit the patient to tracheostomy as OTI can then be difficult to wean off and thus becomes an ethical issue. In addition, general anesthesia is related to respiratory muscle impairment associated with a supine position. Conversely, the finding that standardized use of IV midazolam as conscious sedation is safe and effective during FTP, in our opinion, is crucial to support the argument that this treatment strategy should be used to allow reduction of the procedure-related side effects. A recent clinical review demonstrated that the risk of respiratory complications and procedure-related mortality with conscious sedation is low, even in patients with mild to moderate pulmonary dysfunction [7].

After FTP with NPPV, retained secretions can be difficult to clear, causing pulmonary or ventilatory impairment and difficulty weaning from NPPV. Several clinical reviews suggest frequently performing air-stacking exercises or applying mechanical insufflation–exsufflation (MI-E), which can provide positive pressure on the airway followed immediately by negative pressure. The use of mechanically-assisted cough (MAC) can improve expectoration and reduce adverse events linked to secretions aspiration [8].

39.9 Complications

All complications of FTP during NPPV [2] are clearly detailed.

Major complications can be divided into the following:

- Procedure-related (i.e., local wound infections, peritonitis).
- NPPV-related (i.e., pneumoperitoneum).

Minor complications are mostly represented by disturbances of intestinal transit (i.e., minor bleeding at the G-tube site, mechanical obstruction due to tube migration, dislodged tooth crown) and laryngospasm (i.e., upper-respiratory tract infection, G-tube site cellulitis).

Other less-frequent complications can be as follows:

- Desaturation (2 cases found in our registers), which can be resolved by increasing the NPPV settings.
- Gastric hemorrhage, which can be treated with embolization.

39.10 Survival and Prognosis

It is crucial to highlight that survival is mainly related to NMD progression rather than to the FTP procedure.

FTP has high long-term success rates as mortality and morbidity are low. The techniques used for FTP (PEG, RIG, or PRG) are not significantly different from one another in terms of their rate of complications. FTP has a clinical impact on weight stabilization and drug administration [8].

A large prospective study demonstrated that the two main poor prognostic factors of FTP are

- Age of bulbar ALS onset.
- Nutritional status at FTP-indication-time.

Preoperative respiratory status is known to influence prognosis, but the use of VC or FVC >50% as an indication for FTP is controversial. Several studies show that patients with FVC < 30% of predicted undergoing FTP while receiving noninvasive respiratory care experienced no major complications when compared to the patients receiving invasive respiratory support while the use of conscious sedation, despite general anesthesia, decreased the risk of deterioration of respiratory and bulbar functions, reducing the recurrence of OTI. This data indicates the need to explore a wider range of VC values predicted for feasible gastrostomy in ALS patients [9–11].

On the other hand, it's also important to note that preoperative NPPV-dependent patients experience the worst result, with a significantly higher 30-day mortality rate. In fact, whereas the implementation of NPPV as low-level bi-level PAP during FTP can prevent respiratory failure during the procedure for a relatively mild non-invasive routine using NPPV patients, full settings of noninvasive ventilatory support are required for ventilator-unwearable continuous noninvasive ventilatory support users as well as for others who have VC < 30% of normal, for safety. [10–12].

Other retrospective studies address that recurrent accumulation of airway secretions significantly worsens prognosis after EPT in routine NPPV users, ALS patients, highlighting that adequate peri-operative management of airway secretions is crucial in this context.

The importance of NPPV support and MI-E during FTP was also noted by Allen et al., who demonstrated that open gastrostomy with continuous NPPV support in patients with VC < 10% had no respiratory complications, while four subjects in whom FTP was delayed without NPPV experienced respiratory failure [10, 12].

39.11 Conclusion

FTP is generally recommended in NMD patients to prevent complications such as pneumonia caused by aspiration. Among all FTP methods, PEG is the accepted standard and the most used method. However, the appropriate time for insertion is still controversial. The actual indications are the low nutritional status leading to 10% weight loss and the worsening of respiratory function, while FVC is still >50% of predicted. Several studies showed that FTP can be safely performed in patients in conjunction with NPPV support, and subjects experience fewer complications and adverse events. Retained secretions must be effectively cleared.

References

1. Löser C, Aschl G, Hébuterne X, Mathus-Vliegen E, Muscaritoli M, Niv Y, Rollins H, Singer P, Skelly R. ESPEN guidelines on artificial enteral nutrition – percutaneous endoscopic gastrostomy (PEG). Clin Nutr. 2005;24:848–61.
2. Banfi P, Volpato E, Valota C, D'Ascenzo S, Bani Alunno C, Lax A, Nicolini A, Ticozzi N, Silani V, Bach JR. Use of noninvasive ventilation during feeding tube placement. Respir Care. 2017;62:1474–84.
3. Andersen PM, Abrahams S, Borasio GD, et al. EFNS guidelines on the clinical Management of Amyotrophic Lateral Sclerosis (MALS) – revised report of an EFNS task force. Eur J Neurol. 2011;19:360–75.
4. Kim EY, Kang SW, Suh MR, Jung J, Park J, Choi WA. Safety of gastrostomy tube placement in patients with advanced amyotrophic lateral sclerosis with noninvasive ventilation. J Parent Enteral Nutrit. 2021;45(6):1338–46. https://doi.org/10.1002/jpen.2018.
5. Sancho J, Servera E, Chiner E, Bañuls P, Gómez-Merino E, Sancho-Chust JN, Marín J. Noninvasive respiratory muscle aids during PEG placement in ALS patients with severe ventilatory impairment. J Neurol Sci. 2010;297:55–9.
6. Gregory S, Siderowf A, Golaszewski AL, McCluskey L. Gastrostomy insertion in ALS patients with low vital capacity: respiratory support and survival. Neurology. 2002;58:485–7.
7. Burkhardt C, Neuwirth C, Sommacal A, Andersen PM, Weber M. Is survival improved by the use of NIV and PEG in amyotrophic lateral sclerosis (ALS)? A post-mortem study of 80 ALS patients. PLoS One. 2017;12:e0177555.

8. Strijbos D, Hofstede J, Keszthelyi D, Masclee AAM, Gilissen LPL. Percutaneous endoscopic gastrostomy under conscious sedation in patients with amyotrophic lateral sclerosis is safe. Eur J Gastroenterol Hepatol. 2017;29:1303–8.
9. Hesters A, Amador M del M, Debs R, et al. Predictive factors for prognosis after gastrostomy placement in routine non-invasive ventilation users ALS patients. Sci Rep. 2020; https://doi.org/10.1038/s41598-020-70422-2.
10. Czell D, Bauer M, Binek J, Schoch OD, Weber M. Outcome of percutaneous endoscopic gastrostomy tube insertion in respiratory impaired amyotrophic lateral sclerosis patients under non-invasive ventilation. Respir Care. 2012; https://doi.org/10.4187/respcare.02024.
11. Gaspar R, Ramalho R, Coelho R, Andrade P, Goncalves Miguel R, Macedo G. Percutaneous endoscopic gastrostomy placement under NIV in amyotrophic lateral sclerosis with severe Ventilatory dysfunction: a safe and effective procedure. GE Port J Gastroenterol. 2021;30(1):61–7.
12. Allen JA, Chen R, Ajroud-Driss S, Sufit RL, Heller S, Siddique T, Wolfe L. Gastrostomy tube placement by endoscopy versus radiologic methods in patients with ALS: a retrospective study of complications and outcome. Amyotrophic Lateral Scler Frontotemporal Degeneration. 2013;14:308–14.

Abdominal Radiological Procedures: Deep Sedation and Noninvasive Ventilation in Patients with Neurodegenerative Disorders

40

Caterina Barbaglio, Elisabetta Roma, Fabiane Barboza, Elisa DeMattia, Antonio Rampoldi, and Andrea De Gasperi

40.1 Introduction

Interventional radiology for abdominal visceral or vascular procedures encompasses a wide range of elective and emergency interventions: anaesthesiologists are more and more frequently involved to increase intraoperative safety and perioperative pain control, particularly in frail or unstable patients [1]. Emergency procedures performed by the interventional radiologist (IR) are on the rise and include, among others, drainage of the biliary tree or of abdominal abscesses, control of gastrointestinal haemorrhages, embolisation of acute vascular blushing and transjugular intrahepatic portosystemic shunts (TIPS). Patients requiring emergency procedures who have haemodynamic instability or possible ventilatory complications or in case of complex elective interventions (e.g., TIPS) are usually managed with orotracheal intubation and mechanical ventilation, to secure the airways and to allow the anaesthesiologist to have free hands in the case of a critical event. On the other hand, among the elective procedures requested from IRs, more and more frequently are

C. Barbaglio
Servizio Anestesia e Rianimazione 2, ASST GOM Niguarda, Milan, Italy
e-mail: caterina.barbaglio@ospedaleniguarda.it

E. Roma
Centro Clinico NEMO – Fondazione Serena, Milan, Italy
e-mail: elisabetta.roma@centrocliniconemo.it

F. Barboza · E. DeMattia · A. Rampoldi
Radiologia Interventistica, ASST GOM Niguarda, Milan, Italy
e-mail: fabiane.barbosa@ospedaleniguarda.it; elisa.demattia@centrocliniconemo.it; antonio.rampoldi@ospedaleniguarda.it

A. De Gasperi (✉)
Former Head of the Servizio Anestesia Rianimazione 2, ASST GOM Niguarda, Milan, Italy

© The Author(s), under exclusive license to Springer Nature Switzerland AG 2025

K. Panda et al. (eds.), *Noninvasive Ventilatory Approaches in Interventional Procedures*, Noninvasive Ventilation. The Essentials,
https://doi.org/10.1007/978-3-032-05328-2_40

percutaneously inserted gastrostomy (PIG) for enteral nutrition [2–4] in patients with a severe decline in neurological status or, more often, for neuromuscular/neurodegenerative diseases (amyotrophic lateral sclerosis [ALS] and muscular dystrophies among others) [5]. These latter conditions, which involve motor neurons, are characterised by devastating muscle wasting and severe weakness and evolve, often very rapidly, to progressive dysphagia and respiratory impairment. The main causes are respiratory muscle impairment/failure and recurrent episodes of choking and aspiration leading to respiratory tract infections [5].

40.2 Abdominal Interventional Radiology and Patients with Neurodegeneration: The Challenge for the Anaesthesiologist

Gastrostomy and mechanical ventilation in patients with ALS are now considered relevant options to provide the best support [6–10]. The indications and timing of gastrostomy, reviewed elsewhere, are still controversial and beyond the scope of this work. Gastrostomy can be considered at the onset of non-invasive ventilation (NIV) usage, or according to the severity of dysphagia and the specific neuromuscular disorder. Initiation of NIV is thus key in the patient's trajectory [8]. According to Banfi et al. [8], many patients with non-bulbar ALS have severe respiratory orthopnoea and require NIV support to sleep in a reclined position; however, they often have no bulbar innervated muscle involvement and are able to swallow and protect their airways. Thus, having optimised non-invasive respiratory management, the timing of gastrostomy could be driven by dysphagia alone; this is an appropriate recommendation according to some experts [8, 9].

There are two main approaches for PIG [2–4, 11, 12]: radiologically inserted gastrostomy (RIG), first described in the early 1980s [3] and reported in the Society for Interventional Radiology Practice Guidelines [4], and the transoral technique, usually performed by an endoscopist during a formal upper gastroscopic procedure (i.e. percutaneous endoscopic gastrostomy [PEG]). The reports dealing with the best approach for PIG are conflicting: periprocedural complications, costs, and the need for anaesthesiology consultation for deep sedation are among the reported issues [2]. According to the ProGas Study Group [11], the choice of either PEG or RIG should be primarily based on local facilities and expertise: a multidisciplinary approach has been considered a mandatory standard in this setting. In a recent experience reported by Strijbos et al. [12], PEG and RIG were equal in terms of procedure-related and 30-day mortality. On the other hand, Haber et al. [2] concluded in favour of RIG due to fewer anaesthesiology consultations, shorter procedures and no relevant differences in the incidence of minor or major complications. Regardless of the choice, the use of PIG is on the rise in patients with ALS or other severe neuromuscular disorders. In fact, the combination of NIV and appropriate nutrition (possible with the gastrostomy) is associated with a trend towards better survival in patients with ALS when compared with the implementation of any single intervention [6–11]. Although RIG is often performed without sedation, pain control and supported ventilation [2], patients with serious degenerative neurological diseases and proposed for gastrostomy for enteral nutrition worry about 'feeling pain and discomfort during the procedure'. This is why procedures performed under deep sedation and with the support of NIV are considered of great value according to the views of patients, families and caregivers [13]: the very frail neuropsychological profile of these patients deserves attention and empathy. In AAs' experience, RIG is the preferred interventional option because it has long been performed under deep sedation and with NIV [13]. In fact, with appropriate and tailored solutions, NIV during RIG constitutes an important intraoperative safety issue, together with deep sedation provided by a dedicated anaesthesiologist [13]. At least in Italy and up to now, anaesthesia-related costs have not been an issue; procedural time, using appropriate pharmacological protocols, is not significantly prolonged and the patient's comfort and safety are ensured.

40.3 Deep Sedation and NIV to Perform RIG: How We Do It

Preprocedural evaluation, usually performed 1 week before the gastrostomy, should include a multidisciplinary assessment involving radiologists, anaesthesiologists, the physician (usually a neurologist or a pneumonologist) who is in charge of the patient and respiratory therapists (RT). Tailoring the procedure to the patient is key to a successful procedure in such a fragile setting.

The patient's informed consent for the anaesthesia procedure has to be separated from the patient's consent for the radiological procedure. The approach should be personalised and discussed with the patient, his/her family and the physician in charge. It should be easy to be understood, complete but not redundant, and should include advantages and disadvantages of the deep sedation for the procedure and the risk of urgent/emergent interventions (mainly intubation and emergency surgery in case of periprocedural complications); these latter complications should be well explained by the proceduralist.

Deep sedation, not very different from formal general anaesthesia using an ad hoc face mask (total face mask) instead of intubation [13, 14], is a pivotal part of the procedure. Paravertebral block [15] has been proposed as an alternative to sedation to provide analgesia while minimising risks, but, even if attractive, it is far from practical, and it is not always well accepted by the patients. Beyond pain relief and stress management, the main aims of deep sedation are (i) to provide the maximum comfort to the patient, (ii) to maximise the patient's adaptation to NIV, (iii) to speed up the work of the proceduralist, (iv) to avoid cardiorespiratory reactivity during the procedure, and (v) to keep postprocedural respiratory complications to a minimum [13]. Gastric distension after air insufflation, which is mandatory to perform RIG, could cause discomfort, agitation, altered ventilation, acute tachycardia, and arterial hypertension in the case of the orthosympathetic response or, on the contrary, hypotension and bradycardia should the parasympathetic response prevail.

Benzodiazepines (midazolam), opioids (fentanyl, meperidine, remifentanil) and propofol are the drugs of choice for the induction and maintenance of deep sedation.

The use of ketamine has occasionally been reported in this setting. Dexmedetomidine has been approved for sedation outside the intensive care unit, and its use is now rapidly expanding [13, 14]. Ad hoc intraprocedural monitoring is mandatory and should include heart rate (HR), respiratory rate (RR), non-invasive blood pressure (NIBP), arterial oxygen saturation (SaO2) and microstream end tidal carbon dioxide (EtCO2) [13, 14].

Impaired respiratory muscle strength, possibly amplified in patients with ALS by the supine position and gastric distension, and the respiratory depression induced by sedative drugs are among the risk factors for postprocedural respiratory complications. NIV and particularly pressure-supported ventilation (PSV) are proposed more and more frequently for partial or total support during the procedure, often with personalised ventilatory parameters for an optimal patient–machine interaction [13, 14, 16–18]. Under deep sedation, consciousness as well as ventilatory drive are partially or totally impaired/depressed. Because sedation is a continuum, the individual physiological response of each patient might not be predictable. Assistance using external airway manipulation (chin lift and jaw thrust) may be needed during NIV to keep the maximum adherence of the mask to the face and to avoid air leaks and hypoventilation: the main goal is to maintain the patient's airway and appropriate spontaneous, supported or controlled tidal volumes, according to the tailored ventilator set during the preprocedural ventilatory training [8, 9, 13]. The RT plays a pivotal role in preprocedural training [8, 9] because they help to develop the appropriate personalised setting of PSV that is used during intraprocedural artificial ventilation, particularly with pressure-supported NIV. In fact, adaptation to NIV and mechanical in-exsufflation before the procedure has a key role for both a successful and smooth intraprocedural course and a postprocedural period without respiratory complications [8, 9, 17, 19, 20]. Ventilatory patterns and preprocedural optimisation of NIV together with ventilatory training (overnight vs 24/24) and in-exsufflation exercises are discussed with the pneumonologist and RT [8, 9, 17, 19, 20]. The best NIV setting obtained during ward training while maintaining the procedural position—a semi-recumbent supine decubitus, keeping the head up 20°–30°—is recorded and used during RIG when almost all the patients become totally ventilator dependent (full ventilatory support). According to Banfi et al. [8], they require either high span (15–25 cm H_2O) bi-level PAP or intermittent positive-pressure ventilation at full ventilatory support settings. Portable ventilators are used with active circuits in volume-control mode, with the exhaled tidal volume ranging from 10 to 12 ml/kg body weight or pressure pre-set at 17–25 cmH_2O. PSV is the ventilatory mode usually set to have a backup mandatory ventilation with tidal volume close to 10 ml/kg body weight, PEEP at 5–7 cmH_2O, respiratory rate at 14/min and FiO_2 at 40%. Overall, the median duration of the RIG procedure is usually 20 minutes (range 15–30 minutes). The median recovery time using propofol-based total intravenous anaesthesia is usually 2–5 minutes [13, 14]. Observation in a dedicated recovery room usually lasts 10–15 minutes, with the assistance of the RT and the anaesthesiologist. When stable, awake, and pain-free, the patient is transferred to the ward on NIV, with the assistance of the RT and with HR, NIBP and SaO_2 monitoring.

40.4 Conclusions

Gastrostomy using percutaneous techniques (PEG or RIG) is increasingly required in patients with neuromuscular disorders to implement appropriate enteral feeding programmes. Gastrostomy alongside NIV can improve the short-term and midterm outcomes. The key to managing the minimally invasive but stressful interventional procedure successfully is a multidisciplinary approach, aiming for a personalised periprocedural treatment that includes deep sedation and assisted/controlled NIV. In patients with neuromuscular disorders, deep sedation under NIV is the result of a multidisciplinary effort aimed at achieving successful personalised preprocedural NIV training, implemented by the physicians in charge and RT. During the procedure, anaesthesiologists have to maintain an equilibrium between the depth of sedation and a safe and stable physiological profile. The expected results are the safety of the procedure, reduced patient stress and anxiety and easing the work of the proceduralist. Ample collaboration, prudence, respecting the wishes of patients with neuromuscular disorders and their relatives, and a strong commitment from the entire multidisciplinary team are crucial in this very unique, delicate setting. The best available evidence for the quality of such an approach is the satisfaction and relief expressed by the patients and their relatives after the procedure.

References

1. De Gasperi A, Corti A, Corso R, et al. Transjugular intrahepatic portosystemic shunt (TIPS): the anesthesiological point of view after. 150 procedures managed under total intravenous anesthesia. J Clin Monit Comput. 2009;23:341–6.
2. Haber Z, Charles HW, Gross J, et al. Percutaneous radiologically guided gastrostomy tube placement: comparison of antegrade transoral and retrograde transabdominal approaches. Diagn Interv Radiol. 2017;23:55–60.
3. Wills JS, Oglesby JT. Percutaneous gastrostomy. Radiology. 1983;149:449–53.
4. Itkin M, DeLegge MH, Fang JC, et al. Multidisciplinary practical guidelines for gastrointestinal access for enteral nutrition and decompression from the Society of Interventional Radiology and American Gastroenterological Association (AGA) institute, with endorsement by Canadian Interventional Radiological Association (CIRA) and Cardiovascular and Interventional Radiological Society of Europe (CIRSE). J Vasc Interv Radiol. 2011;22:1089–106.
5. Wijesekera LC, Leigh PN. Amyotrophic lateral sclerosis. Orphanet J Rare Dis. 2009;4:3. https://doi.org/10.1186/1750-1172-4-3.
6. Barc K, Kuzma Kozakiezicz M. Gastrostomy and mechanical ventilation in amyotrophic lateral sclerosis: how best to support the decision-making process? J Neurol Neurosurg. 2020;54:366–77.
7. McGeachan AJ, Hobson EV, Al-Chalabi A, et al. Supportive and symptomatic management of amyotrophic lateral sclerosis. Nat Rev Neurol. 2016;12(9):526–38.
8. Banfi P, Volpato E, Valota C, et al. Use of noninvasive ventilation during feeding tube placement. Respir Care. 2017;62:1474–84.
9. Bertella E, Banfi P, Paneroni M, et al. Early initiation of night-time NIV in an outpatient setting: a randomized non inferiority study in ALS patients. Eur J Phys Rebabil Med. 2017;53:892–9.
10. Sheers N, Berlowitz DJ, Rautela L, et al. Improved survival with an ambulatory model of non-invasive ventilation implementation in motor neuron disease. Amyotroph Lateral Scler Frontotemporal Degener. 2014;15:180–4.

11. PROGAS Study Group. Gastrostomy in patients with amyotrophic lateral sclerosis (ProGas): a prospective cohort study. Lancet Neurol. 2015;14:702–9.
12. Strijbos D, Keszthelyi D, Gilissen LPL, Lacko M, Hoeijmakers JGJ, Van der Leij C, De Ridder RJJ, De Haan MW, Masclee AAD. Percutaneous endoscopic versus radiologic gastrostomy for enteral feeding: a retrospective analysis on outcomes and complications. Endoscopy Internat Open. 2019;07:E1487–95.
13. Roma E, Falcier RF, et al. NIV for minimally invasive Interventional procedures: percutaneous gastric Tube Insertion (PRG) and Radiologically inserted gastrostomy. In: Esquinas AM, Papadakos Porhomayon J, et al., editors. Noninvasive ventilation in anesthesiology and perioperative medicine. Nova Science Publisher; 2022. Chap 41. p. 343–54.
14. Cristalli A, De Gasperi A. Deep sedation and anesthesia for advanced gastrointestinal endoscopy: challenging a continuum. In: Mutignani M, editor. Endotherapy in biliopancreatic diseases: ERCP meets EUS. Springer Nature Switzerland AG; 2020. p. 65–80. https://doi.org/10.1007/978-3-030-42569-2_7. Chap 7.
15. Porter S, McClain R, Robards C, Paz-Fumagalli R, Clendenen S, Logvinov I, Hex KO, Palmucci C, Oskarsson B. Paravertebral block for rardiologically inserted gastrostomy tube placement in amyotrophic lateral sclerosis. Muscles Nerve. 2020;62(1):70–5.
16. Bourke SC, Tomlinson M, Williams TL, et al. Effects of non-invasive ventilation on survival and quality of life in patients with amyotrophic lateral sclerosis: a randomised controlled trial. Lancet Neurol. 2006;5:140–7.
17. Sancho J, Servera E, Chiner E, Bañuls P, Gómez-Merino E, Sancho-Chust JN, Marín J. Noninvasive respiratory muscle aids during PEG placement in ALS patients with severe ventilatory impairment. J Neurol Sci. 2010;297:55–9.
18. Hinkelbein J, Lamperti M, Akeson J, Santos J, Costa J, De Robertis E, Longrois D, Novak-Jankovic V, Petrini F, Struys MRF, Veyckemans F, Fuchs-Buder T, Fitzgerald R. European Society of Anaesthesiology and European Board of Anaesthesiology guidelines for procedural sedation and analgesia in adults. EUR J Anesthesiol. 2018;35:6–24.
19. Birnkrant DJ, Panitch HB, Benditt JO, Boitano LJ, Carter ER, Cwik VA, Finder JD, Iannaccone ST, Jacobson LE, Kohn GL, Motoyama EK, Moxley RT, Schroth MK, Sharma GD, Sussman MD. American College of Chest Physicians Consensus Statement on the respiratory and related management of patients with Duchenne muscular dystrophy undergoing anesthesia or sedation. Chest. 2007;132:1977–86.
20. Vitacca M, Montini A, Lunetta C, Banfi P, Bertella E, De Mattia E, Lizio A, Volpato E, Lax A, Morini R, Paneroni M, the ALS RESPILOM Study Group. Impact of an early respiratory care program with NIV adaptation in patients with ALS. Eur J Neurol. 2018;25:556e33.

Part VIII

Summary of Practical Recommendations and Educational Programs

NIV: Summary of Clinical Results and Practical Recommendations

41

Karolina Zawada-Drozd and Wojciech Drozd

41.1 Technical Aspects

Noninvasive respiratory support encompasses strategies such as standard oxygen therapy, noninvasive ventilation (NIV), continuous positive airway pressure (CPAP) and high-flow nasal cannula (HFNC) therapy.

Standard oxygen therapy can be delivered with the use of different interfaces. The most common interfaces are simple oxygen masks, nasal cannulas, partial rebreather masks, non-rebreather masks, air-entrainment masks, face tents, and tracheostomy collars.

A variety of interfaces for NIV or CPAP is also available, including nasal masks, oronasal masks, full-face masks, nasal pillows, or helmets.

HFNC was initially used in patients in the periprocedural period, in intensive care units (ICUs), and in the process of weaning from invasive ventilation but is currently widely used in the treatment of acute respiratory failure outside ICUs. HFNC delivers high F_IO_2 in conjunction with higher flows than the standard nasal cannula. Comfortable silicone nasal cannulas are used in this method of ventilatory support.

Appropriate assessment of clinical condition, choice of support modality and interface are of key importance in achieving therapeutic success.

The selection and fitting of an NIV interface should be individualized, taking into consideration various factors such as appropriate adjustment of the mask (facial shape, presence of facial injuries, use of intragastric probes), the patient's comfort

K. Zawada-Drozd (✉)
Silesian Medical University in Katowice, Department of Pneumonology, Katowice, Poland

W. Drozd
Brothers Hospitallers of Saint John of God Hospital, Katowice, Poland

© The Author(s), under exclusive license to Springer Nature Switzerland AG 2025

K. Panda et al. (eds.), *Noninvasive Ventilatory Approaches in Interventional Procedures*, Noninvasive Ventilation. The Essentials,
https://doi.org/10.1007/978-3-032-05328-2_41

(necessary to obtain the appropriate degree of patient cooperation), severity of respiratory failure, and risk of aspiration.

41.2 NIV Interface

The choice of interface can be the most difficult part of the process.

Nasal masks are often used in the treatment of sleep apnea, only covering the nose, which is an option for patients who feel claustrophobic while using full-face masks. However, they may not be suitable for patients with high ventilatory needs or those who breathe through their mouth during sleep.

Nasal pillows are small, soft prongs that are inserted into the nostrils. They are well-tolerated by patients but might not deliver adequate pressure support in severe respiratory failure.

Full-face masks cover both the mouth and nose and are commonly used in acute care settings or in patients breathing through their mouth, as they allow for the use of higher respiratory pressures. However, they may increase the risk of aspiration and cause claustrophobia.

Total face masks cover the entire face. Their use is associated with fewer pressure sores but may cause discomfort due to the size.

Helmets covering the entire head can reduce the risk of intubation in certain groups of patients with acute respiratory distress syndrome (ARDS) compared to face masks.

The interest and experience in noninvasive ventilation-assisted techniques have continued to grow over the past two decades. The last 3 years of the COVID-19 pandemic have contributed to the widespread use of these methods both in ICUs and outside acute settings.

NIV has transformed the management of various respiratory conditions over the last few decades. Its results are best supported by clinical studies in the treatment of respiratory failure in the course of chronic obstructive pulmonary disease (COPD), acute respiratory failure, and sleep-disordered breathing.

41.3 NIV Indications

Studies performed in the population with COPD have demonstrated that application of NIV in patients with hypercapnic acute respiratory failure leads to reduced intubation rates [1]. Home NIV application impacts long-term outcomes, leading to a substantial reduction in hospital readmission rates due to COPD exacerbations [2].

NIV and the role of NIV in managing acute respiratory failure is compelling. NIV has been shown to reduce the rate of endotracheal intubation, particularly in patients suffering from cardiogenic pulmonary edema and acute hypercapnic respiratory failure in the course of COPD. Its use is associated with an increase in patients' comfort, contributing to better adherence [3].

41.3.1 NIV and Sleep

In congestive heart failure patients with Cheyne-Stokes respiration, NIV has been shown to improve not only sleep-disordered breathing but also left ventricular function, resulting in improved patient symptoms and reduced hospitalization rates [4].

Use of NIV in the treatment of sleep-disordered breathing, including obstructive sleep apnea (OSA), central sleep apnea (CSA), and obesity hypoventilation syndrome (OHS), reduces daytime sleepiness and improves overall quality of life [5]. Studies also suggest better cardiovascular outcomes associated with the use of NIV in patients with OSA [6].

Multiple studies have reported reduced lengths of hospital stay and ICU admissions resulting from NIV implementation [7]. NIV may reduce mortality rates, most probably due to the avoidance of complications associated with invasive ventilation [7].

The use of NIV allows for shortening the period of invasive ventilation and the length of ICU stay. In patients who underwent tracheostomy due to extubation failure, NIV can support decannulation (in-hospital as well as in special weaning centers) [8]. Similarly, use of HFNC is associated with better results than the standard spontaneous breathing trial [9].

Unfortunately, clinical data on ventilatory support during invasive diagnostic and therapeutic procedures are still scarce. The available data indicate high effectiveness of noninvasive ventilatory support in the prevention of acute respiratory failure or exacerbation of chronic respiratory failure in high-risk patients.

Acute respiratory failure or exacerbation of chronic respiratory failure is one of the most important risk factors for diagnostic and therapeutic procedures, especially in patients with already reduced respiratory reserve. Sedation, administered to improve patient comfort and compliance, may exacerbate underlying conditions, leading to hypoxemia and/or hypercapnia and cause premature termination of the procedure [10].

Invasive procedures are often required in patients who already are in poor clinical condition due to respiratory failure and are considered one of the ways to improve their respiratory state (e.g., bronchoscopic airway clearance therapy).

NIV is a cornerstone for the treatment of acute respiratory failure in various clinical settings. NIV can be successfully implemented during the procedure and in the periprocedural period to improve ventilation and oxygenation and avoid general anesthesia or complications such as endotracheal intubation and invasive ventilation.

One of the most common methods is preoxygenation (e.g., before difficult intubation, electroconvulsive therapy) aimed at reducing the risk of desaturation.

During preoxygenation, conventional oxygen therapy, bag ventilation, high-flow nasal cannula, or noninvasive ventilation may be used.

Ear, nose, and throat (ENT), upper respiratory tract surgeries, and dental procedures can be performed under local anesthesia, which reduces the length of hospital stay with a similar risk for the patient [11], optimizes the treatment area, and reduces the risk of anesthesia-related complications [12]. Tubeless anesthesia via HFNO can be a good alternative to conventional anesthesia in selected patient populations, if performed by trained professionals. To establish a safe surgical environment with tubeless anesthesia, appropriate backup plans, including endotracheal intubation and high-frequency jet ventilation (HFJV), should be available [13].

In psychiatry, preoxygenation and hyperventilation (with bag mask and oxygen) in electroconvulsive therapy (ECT) may improve not only safety but also seizure quality [14]. Unfortunately, there are no controlled clinical trials that would provide a reliable hyperventilation protocol for ECT settings [15].

There are ongoing clinical trials on the use of preoxygenation in this indication [16]. Patients with risk factors for respiratory failure development (including morbidly obese individuals) should be carefully monitored. In case of desaturation, head-up position, use of apneic oxygenation, noninvasive ventilation, HFNC, and supraglottic airway devices are recommended to improve oxygenation and procedure safety [17].

Methods of noninvasive ventilation support have also been used during neurosurgical procedures. In procedures requiring the maintenance of consciousness and the patient's cooperation (awake craniotomy), airway management is crucial. The choice of method depends on the clinical condition, comorbidities, and the course of monitoring. In case of deterioration of respiratory function, non-invasive methods such as HNFC, CPAP, and NIV may often help to avoid further complications [18, 19].

Endoscopic procedures in gastroenterology, pneumonology, and cardiology such as gastroscopy, colonoscopy, bronchofibroscopy, or transesophageal echocardiography are usually performed for diagnostic or interventional reasons. Frequently, local anesthesia or sedation is necessary. Endoscopic procedures are increasingly performed in patients characterized by a high risk of respiratory failure. Exacerbation of ventilation may be associated with oversedation, which is observed in elderly patients with numerous comorbidities. Recently, periprocedural noninvasive techniques have been implemented to improve oxygenation and avoid complications.

Ventilatory support with individually selected interfaces has been delivered during prolonged transesophageal cardiac examinations, therapeutic interventions, and bronchoscopic maneuvers and in the management of difficult airways [20].

NIV has been proven to be a useful and safe tool that facilitates bronchofibroscopy in patients with severe pulmonary diseases.

Currently, prospective studies are required to establish guidelines for the procedure and to define the optimal support modalities [21].

According to Pieri et al. [12], oxygenation strategy during bronchoscopy should be chosen according to the procedure, respiratory and circulatory system function, oxygen requirement during the procedure, and the risk of exacerbation. In patients with mild-to-moderate oxygen requirement, HFNC is preferred over passive oxygen therapy, while CPAP or NIV is a better choice in patients with more advanced respiratory failure.

Considering the need for deeper sedation during some endoscopic procedures, respiratory drive depression may be expected.

The preliminary study revealed that CPAP administered via a tight-fitting mask may be an effective tool to reduce the incidence and duration of obstructive apneic events as well as oxygen desaturation during lower endoscopy procedures with sedation based on propofol and fentanyl [22].

Also, meta-analysis of eight randomized controlled studies and one longitudinal study revealed that the use of HFNO during endoscopy led to a lower incidence of desaturation and a reduction of sedation-related adverse events without significant impact on duration of the procedure [23].

In invasive cardiology and cardiac surgery, deep sedation with NIV may be a reasonable and safe alternative to general endotracheal anesthesia in patients requiring prolonged transesophageal echocardiography during left atrial appendage closure [24].

NIV application can also reduce the need for endotracheal reintubation in patients after cardiothoracic treatment [25].

41.4 Thoracic Surgery

Conscious sedation and local anesthesia are increasingly used in less invasive thoracic surgery procedures, e.g., pleuroscopy.

Considering that thoracic surgery may significantly affect respiratory function, NIV can be of benefit in various clinical scenarios:

- In the preoperative period to optimize the respiratory status of patients with chronic respiratory disease.
- In the postoperative period to reduce complications like pneumonia, respiratory failure, and the need for reintubation, particularly in patients with COPD or individuals with poor lung function,
- In chest trauma surgery to help manage pain-related hypoventilation and prevent acute respiratory distress syndrome (ARDS) [26].

41.5 Infants

Use of NIV can improve outcomes in infants with RDS—lung-protective management includes initiation of noninvasive respiratory support from birth, balanced use of oxygen, and appropriate pharmacotherapy. Methods of ongoing noninvasive respiratory support may help reduce chronic lung disease with a reduction of lung injury incidence [27]. Meta-analyses of trials comparing NIV with CPAP in infants demonstrate that postextubation NIV is superior to CPAP in the prevention of respiratory failure resulting in the need for additional ventilatory support [28].

41.6 NIV Interface and Complications

Despite these positive results, some controversies persist in NIV use. Although NIV is generally considered safer than invasive ventilation, it carries its own risks:

- The success of NIV significantly depends on the interface selection, as ill-fitting masks can cause discomfort, skin necrosis, or pressure sores. They may also lead to air leaks, negatively impacting the efficacy of ventilation.
- NIV can lead to gastric insufflation, especially at high pressures, causing abdominal distension, nausea, and, in severe cases, vomiting, which can increase the risk of aspiration, particularly in semi-conscious or unconscious patients.
- Patients receiving NIV can experience eye irritation or conjunctivitis due to leakages of air from the mask, especially with oronasal or full-face masks.
- While NIV aims to relieve respiratory muscle fatigue, inappropriate settings can paradoxically cause or exacerbate this condition—especially if inspiratory pressures are insufficient or if the machine's triggering is not synchronized with the patient's effort.

41.7 NIV Limitations

Also, while NIV has wide applications, it is not suitable in every clinical scenario:

- Patients with severe respiratory acidosis may not respond well to NIV; therefore, they require thorough monitoring of vital signs to not overlook the need for endotracheal intubation.
- In cases of respiratory arrest, NIV is not the appropriate intervention—these situations require immediate intubation and invasive mechanical ventilation.
- Use of NIV usually requires patient cooperation.
- Patients with facial deformities, recent facial trauma, or surgery may not be suitable for NIV as the mask may not fit properly, leading to ineffective ventilation and potential harm.
- NIV requires specific equipment and trained healthcare providers; its effectiveness can be limited in settings where these resources are not available.

To recapitulate, despite many advancements in the use of NIV in various clinical settings, understanding the risks and limitations of this modality is vital. Tailoring the use of NIV to each patient's unique needs is the key to treatment optimization.

41.8 NIV in the Periprocedural Period

The use of noninvasive respiratory support methods should be considered during the procedure and periprocedural period in any case of a patient with risk factors of respiratory failure development or individuals who have already developed respiratory failure but remain conscious and hemodynamically stable and do not require general anesthesia or invasive mechanical ventilation.

41.9 NIV Monitoring

Individuals without a history of respiratory tract diseases should also be carefully monitored to ensure rapid intervention in the event of respiratory failure.

The technique of respiratory support should be based on an individualized assessment of the patient's condition, comorbidities, type, and degree of respiratory failure. An individualized approach to the choice of the patient's interface is advised.

In places where invasive procedures are performed, access to various methods of respiratory support should be ensured, and the staff should be trained in their use in clinical practice.

Initial ventilatory settings should be patient-specific. However, a common approach is to start with low-pressure support and gradually increase it based on the patient's tolerance and arterial blood gas analysis.

Patients should be closely monitored, especially during the initial hours of NIV application. Regular arterial blood gas analysis is necessary to assess the response to treatment. Patient comfort and cooperation should be continuously evaluated.

Healthcare providers should be adequately trained in NIV application, monitoring, and troubleshooting. Patient education regarding NIV can enhance their comfort, cooperation, and adherence to therapy.

41.10 NIV Future Perspectives

In the future, NIV devices may feature improved synchronization, more adaptive interfaces, and integrated systems for more comprehensive monitoring. These advancements can enhance patient comfort and the effectiveness of NIV.

As our understanding of respiratory physiology and disease deepens, there is a shift towards more individualized ventilation strategies. Future research will help tailor NIV settings to the individual patient, optimizing outcomes.

41.11 Summary

In conclusion, despite increased use of noninvasive ventilatory support, more studies and good-quality data are still needed.

References

1. Osadnik CR, Tee VS, Carson-Chahhoud KV, Picot J, Wedzicha JA, Smith BJ. Non-invasive ventilation for the management of acute hypercapnic respiratory failure due to exacerbation of chronic obstructive pulmonary disease. Cochrane Database Syst Rev. 2017;7(7):CD004104. https://doi.org/10.1002/14651858.CD004104.pub4. PMID: 28702957; PMCID: PMC6483555
2. Frazier W, van Eijndhoven E, Murphy R, Jena AB. Noninvasive ventilation at home reduces mortality in COPD with CRF. Am J Manag Care. 2021;27(9):e308–15. https://doi.org/10.37765/ajmc.2021.88743.
3. Wilson ME, Dobler CC, Morrow AS, Beuschel B, Alsawas M, Benkhadra R, Seisa M, Mittal A, Sanchez M, Daraz L, Holets S, Murad MH, Wang Z. Association of Home Noninvasive Positive Pressure Ventilation with clinical outcomes in chronic obstructive pulmonary disease: a systematic review and meta-analysis. JAMA. 2020;323(5):455–65. https://doi.org/10.1001/jama.2019.22343. PMID: 32016309; PMCID: PMC7042860
4. Abubacker AP, Ndakotsu A, Chawla HV, Iqbal A, Grewal A, Myneni R, Vivekanandan G, Khan S. Non-invasive positive pressure ventilation for acute cardiogenic pulmonary edema, and chronic obstructive pulmonary disease in prehospital and emergency settings. Cureus. 2021;13(6):e15624. https://doi.org/10.7759/cureus.15624. PMID: 34277241; PMCID: PMC8277092
5. Masip J, Peacock WF, Price S, Cullen L, Martin-Sanchez FJ, Seferovic P, Maisel AS, Miro O, Filippatos G, Vrints C, Christ M, Cowie M, Platz E, McMurray J, DiSomma S, Zeymer U, Bueno H, Gale CP, Lettino M, Tavares M, Ruschitzka F, Mebazaa A, Harjola VP, Mueller C, Acute Heart Failure Study Group of the Acute Cardiovascular Care Association and the Committee on Acute Heart Failure of the Heart Failure Association of the European Society of Cardiology. Indications and practical approach to non-invasive ventilation in acute heart failure. Eur Heart J. 2018;39(1):17–25. https://doi.org/10.1093/eurheartj/ehx580. PMID: 29186485; PMCID: PMC6251669
6. Javaheri S, Brown LK, Abraham WT, Khayat R. Apneas of heart failure and phenotype-guided treatments: part one: OSA. Chest. 2020;157(2):394–402. https://doi.org/10.1016/j.chest.2019.02.407. Epub 2019 Apr 29. PMID: 31047953; PMCID: PMC7005380
7. Wang G, Goebel JR, Li C, Hallman HG, Gilford TM, Li W. Therapeutic effects of CPAP on cognitive impairments associated with OSA. J Neurol. 2020;267(10):2823–8. https://doi.org/10.1007/s00415-019-09381-2. Epub 2019 May 20. PMID: 31111204
8. Picard F, Panagiotidou P, Weinig L, Steffen M, Tammen AB, Klein RM. Effect of CPAP therapy on nocturnal blood pressure fluctuations, nocturnal blood pressure, and arterial stiffness in patients with coexisting cardiovascular diseases and obstructive sleep apnea. Sleep Breath. 2021;25(1):151–61. https://doi.org/10.1007/s11325-020-02075-4. Epub 2020 Apr 15. PMID: 32297145
9. Fernando SM, Tran A, Sadeghirad B, Burns KEA, Fan E, Brodie D, Munshi L, Goligher EC, Cook DJ, Fowler RA, Herridge MS, Cardinal P, Jaber S, Møller MH, Thille AW, Ferguson ND, Slutsky AS, Brochard LJ, Seely AJE, Rochwerg B. Noninvasive respiratory support following extubation in critically ill adults: a systematic review and network meta-analysis. Intensive Care Med. 2022;48(2):137–47. https://doi.org/10.1007/s00134-021-06581-1. Epub 2021 Nov 25. PMID: 34825256
10. Burns KE, Meade MO, Premji A, Adhikari NK. Noninvasive positive-pressure ventilation as a weaning strategy for intubated adults with respiratory failure. Cochrane Database Syst Rev. 2013;2013(12):CD004127. https://doi.org/10.1002/14651858.CD004127.pub3. PMID: 24323843; PMCID: PMC6516851
11. Arora G, Arshad Z, Prakash R, Sharma M, Singh GP, Kohli M. High-flow nasal cannula as an alternate weaning strategy: a randomized controlled trial. Cureus. 2023;15(3):e36511. https://doi.org/10.7759/cureus.36511. PMID: 37090360; PMCID: PMC10120274

12. Pieri M, Landoni G, Cabrini L. Noninvasive ventilation during endoscopic procedures: rationale, clinical use, and devices. J Cardiothorac Vasc Anesth. 2018;32(2):928–34. https://doi.org/10.1053/j.jvca.2017.09.038. Epub 2017 Sep 27. PMID: 29317119
13. Tolvi M, Lehtonen L, Tuominen-Salo H, Paavola M, Mattila K, Aaltonen LM. Overstay and readmission in ear, nose, and throat day surgery-factors affecting Postanesthesia course. Ear Nose Throat J. 2021;100(7):477–82. https://doi.org/10.1177/0145561319872165. Epub 2019 Oct 3. PMID: 31581823
14. Aksay SS, Bumb JM, Janke C, Hoyer C, Kranaster L, Sartorius A. New evidence for seizure quality improvement by hyperoxia and mild hypocapnia. J ECT. 2014;30(4):287–91. https://doi.org/10.1097/YCT.0000000000000109. PMID: 24625713
15. Min SH, Seo JH. Tube or tubeless: an anesthetic strategy for upper airway surgery. Anesth Pain Med (Seoul). 2023;18(2):123–31. https://doi.org/10.17085/apm.23014. Epub 2023 Apr 4. PMID: 37183280; PMCID: PMC10183614
16. Gómez-Arnau J, de Arriba-Arnau A, Correas-Lauffer J, Urretavizcaya M. Hyperventilation and electroconvulsive therapy: a literature review. Gen Hosp Psychiatry. 2018;50:54–62. https://doi.org/10.1016/j.genhosppsych.2017.09.003. Epub 2017 Sep 23. PMID: 29054017
17. Chi SY, Han Y, Li WX, Wang G. Ventilatory management in shared airway surgery: current status, challenges, and future directions. Zhonghua Yi Xue Za Zhi. 2022;102(21):1568–73. https://doi.org/10.3760/cma.j.cn112137-20220118-00121. Chinese. PMID: 35644956
18. Karim HMR, Esquinas AM. High-flow nasal cannula oxygen therapy for modified electroconvulsive therapy. Eur J Anaesthesiol. 2020;37(1):56–7. https://doi.org/10.1097/EJA.0000000000001076. PMID: 31794531
19. Koyama Y, Tsuzaki K, Suzuki T, Ozaki M, Saito S. Prevention of oxygen desaturation in morbidly obese patients during electroconvulsive therapy: a narrative review. J ECT. 2020;36(3):161–7. https://doi.org/10.1097/YCT.0000000000000664. PMID: 32040021
20. Yamamoto F, Kato R, Sato J, Nishino T. Anaesthesia for awake craniotomy with non-invasive positive pressure ventilation. Br J Anaesth. 2003;90(3):382–5. https://doi.org/10.1093/bja/aeg068. PMID: 12594155
21. Lee SS, Berman MF. Use of the Draeger Apollo to deliver Bilevel positive pressure ventilation during awake frontal craniotomy for a patient with severe chronic obstructive pulmonary disease. A A Case Rep. 2015;5(11):202–5. https://doi.org/10.1213/XAA.0000000000000216. PMID: 26588034
22. Skoczyński S, Minarowski Ł, Tobiczyk E, Oraczewska A, Glinka K, Ficek K, Mróz R, Barczyk A. Noninvasive ventilation-facilitated Bronchofiberoscopy in patients with respiratory failure. Adv Exp Med Biol. 2019;1160:53–64. https://doi.org/10.1007/5584_2019_375. PMID: 30989590
23. Pelaia C, Bruni A, Garofalo E, Rovida S, Arrighi E, Cammarota G, Navalesi P, Pelaia G, Longhini F. Oxygenation strategies during flexible bronchoscopy: a review of the literature. Respir Res. 2021;22(1):253. https://doi.org/10.1186/s12931-021-01846-1. PMID: 34563179; PMCID: PMC8464093
24. Fogarty M, Orr JA, Sakata D, Brewer L, Johnson K, Fang JC, Kuck K. A comparison of ventilation with a non-invasive ventilator versus standard O_2 with a nasal cannula for colonoscopy with moderate sedation using propofol. J Clin Monit Comput. 2020;34(6):1215–21. https://doi.org/10.1007/s10877-019-00426-5. Epub 2019 Nov 23. PMID: 31760586
25. Khanna P, Haritha D, Das A, Sarkar S, Roy A. Utility of high-flow nasal oxygen in comparison to conventional oxygen therapy during upper gastrointestinal endoscopic procedures under sedation: a systematic review and meta-analyses. Indian J Gastroenterol. 2023;42(1):53–63. https://doi.org/10.1007/s12664-022-01308-6. Epub 2023 Feb 13. PMID: 36780095; PMCID: PMC9924186
26. Chiumello D, Coppola S, Froio S, Gregoretti C, Consonni D. Noninvasive ventilation in chest trauma: systematic review and meta-analysis. Intensive Care Med. 2013;39(7):1171–80. https://doi.org/10.1007/s00134-013-2901-4. Epub 2013 Apr 10. PMID: 23571872
27. Zangrillo A, Mazzone P, Votta CD, Villari N, Della Bella P, Monaco F. Prolonged transesophageal echocardiography during percutaneous closure of the left atrial appendage without gen-

eral anesthesia: the utility of the Janus mask. Can J Anaesth. 2016;63(8):962–5. https://doi.org/10.1007/s12630-016-0659-1. English. Epub 2016 Apr 26. PMID: 27117991
28. Zhu G, Huang Y, Wei D, Shi Y. Efficacy and safety of noninvasive ventilation in patients after cardiothoracic surgery: a PRISMA-compliant systematic review and meta-analysis. Medicine (Baltimore). 2016;95(38):e4734. https://doi.org/10.1097/MD.0000000000004734. PMID: 27661021; PMCID: PMC5044891

NIV: Educational Programs

42

Maciej Dyrbuś and Antonio M. Esquinas

42.1 Introduction

Noninvasive ventilation (NIV), first introduced into clinical practice more than 30 years ago, is one of the most valuable tools in the management of respiratory failure, which allows not only to improve patients' outcomes, but also to substantially improve the quality of life in those patients [1]. The success of NIV therapy is dependent not only on an appropriate patient selection and optimal settings of the device itself but also on patient and caregiver education, which are crucial for obtaining a final success. Patient education is vital for ascertaining appropriate adherence to NIV therapy and successful management of potential complications. Similarly, caregiver education can significantly impact NIV therapy outcomes, including reduced work burden and stress. In this chapter, we will discuss the importance of patient and caregiver education in NIV management, the content of education programs, and the benefits of these programs for both patients and caregivers. We will also address the implementation of educational programs, including strategies for tailoring programs to meet the needs of diverse patient populations and evaluating their effectiveness. By providing a comprehensive review of NIV educational programs, this chapter aims to promote the integration of patient and caregiver education into routine NIV management, ultimately improving patient outcomes and quality of life. Although to date, no relevant, optimally randomized original data can be found while browsing the publicly available databases on the

M. Dyrbuś (✉)
3rd Department of Cardiology, School of Medical Sciences in Zabrze, Medical University of Silesia, Katowice, Poland

A. M. Esquinas
Fellow NIV, Director NIV Fellowship Program & International Non Invasive Ventilation College of Experts Intensive Care Unit; Hospital Morales Meseguer, Murcia, Spain

© The Author(s), under exclusive license to Springer Nature Switzerland AG 2025
K. Panda et al. (eds.), *Noninvasive Ventilatory Approaches in Interventional Procedures*, Noninvasive Ventilation. The Essentials,
https://doi.org/10.1007/978-3-032-05328-2_42

field of education in noninvasive ventilation, it probably reflects that structured education and training programs are still a rather novel strategy and thus have not yielded measurable outcomes yet.

42.2 Patient Education

Patient education is an essential component of NIV management. Patients who are well-informed about NIV and its benefits are less likely to experience NIV failures, while being much more likely to adhere to the therapy and experience improved outcomes [1]. Education should already begin before the time of NIV initiation and be continued on the first days of NIV and further throughout the patient's care. The content of patient education programs should be tailored to the patient's needs, including their level of health literacy, background, and comorbidities.

In general, patients qualified for NIV are most often subjects with respiratory failure; thus, the attention of the team monitoring the patient should be placed on delivering optimal ventilation as a priority. The management of comorbidities requires additional resources, and therefore, each step performed in delivering a proper education to patients might reduce the burden of work in those subjects.

Each patient on NIV should be educated on the indications for the therapy, including acute exacerbations of chronic obstructive pulmonary disease (COPD), cardiogenic pulmonary edema, acute respiratory failure, and neuromuscular diseases. Patients should also be informed about the benefits of NIV, including improved respiratory function, reduced dyspnea, and decreased risk of intubation and mechanical ventilation. The improved knowledge on the indications might not only result in the patients' higher confidence in the administered therapy, but also increase the potential adherence to this therapy. Patients who are educated about the most efficacious breathing patterns, reducing the work of breathing and mitigating dyspnea, are less prone to episodes of hypoventilation and demonstrate lower levels of anxiety and stress [2]. Another important issue requiring education is the subject of proper use and maintenance of NIV equipment, which is critical for successful NIV therapy. Patients should be instructed on how to correctly apply all elements of the equipment, as well as how to maintain an appropriate cleanliness, in order to prevent infection and maintain proper functioning of the system. Moreover, as the patients ventilated in the chronic setting might often face significant troubles with attending in-person visits, they must be well educated on how to troubleshoot the most prevalent issues with NIV therapy, such as mask discomfort, air leaks, or skin irritation. Furthermore, a structured NIV training would allow a successful use of NIV in stressful situations when patients are facing acute respiratory failure decompensation, with the potential to delay or even avoid invasive ventilation.

All aforementioned strategies are aimed at improving patient adherence and satisfaction with NIV therapy. Importantly, patients should also be instructed on the potential consequences of non-adherence, such as increased risk of escalation to invasive ventilation, hospitalization, and a higher risk of death.

Finally, as the prevalence of unhealthy lifestyle habits in patients using NIV is high, lifestyle modifications, such as smoking cessation, weight loss, and physical activity, are extremely important in order to improve their outcomes. Patients should be educated on the importance of lifestyle modifications and provided with resources and support to help achieve their goals.

42.3 Caregiver Education

Caregivers play a vital role in NIV management, providing continuous support to patients on NIV therapy. Recent years have seen a dramatic increase in the tendency to form multidisciplinary teams focused on supporting patients ventilated with NIV. The present multidisciplinary teams most usually consist of emergency ward specialists, pulmonologists, anesthesiologists, nurses, respiratory physiotherapists, although they might often be expanded by inclusion of dieticians, psychologists, and members of any other subspecialty managing a particular patient. The appropriate education of all team members is essential in ensuring the successful implementation and management of NIV therapy, as caregivers who are well-informed about NIV therapy and its management are better equipped to provide optimal support to patients, reducing patients' stress and, by maintaining an optimal management of patients, reducing the burden of work in their clinics. As with patients' education, each member of the team, from the moment of qualification to NIV, should be well aware of all potential benefits and risks associated with the procedure, in order to guide decision-making during ventilation.

In brief, the contents of caregiver education programs should not only include all information essential for the patient but also contain additional information on how to implement those resources. Among them, the most important are indications for NIV, the recommendations on proper use and maintenance of NIV equipment, troubleshooting of the common problems, and an emphasis on the importance of adherence to NIV therapy. Another important aspect required from all members of the caregiving team is the knowledge of how to overcome the most frequent, perilous medical conditions occurring in patients ventilated with NIV, including exacerbation of hypoxemic or hypercapnic respiratory failure. Finally, in case of NIV failure, there is a need to define the structured strategy of escalation to invasive ventilation, with the team members experienced in intubation and maintenance of invasive respiratory care. In the Spanish prospective observational cohort study, performed in patients requiring NIV for acute hypoxemic respiratory failure (AHRF) in conventional wards, the factors influencing the NIV efficacy were analyzed [3]. Apart from the clinical factors influencing the outcome of the patients, such as baseline pH and APACHE score, the lack of personnel training was identified to independently increase the risk of NIV failure. Among the detected errors, insufficient mask fitting leading to excessive air leaks, lack of knowledge on how to properly handle the ventilator alarms, and how to titrate the flow of gases are worth noting. In another study, it has been demonstrated that the personnel declared discomfort when needing to deliver NIV, due to their lack of skill and education [4]. Such results clearly indicate that the positive outcome of patients is clearly dependent on the education of the caring team.

With no doubt, there is an unmet need to provide continuous education to nurses, who play a pivotal role in coordinating patient care and who substantially contribute to a collaborative and cost-effective approach for patients ventilated noninvasively. To ascertain that NIV treatment is successful, it is important to have specialized nurses and respiratory therapists who are exclusively trained in managing ventilator settings, assisting patients in adapting to the respiratory equipment, and regularly monitoring the patient's response to NIV. The presence of specialized healthcare professionals helps maintain focus on NIV treatment and prevent any desynchronization or therapeutic failure.

One of the most important and clinically approachable aspects of caregivers' education should be the focus on hands-on training, including training with simulators. In interventional medicine, the use of simulation-based training has become increasingly prevalent, as it allows the replication of real-life experiences by providing guided, immersive experiences that closely resemble various aspects of real-world cases. There are multiple studies, including systematic reviews and meta-analyses, which demonstrated its effectiveness in terms of knowledge and skill acquisition [5–7]. Although in patients with NIV, the results clearly demonstrating improvement in patients' outcome owing to the implementation of simulation training are scarce, there are a few NIV simulators that can be utilized to evaluate a user's ability to configure ventilator settings and understand and properly respond to the patient's pathophysiology and ventilation tolerance [8].

One of the perfect examples of the benefits of approaches utilizing simulators is the study by Spadaro et al., who aimed to compare the efficacy of computer-based and mannequin-based approaches in the training of residents on MV [9]. This prospective, single-blind study randomized 50 training residents, who after having attended a lecture on respiratory pathophysiology were randomly assigned to either the mannequin- or computer screen-based simulator group. Both groups underwent training on five different acute respiratory failure scenarios of various etiologies and, afterwards, further testing on patient management by simulating acute respiratory distress syndrome. The final evaluation revealed that only the scores of the group trained on mannequins significantly improved between the baseline and final training session.

Finally, each caregiver should optimally be instructed not only on what each patient should be instructed when facing a particular challenge, but—often more importantly—how to deliver the information to the patient to maintain a patient-centered strategy of mutual trust and engagement. Moreover, as caregiving can be a stressful and challenging experience, particularly for those caring for chronically ill patients, strategies for managing caregiver stress and burnout need to be presented. Optimally, caregivers should be provided with resources and strategies for managing stress and burnout, including support groups and counseling.

The European Respiratory Society has introduced both advanced and basic courses on noninvasive ventilation [10]. Notably, the European Respiratory Society's "Harmonized Education in Respiratory Medicine for European Specialists

(HERMES)" project is a significant endeavor, with the purpose of standardizing education in order to tackle the variation in respiratory health training throughout Europe. Following that, a range of educational initiatives has been created for diverse audiences. Also, the International School of Noninvasive Ventilation, a panel constituting world experts on NIV, organizes regular training and lectures aimed at spreading practical insights on optimal management of patients ventilated noninvasively [11]. Worth noting are also initiatives undertaken by the national scientific societies—for instance, the Polish Society of Lung Diseases has introduced dedicated training programs on NIV for various caregiving participants, including courses for physicians, nurses, and physiotherapists, which are then subdivided on the basis of experience and skills into advanced and beginner levels [12].

42.4 Educational Program Implementation

A successful implementation of educational programs requires careful planning and consideration of the needs of patients and caregivers. Strategies for program implementation should include identifying the target population, selecting appropriate educational materials, and incorporating patient and caregiver feedback into program development. A proposed scheme of NIV educational program initiation is presented in Fig. 42.1.

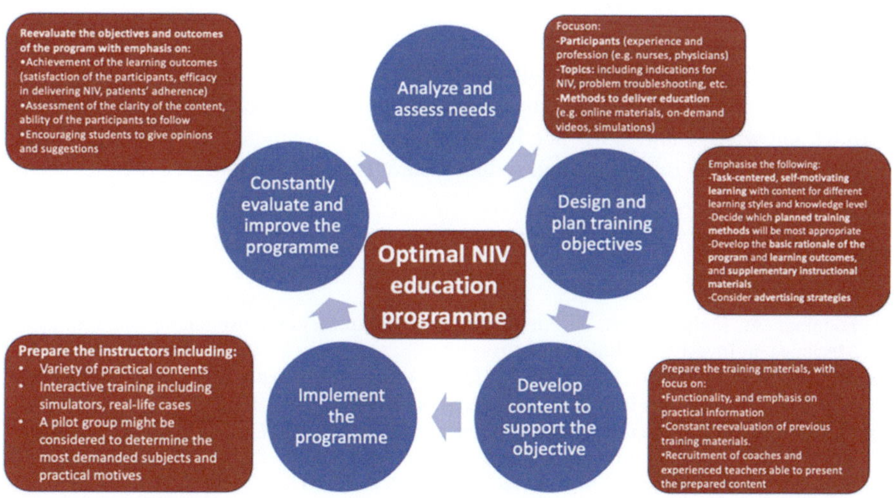

Fig. 42.1 Cycle of an optimal noninvasive ventilation (NIV) education program. Each phase of the program—analysis of the needs, planning of the objectives, development of content, its implementation, and continuous evaluation—is accompanied by the considerations aimed at enhancing educational effectiveness. These include tailoring the program to participant needs and experience, using optimal training methods, adjusting teaching strategies, and regularly reviewing and adapting the program based on feedback and outcomes

The following systematic approach can be used as a guide for the implementation of a successful educational NIV program:

1. *Needs assessment*, which should be conducted to identify the specific needs of patients and caregivers. This will help in developing program content addressing the gaps in knowledge and experience.
2. *Program planning*, based on the results of the needs assessment, with emphasis on determining objectives, content, and delivery methods.
3. *Program development*, based on evidence-based guidelines and best practices, reviewed and prepared by healthcare professionals with experience in NIV therapy and conveying the practical information to the trainees.
4. *Program implementation*, with the involvement of healthcare providers, including physicians, nurses, and physiotherapists. Healthcare providers should ascertain that patients and caregivers have access to the educational materials and are provided with sufficient time to participate in the program.
5. *Program evaluation*, with emphasis on the achievement of the objectives. The following are some of the evaluation endpoints that can be used:
   - *Patient and caregiver satisfaction.*
   - *Adherence rates* (measurable, e.g., as the number of hours of NIV use per day).
   - *Hospital readmission rates* before and after initiation of educational programs.
   - *Mortality rates*: before and after initiation of educational programs.
   - *Cost-effectiveness*: on the basis of objective endpoints listed above.

In summary, program implementation and evaluation are essential in ascertaining the effectiveness of NIV educational programs. By investing in NIV educational programs, healthcare providers can ensure that patients and caregivers are equipped with the knowledge and skills needed to successfully manage NIV therapy, leading to improved patient outcomes and reduced caregiver burden and stress.

References

1. Esquinas A. Fundamentos de Metodologia y Organizacion Hospitalaria en Ventilacion Mecanica no Invasiva. 3° Edicion. 2016
2. Nicolini A, Piroddi IMG, Barlascini C. How to enhance experience and skill of non invasive ventilation: suggestions from the literature. Short Breath. 2015;4:19–25.
3. Lopez-Campos JL, Garcia Polo C, Leon Jimenez A, Arnedillo A, Gonzalez-Moya E, Fenandez Berni JJ. Staff training influence on non-invasive ventilation outcome for acute hypercapnic respiratory failure. Monaldi Arch Chest Dis. 2006;65:145–51.
4. Plumb J, Juszczyszyn M, Mabeza G. Non-invasive ventilation (NIV) a study of junior doctor competence. Open Med Educ J. 2010;3:11–7.
5. Seam N, Lee AJ, Vennero M, Emlet L. Simulation training in the ICU. Chest. 2019;156(6):1223–33.

6. Tonapa SI, Mulyadi M, Ho KHM, Efendi F. Effectiveness of using high-fidelity simulation on learning outcomes in undergraduate nursing education: systematic review and meta-analysis. Eur Rev Med Pharmacol Sci. 2023;27(2):444–58.
7. Huang GC, McSparron JI, Balk EM, et al. Procedural instruction in invasive bedside procedures: a systematic review and meta-analysis of effective teaching approaches. BMJ Qual Saf. 2016;25(4):281–94.
8. Chatwin M, Hare A, Kurosinski P, et al. Evaluation of the educational outcomes of simulation-based training (SBT) for NIV. 2.2 Noninvasive Ventilatory Support. 2015.
9. Spadaro S, Karbing DS, Fogagnolo A, et al. Simulation training for residents focused on mechanical ventilation: a randomized trial using mannequin-based versus Computer-based simulation. Simul Healthc. 2017;12(6):349–55.
10. https://www.ers-education.org/home/ – Official Website of the ERS (European Respiratory Society) – which organizes various courses and training programmes on optimal management of patients ventilated noninvasively.
11. https://escuela-internacional-de-ventilacion-mecanica-no-invasiva.webnode.es/ – Official Website of the International School of Non Invasive Mechanical Ventilation, which organizes regular courses on NIV.
12. https://ptchp.org/edukacja/terminarz-szkolen/ – Official Website of the Polish Society of Lung Diseases, which organizes training programmes for caregivers on different levels of experience and skills.

MIX
Papier aus verantwortungsvollen Quellen
Paper from responsible sources
FSC® C105338

If you have any concerns about our products,
you can contact us on
ProductSafety@springernature.com

In case Publisher is established outside the EU,
the EU authorized representative is:
Springer Nature Customer Service Center GmbH
Europaplatz 3, 69115 Heidelberg, Germany

Printed by Libri Plureos GmbH
in Hamburg, Germany